Conceptual Foundations of
Professional
Nursing Practice

Conceptual Foundations of
Professional
Nursing Practice

JOAN L. CREASIA, PhD, RN

Professor and Dean,
College of Nursing,
University of Tennessee,
Knoxville, Tennessee

BARBARA PARKER, PhD, RN, FAAN

Professor of Nursing;
Director, Center for Nursing Research,
School of Nursing,
University of Virginia,
Charlottesville, Virginia

Second Edition

with 60 illustrations

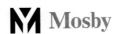 Mosby

St. Louis Baltimore Boston Carlsbad Chicago Naples New York Philadelphia Portland
London Madrid Mexico City Singapore Sydney Tokyo Toronto Wiesbaden

Vice President and Publisher: Nancy L. Coon
Executive Editor: N. Darlene Como
Senior Developmental Editor: Laurie Sparks
Project Manager: Deborah L. Vogel
Production Editor: Judith Bange
Designer: Pati Pye
Manufacturing Supervisor: Karen Lewis
Cover Art: Elizabeth Rohne Rudder

Second Edition

Copyright © 1996 by Mosby–Year Book, Inc.

Previous edition copyrighted 1991

Printed in the United States of America
Composition by Top Graphics
Lithography by Top Graphics
Printing/binding by R.R. Donnelley & Sons Company

Mosby–Year Book, Inc.
11830 Westline Industrial Drive
St. Louis, Missouri 63146

Library of Congress Cataloging in Publication Data

Conceptual foundations of professional nursing practice / edited by
  Joan L. Creasia, Barbara Parker. — 2nd ed.
      p.   cm.
  Includes bibliographical references and index.
  ISBN 0-8151-1406-0
  1. Nursing—Practice.   2. Nursing.   I. Creasia, Joan L.
  II. Parker, Barbara, RN.
  RT86.7.C66   1996
  610.73—dc20   96-1669
                                                              CIP

96 97 98 99 00 / 9 8 7 6 5 4 3 2 1

Contributors

Barbara Brodie, PhD, RN, FAAN
Professor,
School of Nursing,
University of Virginia,
Charlottesville, Virginia

Sara T. Fry, PhD, RN, FAAN
Henry R. Luce Professor of Nursing Ethics,
School of Nursing,
Boston College,
Chestnut Hill, Massachusetts

Joan Garity, EdD, RN
Assistant Professor,
College of Nursing,
University of Massachusetts–Boston,
Boston, Massachusetts

Audrey G. Gift, PhD, RN, FAAN
Associate Professor and Assistant Director,
Center for Nursing Research,
School of Nursing,
University of Pennsylvania,
Philadelphia, Pennsylvania

Patty J. Hale, PhD, RN
Assistant Professor,
School of Nursing,
University of Virginia,
Charlottesville, Virginia

Sylvia E. Hart, PhD, RN
Professor Emeritus,
College of Nursing,
University of Tennessee,
Knoxville, Tennessee

Cheryl Bland Jones, PhD, RN
Assistant Professor,
School of Nursing,
University of Virginia,
Charlottesville, Virginia

Kathryn Hopkins Kavanagh, PhD, RN
Associate Professor,
School of Nursing,
University of Maryland–Baltimore,
Baltimore, Maryland

Arlene W. Keeling, PhD, RN
Assistant Professor,
School of Nursing,
University of Virginia,
Charlottesville, Virginia

Marian M. Larisey, PhD, RN
Associate Professor and Chair,
Medical University of South Carolina RN-BSN
    Satellite Program at Francis Marion
    University,
Florence, South Carolina

Donna M. Mahrenholz, PhD, RN
Associate Professor and Director,
Nursing Management and Policy Program,
School of Nursing,
Yale University,
New Haven, Connecticut

Gail O. Mazzocco, EdD, RN
Assistant Professor and Coordinator,
Western Maryland Outreach
(Program of the University of
    Maryland–Baltimore School of Nursing),
Cumberland, Maryland

Patricia McMullen, JD, MS, CNP
Associate Professor,
Uniformed Services University of the Health
    Sciences,
Rockville, Maryland

Teresa L. Panniers, PhD, RN, CRNP
Assistant Professor,
School of Nursing,
University of Maryland–Baltimore,
Baltimore, Maryland

Anne Griswold Peirce, PhD, RN
Professor and Dean,
School of Nursing,
University of Mississippi Medical Center,
Jackson, Mississippi

Nathaniel W. Peirce, EdD
Educational Consultant,
Norfolk, Virginia

Nayna Philipsen, PhD, JD, RN
Senior Compliance Analyst,
Board of Physician Quality Assurance,
Baltimore, Maryland

C. Fay Raines, PhD, RN
Professor and Dean,
College of Nursing,
University of Alabama–Huntsville,
Huntsville, Alabama

Sandra J. Sundeen, MS, RN
Chief Nurse, Mental Hygiene Administration,
Department of Health and Mental Hygiene,
Baltimore, Maryland

Karen MacDonald Thompson, MS, RN
Research Assistant, Doctoral Student,
School of Nursing,
University of Virginia,
Charlottesville, Virginia

Janet B. Younger, PhD, RN
Professor and Associate Dean for the
    Undergraduate Program,
Medical College of Virginia School of Nursing,
Virginia Commonwealth University,
Richmond, Virginia

Consultants

Sharon E. Beck, DNSc, RN
Assistant Hospital Director–Nursing
    Education/Performance Improvement,
Temple University Hospital,
Philadelphia, Pennsylvania

Ann Martinen Doordan, PhD, RN, CRRN
Associate Professor,
School of Nursing,
San Jose State University,
San Jose, California

Margaret A. Droste, PhD, RN
Assistant Professor,
Department of Nursing,
Webster University,
St. Louis, Missouri

Laura M. Inouye, EdD, RN
Associate Dean,
School of Health,
Division of Nursing,
California State University–Dominguez Hills,
Santa Ana, California

Mary N. McAlindon, EdD, RN, CNAA
Assistant to the Vice President,
McLaren Health Care Corporation,
Flint, Michigan

Cheryl McKenzie, MN, RN,C, FNP
Associate Professor,
Department of Nursing,
Northern Kentucky University,
Highland Heights, Kentucky

Bonnie C. Pearson, MEd, RN
Associate Professor,
College of Nursing,
University of Alabama–Huntsville,
Huntsville, Alabama

Anita B. Singleton, EdS, RN
Associate Professor,
Nursing Department,
Missouri Southern State College,
Joplin, Missouri

Preface

Nursing has undergone significant changes and faced many challenges during the past few decades in its quest for professionalism in practice. One of the most influential forces has been the American Nurses' Association (ANA) 1965 recommendation that the minimum educational preparation for professional nurses be at the baccalaureate level. Although this recommendation was not fully embraced by the nursing community, it did serve to heighten awareness of the need for additional education. This prompted many nurses who received their basic education in an associate degree or a diploma program to return to school for a baccalaureate degree in nursing. The first edition of *Conceptual Foundations of Professional Nursing Practice* was designed for RN students in upper-division BSN completion programs who varied in their years of practice and clinical focus.

During the 5 years since publication of the first edition, we became aware that our book was being used, not only in RN-BSN completion programs, but also in foundational courses in basic baccalaureate programs, and in core courses in graduate nursing programs. This information, along with comments and suggestions from our readers, influenced the selection of content for the second edition.

Because concepts included in the first edition such as stress, coping, pain, crisis, social support, and so forth, are covered in detail in other texts, they were omitted from the second edition. The section on major life themes, which included sexuality, parenting, loss, and aging, was omitted for the same reason. New chapters on nursing history, education, socialization, health care delivery issues, caring, critical thinking, change, and research were added, as was a separate chapter on the nursing process. These chapters, along with the ones retained from the first edition, make the book more relevant for use in both undergraduate and graduate nursing programs.

ORGANIZATION

The second edition of *Conceptual Foundations of Professional Nursing Practice* comprehensively explores issues and concepts that influence professional practice and the delivery of nursing care. The book is divided into three parts: the context, dimensions, and themes of professional nursing practice. Part I, The Context of Professional Nursing Practice, begins with an exploration of historical events that shaped nursing practice and education. This is followed by an examination of issues related to professional socialization and role taking in nursing. Subsequently, an examination of the nursing process as a framework for practice; an overview of individual, family, and community client systems; and frameworks and theories that provide structure for the discipline of nursing are presented. Part I concludes with a description of the health care environment where nurses practice and highlights current issues in health care delivery, such as cost, quality, and access.

Part II, Dimensions of Professional Nursing Practice, focuses on political, economic, and legal forces that have an impact on current practice. Ethical principles and moral beliefs that are integral to nursing practice decisions are examined, and culturally sensitive approaches to effectively manage and treat our diverse clients are discussed. Part III, Themes in Professional Nursing Practice, includes concepts that are applicable to a variety of clients and clinical practice settings. Such concepts include caring, health and health promotion, teaching and learning, communication, critical thinking, and change. Chapters on nursing research and information technology describe the state of the art and highlight issues for further consideration.

APPROACH

The rapid changes occurring in the health care delivery system provide both opportunities and challenges for nursing. Both advanced technological developments and health policy issues play a major role in the planning and delivery of comprehensive nursing care. The focus on health promotion for individuals, families, and communities and efforts to control health care costs have given rise to alternative forms of health care delivery and innovative reimbursement models. In addition, increased acuity of hospitalized clients and limited hospital stays have resulted in a greater demand for home and community health services. These changes have political, legal, and economic implications that must be incorporated into the educational foundation and professional practice of nursing. Chapters from the first edition that are included in the current edition were revised and updated to reflect these changes, with particular attention given to the ongoing evolution of nursing as a profession.

With the trend toward advanced education in nursing, a highly diverse student body is emerging. Second-career men and women with valuable life experiences and students returning for renewed nursing careers are now commonplace in many nursing education programs. Non-nurses, often with degrees in other fields, are seeking entry into basic nursing programs or accelerated graduate programs. As a result, the student population as a whole tends to be more heterogeneous than the traditional college student, in terms of both age and experience. These students, often classified as adult learners, have an increased capacity for critical thinking and self-directed learning. Thus it is meaningful to develop a conceptual approach to nursing practice that encourages critical thinking and is applicable to assorted client groups and clinical settings. This book offers such an approach and can be used effectively to teach nursing concepts to today's students.

As editors, we have struggled with the terminology used to describe the recipients of nursing care. Although philosophically we prefer the term "client" with its connotation of partnership in nursing care, there were times when this terminology became cumbersome or inaccurate, as in reference to "patient's bill of rights," for example. Thus the reader will find both "client" and "patient" used, at times interchangeably. We believe the difficulty in determining the appropriate term is a reflection of the changing nature of nursing practice and the health care system.

SPECIAL FEATURES

For the purpose of focusing the reader's attention, each chapter begins with learning objectives. The Profile in Practice features a nurse whose practice reflects the focus of the chapter. Each chapter is developed in a similar format. An overview of the concept is followed by definitions of key terms, an in-depth discussion of the concept, and application of the concept to nursing. Research findings and material from current literature are integrated throughout the chapter. Significant facts and issues are highlighted at the end of the chapter as Key Points. Critical Thinking Exercises provide opportunities for the student to examine the content and apply it to nursing. A comprehensive and current reference list offers the opportunity to pursue further reading on the subject.

As each concept unfolds, the reader is challenged to discover new knowledge or reframe prior learning on a more conceptual and universally applicable level. Using this knowledge to enhance current and future nursing practice remains the final challenge.

Joan L. Creasia
Barbara Parker

Acknowledgments

We are deeply grateful to the many persons who have helped us bring this work to completion. Our special thanks go to the talented contributors who shared their knowledge, experience, and expertise in a form that is of immeasurable value to professional nurses, nursing students, and nurse educators. We appreciate the efforts of anonymous reviewers and colleagues who spent many hours critiquing the manuscript and offering suggestions for refinement. Special thanks go to Dr. Janet Wyatt for her extraordinary assistance with the *Instructor's Manual*.

The working relationship we shared as coauthors during the development of the first edition continued from afar through development of the second edition. Once again, writing this book was a valuable and rewarding experience. Our working relationship, in addition to the support and encouragement of our families, enabled us to achieve our goal. We gratefully acknowledge our supportive husbands, Don Creasia and Dale Schumacher, and our children and their partners: Paul and Karen Creasia Yarrish; Tracey Creasia; Andrea Schumacher and Bill Leconte; Meg Schumacher and John Boyd; and Peter Schumacher and Carol Brueggemeier.

Joan L. Creasia
Barbara Parker

Contents

part I

THE CONTEXT OF PROFESSIONAL NURSING PRACTICE

The background, circumstances, frameworks, conditions, and settings of nursing practice collectively reflect its context. In this section the reader is invited to explore the evolution of nursing as a practice discipline, obtain a new awareness of the extent of the nurse's role, identify issues that cut across all areas of nursing practice, and gain an appreciation of the milieu within which nursing care is delivered.

The context of professional nursing practice constitutes those elements, both internal and external to the nurse, that are integral to the delivery of nursing care. This section begins with an overview of nursing practice and education. These chapters are presented along a historical time line, not only to illustrate the development of the profession, but also to provide an understanding of how nursing practice and education evolved to their present forms. A critical analysis of professional socialization further promotes an understanding of the evolution of nursing as a practice discipline. A discussion of the array of roles nurses commonly assume, such as caregiver and teacher, and advanced practice roles, such as nurse practitioner and clinical nurse specialist, provides an appreciation of the scope of nursing practice and the complexity of the health care system. Chapters on the nursing process and nursing theories and frameworks describe the infrastructure on which nursing care is designed, implemented, and evaluated. Also included is a discussion of individual, family, and community client systems as the recipients of nursing care. Finally, a discussion of issues in health care delivery highlight the nursing practice environment and illustrate the movement of nursing beyond traditional boundaries to new frontiers.

History of the Foundations of American Professional Nursing

1

Barbara Brodie and Arlene W. Keeling

 ## Objectives

At the completion of this chapter, the reader will be able to:

- Describe the social, political, and governmental influences on the development of professional nursing in America from the late nineteenth to the twentieth century.

- Describe the evolution of nurse's training from hospital-based programs to collegiate programs.

- Discuss the impact of war on the profession.

- Discuss the movement toward nursing licensure.

- Describe the history of discrimination against men and African-Americans in nursing.

Profile in Practice

Sandra Taylor, PhD, RN
Associate Professor,
Norfolk State University,
Norfolk, Virginia

I have always been interested in history and reading to learn about other people's lives. I first became interested in nursing history when I was in the doctoral program at the University of Virginia. We had a course in nursing history, and I chose to write a paper on the role of African-American nurses in the Public Health Department in Richmond, Virginia. I chose this topic because I remember my parents speaking very highly about the IVNA (Instructional Visiting Nurses Association) when I was growing up as an African-American in Richmond.

In researching this topic, I discovered four Negro nurses who provided public health care for the entire Negro population of Richmond. The nurses were leaders in their community and symbolized a "higher life," demonstrating that women could overcome poverty, racism, and ignorance. They had pride in themselves and in their abilities, and they served as exemplary role models for the women and children of the community. Their struggle for respect, recognition, and acceptance was an example of the nursing profession's similar struggles.

Knowing about their struggles inspires me in my daily practice, and I can see the value of learning more about the history of our profession. I think of them and their struggles when I run into similar barriers, and I try to teach my students to not be afraid of what has caused pain in the past, but to use it to broaden our horizons, and to use what we have learned to help other emerging minority groups.

A challenge I have encountered in presenting this research is that, at times, people are offended by my use of the word *Negro*. I explain to them that this was the term used at the time and that to accurately reflect these nurses' experiences, we must be faithful to the historical context of their times.

"No occupation can be intelligently followed or understood unless it is, at least to some extent, illumined by the light of history . . ."
Dock & Stewart, 1931, p. 3

The development of nursing theory is a recent phenomenon in the history of the profession. For over a century, the foundation of clinical nursing was built on a rich empirical basis of practice. To understand what led the profession to subject its clinical practice to scientific and philosophical scrutiny, the development of the profession must be traced.

The nursing profession of today is a composite and distillation of over 100 years of development. Its practitioners (and the clinical and ethical dimensions of its practice), its relationship with patients, and its place in society have been forged by powerful social forces that have created the American health care system. More specifically, contemporary nursing has been shaped by society's view of women and care, advances in medical science, the growth of hospitals and public health, changes in the philosophy of science, philanthropic and government initiatives, and the actions of nurse leaders who struggled to transform a domestic vocation into a professional discipline.

ORIGINS

In the last quarter of the nineteenth century, major changes were occurring throughout the United States. The homogeneous population and agrarian, rural culture of the early republic were being replaced by a heterogeneous population and an industrialized, urban culture. Millions of immigrants entered the country seeking new lives and economic opportunities. Joining forces with American-born citizens, they built new cities, promoted the growth of industry, and settled the nation. With each development came new challenges and opportunities for women and men to create new roles and institutions. Caring for the ill and protecting the health of the society offered nursing a major role in the health care revolution of the twentieth century.

Women's Role in Caring

The health of the American family has always been viewed by society as a responsibility of the woman, usually as a function of the role of the mother. Birth, illness, and dying took place in the home under the watchful ministration of women because it was believed that women possessed a maternal instinct that directed them to care for the sick. To care for the ill bereft of family support, Colonial American communities established almshouses, which served as refuges for the needy and poor and as infirmaries for the sick. The nursing and medical care provided to residents of almshouses, however, reflected the low social status of the indigent and the dismal lack of knowledge concerning diseases and their treatment. Physicians avoided almshouses, preferring to practice medicine in the homes of their private patients. What little nursing care that almshouse residents received was provided by other residents or by female prisoners who served their prison time in the infirmary ward. Although a few religious women provided care to the indigent, it was not considered proper for a "decent" woman to enter an almshouse.

The Birth of the Nursing Profession in America

The Civil War (1861 to 1865) provided a strong catalyst for the movement of women from their homes into nursing. The war created a great demand for nursing services to care for the sick and wounded soldiers in both the North and the South. Women, following Florence Nightingale's example in the Crimean War (1851 to 1855), volunteered to serve in hospitals, infirmaries, and on the battlefields, caring for the injured and dying. Their experience proved that nursing was essential to the care of the hospitalized patient and that women were particularly suited for the occupation. Several prominent women and men who had served in hospitals during the war used that experience to begin nursing schools. In 1873, America's first three Nightingale-modeled schools—Bellevue Training School for Nurses in New York City; Connecticut Training School for Nurses in New Haven, Connecticut; and the Boston Training School for Nurses at Massachusetts General Hospital—were established (Dock, 1907).

Loosely following the Nightingale form of apprenticeship training, these nursing schools attracted single women seeking an occupation that promised higher wages and status than was generally available to women. The training programs stressed on-the-job learning, and although the work was physically daunting and the programs demanded loyalty, obedience, and duty from the pupil, nurses' training promised the opportunity for young women to become self-supporting, independent practitioners employed as private-duty nurses in patients' homes.

Physicians and hospital administrators (many of whom were themselves physicians) of these early nursing programs quickly learned that the quality of patient services could be dramatically improved with the use of "pupil nurses" (as they were known in that era). Soon, other hospitals recognized that, with only a modest investment, a training school could be initiated that would provide an intelligent and skillful labor force for their hospitals (Fig. 1-1). The establishment of nursing schools spread rapidly across the nation, and by 1900 there were 432 schools in the United States (Roberts, 1954).

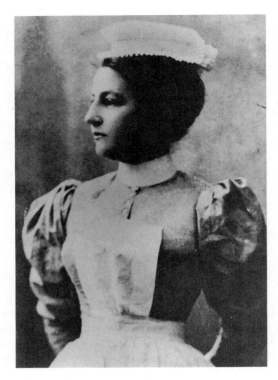

Fig. 1-1   Nurse circa 1903. (From the collection at the Center for Nursing Historical Inquiry, University of Virginia, Charlottesville, VA.)

The birth of nursing coincided with dramatic advances in the medical sciences, including the discovery of anesthesia, Pasteur and Koch's work in bacteriology, and Lister's contribution to antisepsis in surgery. These advances laid the foundation for modern surgery and medicine and, combined with the services of nurses, transformed almshouses from refuges for the destitute to hospitals that provided adequate care and healing. Although they were still primarily used by the poor, by the 1890s hospitals were becoming important in the education and practice of physicians. Physicians soon learned that hospitals with training schools for nurses helped attract paying patients. In addition, the presence of nurses in training also assured the physicians an environment in which their orders were carefully followed (Rosenberg, 1987).

The dual purpose of training schools—to provide patient services and to train students—often conflicted. Caring for patients, however, was considered essential in the preparation of a nurse, and much of the training centered on comfort measures and procedures. In addition to providing direct patient care, students were responsible for keeping the hospital organized and clean, and for preparing food for the patients and staff. Their education became a lesser priority. Nursing lectures had to be slipped into the students' busy days, usually in the evening after a 12-hour day. The superintendents recognized the inadequacies of training but were powerless to remedy the situation. To ensure an adequate supply of student workers, admission and educational standards were kept low. Superintendents who attempted to increase the educational content of the program or to seek auxiliary help to relieve students of housekeeping activities faced being reprimanded or discharged.

In 1893 Isabel Hampton, as superintendent of the Johns Hopkins Hospital School of Nursing, brought together, at the Columbian Exposition in Chicago, many of the superintendents of America's largest schools to discuss problems in nursing education. Adopting many of the strategies used at the time by the American Medical Association to upgrade their profession, the nurse leaders initiated a course of action to gain control of nursing education and to raise its standards (Dock & Stewart, 1931).

STEPS TO PROFESSIONALIZATION

The first step in the long struggle to transform nursing from a vocation to a profession was the establishment of the American Society of Superintendents of Training Schools for Nurses of the United States and Canada in 1894. (This society was renamed the National League of Nursing Education [NLNE] in 1912.) This organization served as the focal point for ideas and strategies that were used by nurses across the nation to gain professional status for nursing. The early nursing leaders also recognized that graduate nurses faced multiple problems establishing their role in a society that could not differentiate between a trained and an untrained nurse. The public's growing perception that many of their physical ills could be relieved by modern medicine had created a demand for the services of nurses. Women who "claimed" to be nurses competed with graduate nurses for employment. Vexed by census data that revealed that there were almost 109,000 "untrained nurses and midwives competing with 12,000 graduate nurses," the superintendents took action to rectify this threatening situation (U.S. Bureau of Census, 1900, p. xxiii). In 1896 this same group of leaders formed the Nurses' Associated Alumnae of the United States and Canada (renamed the American Nurses' Association [ANA] in 1912) (Nutting, 1926).

Nurse Registration

The first initiative of the Nurses' Associated Alumnae (and heartily endorsed by the superintendents' group) was the acquisition of legal registration for nurses. The idea had first been discussed by British nurses. However, opposition from Florence Nightingale, who feared that legal certification would weaken the moral training of nurses, slowed the British nurses' registration movement. American nurses, however, believed that the moral underpinnings of nurses' training would not be weakened by state regulations. Rather, they believed, the legal power of the state could be harnessed to develop uniform nursing educational and ethical standards of practice.

The swift passage of new medical practice acts at the turn of the century served as an example to nurses of how medical educators and state medical societies gained legal monopolies over the provision of certain services and strengthened their powers of self-regulation over practice and medical education (Friedman, 1965). By making nursing licensure dependent on the graduates' educational credentials and performance on a qualifying examination, nursing pioneers believed that the individual state licensure boards would force nursing schools to adopt higher educational standards and thus enhance the economic and social standing of the graduate nurse.

In a salient article in the first issue of the *American Journal of Nursing,* Lavinia Dock outlined a rationale for state licensure and methods that nurses could use to activate the political process. Dock, one of nursing's most analytical leaders and foremost historians, cautioned the politically neophyte nurses that in order to succeed, they would need to form medical and social coalitions. Furthermore, she noted that once legal power was attained, "continuous efforts for the rest of time" would be required to assure nursing a professional status in the health care arena (Dock, 1900).

The Nurses' Associated Alumnae quickly moved to establish constituent state organizations so that local nurses could conduct the necessary lobbying for requiring registration. The quest for state laws forced cohesiveness among nurses and provided them with a structure that allowed private-duty nurses and educators to address nursing problems. The quest also taught them ways to align themselves temporarily with special-interest groups who benefitted economically from the closing of small hospitals whose training programs could not meet licensing standards (Tomes, 1983).

In March of 1903, the North Carolina State Nurses' Association was the first to acquire a registration act. Other registration acts were enacted in New Jersey, New York, and Virginia later in the same year. Although lacking in universal educational standards and any definition of nursing practice, the first registration acts defined for the public that a "registered nurse" had attended an acceptable nursing program and had passed a board evaluation examination. The acts also created state nursing boards that could use some force to remedy educational deficits in schools of nursing.

By 1910, 27 states had passed nurse registration acts in spite of the fact that women lacked the right to vote. By 1923 all the states in the United States, plus Hawaii and the District of Columbia, had nurse registration laws (Bullough, 1975).

COMMUNITY HEALTH NURSING

The rapid urbanization and industrialization of the United States at the turn of the century was fueled by the massive influx of immigrants. Between 1890 and 1910 almost 19 million immigrants sought new homes in America, especially in the cities. As a result, urban populations rose by 12 million in cities with over 100,000 inhabitants (Taylor, 1971).

Crowded into squalid tenement districts in ethnic ghettos, immigrants fought to survive and raise their families. In the 1870s concerned American women, worried about the living conditions of the immigrants, employed graduate nurses to visit among the ghetto poor. Under the auspices of private philanthropy, the Boston and Philadelphia Visiting Nurse Societies were founded in the 1880s. The role of the community health nurse, however, was firmly established by the actions of Lillian Wald, a graduate nurse (Buhler-Wilkerson, 1989).

In 1893 New York City not only served as the country's major port of entry, but it also was home to the largest number of immigrants. Wald, a recent graduate of the New York Hospital Training School, was teaching a home nursing class to immigrants on the city's lower East Side when she was asked to visit an ill woman in the tenements. The shock of finding a desperately ill person amidst the residue of a 2-day-old hemorrhage profoundly influenced her life. From that point on, Wald made it her life's work to serve the country's forgotten immigrant and poor families (Wald, 1938).

Securing financial support from wealthy friends, Wald and a fellow nurse, Mary Brewster, moved into an East Side apartment and began offering nursing services to their neighbors. The community's need for nursing care soon necessitated more nurses and a move to larger quarters. In 1895 the famed Henry Street Settlement House and Henry Street Visiting Nurse Services came into existence.

Under Wald's innovative leadership, many creative roles for community nurses were launched. In 1902 Wald offered the services of a nurse to the New York City school board in an experimental program. Wald wanted to demonstrate that the high absenteeism from school because of illness could be reduced. In 1 month, the absenteeism among the children had been reduced so significantly that the city's school board hired the nurse; then in 1903 the school board hired 27 more nurses to work within the system. Within 2 years, school nurses came to be recognized as an essential component of children's health services in cities across the country (Struthers, 1917).

In 1909, community services were further expanded by Wald in a joint project with the Metropolitan Life Insurance Company that sent nurses into the homes of the company's policy holders when they were ill. The financial benefit accrued by the company from the project guided them to contract for similar nursing services with over 400 visiting nurse agencies in the United States and Canada by 1912. Other major insurance companies followed suit and employed nurses to provide health services to their industrial policy owners. This business relationship with insurance companies not only subsidized the growth of community nursing, but also taught nurses the need for patient record keeping, the importance of health statistics, and the relationship of patient costs and the outcome of services rendered (Hamilton, 1989). Metropolitan Life Insurance Company, through pioneer health surveys done with nurses, became the authoritative source of data on the nation's health status (Hamilton, 1992).

Additional community services, such as industrial nursing in 1895, tuberculosis nursing in 1903, and infant welfare nursing arising from the clean milk movement of the 1900s, expanded the numbers and domain of nurses. Mary Gardner, a public health leader and early textbook author, estimated that the 200 public health nurses in 1900 had grown to approximately 3000 by 1912 (Gardner, 1936). The development of public health was important to the nation and to the profession because it brought health care and health teaching to the public and provided graduate nurses more opportunity to use concepts of sanitation, epidemiology, and health education in developing new nursing skills, Just as important, community nurses were enlarging the client domain of nursing to include individuals, families, and communities. Their pioneer activities in health promotion, disease prevention, and advocacy of welfare reform were shaping both the American public health system and the discipline of nursing (Fig. 1-2).

In 1912 the National Organization for Public Heath Nursing (NOPHN) became nursing's first clinical specialty national organization. Lillian Wald named the specialty *public health nursing* in the hope that the newly emerging fields of health nursing and preventive medicine could be linked together to meet the health needs of the public (Brainard, 1922).

The NOPHN worked closely with the Children's Bureau to implement systematic studies of the conditions that contributed to the nation's high infant and maternal mortality and morbidity rates. These studies, and the publicity they received, emphasized the need for better infant and obstetrical care, especially for low-income rural families. As a result, in 1921 Congress approved the Sheppard-Towner Maternal and Infant Act. Forty-five states quickly passed legislation enabling them to qualify for matching federal funds to establish health services to at-risk mothers and children. Nurses proved to be critical to the states' success in bringing health care to families in remote regions of the country (Brodie, 1993).

In 1925, 561 permanent child health and prenatal centers were opened, and a total of 21,935 health-related conferences were given by nurses and physicians. Public health nurses also provided 299,100 instructional home visits and contacted thousands of local physicians to ensure that infants and mothers in need of medical care received help (Meckel, 1990). Opposition, primarily from the American Medical Association, terminated this federal initiative in 1929, but the precedent had been set for the government's involvement in the provision of health care to citizens.

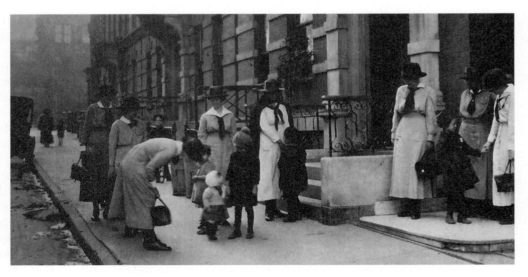

Fig. 1-2   Public health nurses in the 1930s. (Courtesy Visiting Nurse Service of New York City.)

PRIVATE-DUTY NURSING

The belief that student nursing services were desirable for patient care left little opportunity for graduate nurses to find employment in hospitals. The majority of registered nurses therefore worked as private-duty nurses in the homes of families. Working as independent practitioners and committed to individual patient care, graduate nurses enjoyed being independent of hospital restrictions. By the 1920s, however, graduates found that employment opportunities were scarce, and the conditions under which they worked were becoming increasingly difficult. Patients, once plentiful, were now referred to nurses by either physicians or through nurse registries. To ensure their employment, nurses had to be available within hours to be dispatched to patients' homes. Once assigned a patient, the nurse worked in increments of 12 to 24 hours for as many days as necessary, staying in the patient's home. The work, often involving domestic chores, was exhausting and socially isolating. In addition, the pay was poor. Annual earnings of a nurse in the late 1910s averaged about $950, a sum that sustained her but left little to be set aside for future needs (Reverby, 1987).

By 1920 the plight of the private-duty nurse became grimmer. The families who had been able to afford nurses in their homes began to use hospitals when illness occurred. Although they still engaged a private-duty nurse in the hospital when a loved one was critically ill, families used the services of the hospital's student nurse staff once the crisis period had passed. Physicians and hospital administrators supported this decision because not having to pay for private-duty nurses left families better able to pay the bills of the physicians and hospitals (Reverby, 1983).

Advances in medicine during this decade encouraged more people to use hospitals. Instead of adding graduate nurses to their staffs to meet new patient demands, hospital administrators increased their numbers of student nurses. Disturbed by the economic plight of graduate nurses, the NLNE, ANA, and NOPHN authorized a study of the economic status of nursing in 1926. May Ayers Burgess, the statistician who directed the survey, uncovered the widespread underemployment and bleakness of working conditions of most graduates (Burgess, 1928).

A survey of New York State nurses by Janet Geister, a strong advocate of private-duty nurses, confirmed their economic difficulties. She reported that even when work was found, 80 percent of the nurses were only able to obtain 1-day, 12-hour cases. This level of employment provided a weekly salary of $31.26. Nurses' hourly rate now averaged 49 cents, slightly less than the 50 cents an hour that scrubwomen earned (Geister, 1926).

MODERN HOSPITALS

America's appreciation of the benefits of scientific medicine could be seen in the proliferation of hospitals and in the increase in status of the physicians who used them. Between 1925 and 1929, $890 million was spent on the construction of hospitals. Modern obstetrics, with its promise of "twilight sleep" to reduce the pain of childbirth, attracted women to the prospect of delivering in a hospital. Furthermore, the addition of pediatric and psychiatric specialties, physical therapy services, and private rooms enhanced the hospital's image in the eyes of the consumer (Roren, 1930).

While medical care provided in hospitals had become increasingly sophisticated, the inexpensive and unsophisticated labor provided by student nurses still met the needs of most hospital administrators and physicians. it was argued that hiring graduate nurses would not only add to hospital costs, but also would allow graduates an opportunity to become involved in medical and hospital decisions. As one physician-administrator noted, nursing was "only a differentiation of domestic duty" and the graduate nurse a "half-baked social product thrust into the fulfillment of an uncertain social need" (Howard, 1912, p. 76).

Nursing educators, through the NLNE and the state boards of nursing, continued to struggle to convince hospitals that graduate nurses should provide more patient services so that students might be educated in the science of nursing. Even after the publication of the results of the landmark Goldmark Report, a national study of nursing education modeled on the Flexner Report of medical education, little had been accomplished in raising the standards of nursing education and practice (Goldmark, 1923).

The Depression Years

The economic depression that gripped the country in the 1930s drastically altered American life. The sharp decline of the world's economy brought financial, social, and health problems to the nation. Business failures and unemployment spread throughout the country, and by 1932 one out of four working Americans was without a job (Blum, 1981).

Hospital administrators, faced with a drastic reduction in the number of paying patients, were forced to examine the costs of providing care. This examination included the costs of nursing services. Many small hospitals closed or terminated their schools of nursing in an effort to reduce costs. At the same time, large hospitals, especially municipal ones, experienced an influx of patients seeking charitable care. To rectify this situation, Blue Cross, a revolutionary prepaid health insurance plan, was developed by groups of hospitals (Numbers, 1978). Selling health plans to workers able to pay for future services, this program ensured the financial stability of hospitals.

The American Medical Association rejected the plan, characterizing it as being "economically unsound, unethical and inimical to the public interests" (Kimball, 1934, p. 45). In spite of this opposition, Blue Cross proved to be attractive to hospitals and patients, and because it kept community hospitals open, it was formally approved by the American Hospital Association in 1937. As one hospital official noted, "Blue Cross was sired by the Depression and mothered by hospitals out of desperate economic necessity" (Sommers & Sommers, 1961, p. 21). Over 1 million people participated as members of Blue Cross in 1937, providing hospitals with enough income not only to remain open, but also to grow.

Staff Nursing

Nurses' training programs, however, continued to be seen as a financial drain on hospitals. The cost of maintaining these nursing schools proved so expensive that 570 training programs closed in the 1930s. At first, hospitals replaced student nurses with untrained attendants. In time, however, it became evident that graduate nurses were essential to the provision of safe patient care. This recognition on the part of hospital administrators, coupled with the availability of unemployed graduate nurses willing to work for minimum wages, led to the addition of graduate nurses to hospital staffs (Fitzpatrick, 1975).

The transition to a graduate nursing staff, increasing in numbers from 4000 positions in 1929, to 28,000 in 1937, to over 100,000 by 1941, added quality to the nursing care of patients. It also introduced professional tension within the hospital system (Cannings & Lazonick, 1975). Many hospital administrators were accustomed to having student nurses provide patient care. As a result, they considered paying for nursing services "unreasonable." In addition, graduate nurses were viewed as a potential threat to the administrators and physicians because they were far less compliant than students, and their clinical decisions were based on their independent judgment rather than hospital routine.

The graduate nurses, although welcoming the steady employment provided in the hospital and the opportunity to develop new clinical and management skills, experienced their own set of tensions. As independent, private-duty practitioners, they had possessed the power to control the quality of their patient care. Staff nursing, however, required that they function in a bureaucracy, in a role that demanded loyalty to the institution and the physician rather than to the patient. The employment of lower-paid, subsidiary nursing and housekeeping personnel added to the expanding numbers of personnel that the graduate nurse was expected to manage efficiently. For many, the strict institutional control of their practice reminded them of the harsh discipline, regimentation, and exploitation of their student days (Flood, 1981).

Given the economic realities of the Depression, however, both graduates and hospital administrators began an uneasy working alliance. Learning how to interact with professional graduates rather than with a student staff challenged hospital administrators for decades. Well into the 1950s and later, hospital administrators failed to establish personnel policies that befitted a professional group. Instead, as historian Susan Reverby notes in her book *Ordered to Care,* they offered graduates "low pay, long hours, split shifts, authoritarian supervision, and rigid rules" (Reverby, 1987, p. 192).

COLLEGIATE NURSING EDUCATION: THE EARLY YEARS

In 1899, with the offering of a postdiploma hospital economics program at Teachers College, Columbia University, nursing marked its first effort to move into academic institutions. The original program, conceived by Isabel Hampton Robb, was designed, partially taught, and voluntarily funded by NLNE members. The program prepared nurses to manage nursing services and educate pupil nurses. A generous endowment of $200,000 in 1910 by Helen Hartley Jenkins, a trustee of Teachers College, financially established the department and allowed for its expansion. Directed for 40 years by two outstanding educators, Mary Adelaide Nutting and Isabel Stewart, the college offered innovative programs in administration, education, and public health nursing to thousands of nurses from the United States and abroad (Christy, 1969).

Several short-lived basic collegiate programs also opened in the 1890s, but it was the University of Minnesota in 1909 that established the first permanent university-related nursing program in the United States. The inability of hospital training programs to improve the educational experiences for students stimulated leaders to establish university programs, and by 1923 there were 17 schools offering 5-year degree programs. Because of time and financial costs, enrollment in these institutions remained relatively low compared with enrollment in diploma programs. While nursing had made some progress toward undergraduate collegiate status, it lacked the major financial support given to the profession of medicine.

Large foundation endowments, primarily from the Rockefeller, Carnegie, and Commonwealth funds, moved medical education into the mainstream of university education. The famous Flexner Report of 1910 served as the catalyst for this action. Subsequently, through the Rockefeller General Education Board alone, over $91 million was funneled into medical schools (Starr, 1982, p. 121). Nursing leaders, impressed with the ability of medicine to develop into a scientific discipline, sought similar assistance for nursing education. Only the Rockefeller Foundation, however, could be persuaded to endow the establishment of two schools: Yale in 1924 and Vanderbilt in 1930.

Annie Goodrich, noted nursing educator and director of the Army School of Nursing in 1918, was selected to direct an autonomous collegiate school at Yale University. The program was based on the premise that nursing concepts pertinent to acute illness, the psychosocial dimensions of illness, and public health were foundational to nursing practice. Using a "case method" approach to patient care rather than teaching nursing techniques, and assigning nursing students to various clinical agencies for educational experiences, Yale faculty demonstrated what collegiate nursing would become (Sheahan, 1979).

In Cleveland Case Western Reserve University's Department of Nursing Education was endowed in 1923 by Frances Payne Bolton, allowing it to offer an undergraduate program. In 1923 both Case Western Reserve University and Yale University began master's degree programs in nursing education (Faddis, 1973). Catholic University of America began graduate courses in 1932, and the University of Chicago developed a graduate program in 1934 (Baer, 1992). By 1935 there were sufficient numbers of collegiate programs to organize the Association of Collegiate Schools of Nursing. This organization's major mission was to establish collegiate nursing programs in America's universities. Its members believed that nursing would not become a profession until it could generate scientifically sound nursing knowledge (Stewart, 1943).

GOVERNMENT INITIATIVES

A characteristic of twentieth-century America has been the federal government's growing involvement in matters pertaining to the health and welfare of citizens. Since nurses have been consistently involved in this arena, the affairs of nursing have been significantly influenced by the actions of the government. The federal government's first involvement with nursing came as a result of wartime emergencies. Beginning with the Civil War, both the Union and Confederate armies sought the services of women to care for the ill and wounded. During the Spanish-American War in 1898, nurses volunteered to serve with the military to care for thousands of soldiers suffering from yellow fever. This experience persuaded Congress that nurses should be permanent members of the nation's defense forces. As a result, the Army Nurse Corps was begun in 1901, and the Navy Nurse Corps was initiated in 1908.

State governments were also involved with nursing in the early years. At the turn of the century, when nursing sought to protect the public from untrained practitioners and upgrade its educational standards, state governments supported nursing's claim to special knowledge and expertise, and passed legislation requiring nurse registration.

During World War I (1917 to 1919), nursing leaders cooperated with the government to mobilize nurses to serve in the war effort. Innovative programs to increase the supply of nurses, such as the Vassar College nursing program and the Army School of Nursing, were designed by nurses and supported by the government (Koch, 1951; "Vassar Prepatory Course," 1918).

The economic depression of the 1930s created as severe a national emergency as did external wars. The severity and length of the depression threatened the stability of the country and the health of the people. During President Franklin D. Roosevelt's first term (1932 to 1936), the government enacted emergency legislation that created jobs that improved the nation's health and welfare. The Federal Emergency Relief Act and the Works Progress Administration not only provided health and medical care for indigent citizens, but also provided employment for thousands of nurses in hospitals and public health agencies. In addition, the passage of the Social Security Act in 1935, with its welfare benefits for the elderly, extended the government's mandate to assume responsibility for the well-being of its citizens (Stevens, 1971).

World War II

As war spread throughout Europe and the Eastern Hemisphere in 1939, the United States prepared for the possibility of military involvement. When Congress declared war on December 8, 1941, however, inadequate numbers of nurses for military and civilian needs created a dangerous situation. To deal with this crisis, the federal government created two programs to ease the nursing shortage: the American Red Cross volunteer nurse's aides program (1941), and the Cadet Nurse Corps (1943) (Johnston, 1966) (Fig. 1-3).

The American Red Cross nurse's aides program grew out of the country's need for nursing personnel. The loss of professional and nonprofessional staff to the military and to defense industry positions left hospitals and public health agencies in need of auxiliary help to provide care for the citizens on the home front. Through a joint venture with the Office of Civilian Defense and the American Red Cross, over 200,000 women volunteered to become certified nurse's aides and worked under nursing supervision to provide nursing care. This successful experience proved to be an important step in the stratification of nursing's functions into registered, practical, and aide levels (Bullough & Bullough, 1978).

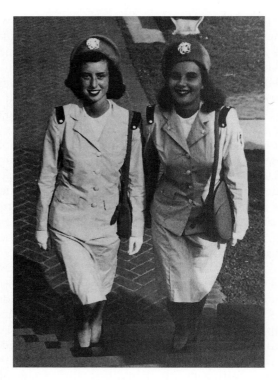

Fig. 1-3   Cadet nurses. (From the collection at the Center for Nursing Historical Inquiry, University of Virginia, Charlottesville, VA.)

The Cadet Nurse Corps was the most significant program sponsored by the federal government to increase the supply of nurses. In 1943 Congresswoman Frances Payne Bolton from Ohio, long a friend of nursing, sponsored a bill that authorized the U.S. Public Health Service to establish the Cadet Nurse Corps. The Cadet Nurse Corps subsidized the education of nursing students who agreed to serve in military or civilian agencies for the duration of the war. This program paid for tuition, fees, and books, and provided a monthly stipend to student nurses throughout their training. Nursing schools that agreed to participate in the program also received funds for instructional facilities and support for faculty seeking postgraduate education.

Although the Cadet Nurse Corps accepted students for only 2 years (July 1943 to October 1945), almost 170,00 cadets entered 1125 participating schools, and two thirds of these students graduated. The Cadet Nurse Corps not only added a large number of nurses to the profession, but it also instigated major changes in nursing education. Government requirements of a 30-month (versus a 36-month) program, a 48-hour student work week of classes and clinical work (versus 56 hours), and the removal of policies that discriminated on the basis of race and marital status allowed faculty an opportunity to redesign nursing education. In addition, because the federal money had to be administered by the schools' nursing directors, the costs of the educational pro-grams and the services the students provided the hospitals became known. Armed with this new information, school directors were better able to negotiate the funds necessary to upgrade programs (Brueggemann, 1992).

Nursing and Minorities

As another method to increase the availability of graduate nurses, the profession turned to two groups that had been excluded from mainstream nursing: African-Amer-icans and men. The racial and gender biases of the era had led to the development of discriminatory or restricted policies regarding the admission and employment of both African-Americans and men. To become nurses, African-American women attended African-American hospital schools of nursing. Men enrolled in male-only schools lo-cated primarily in state and religious hospitals or sanitariums. Although these groups numbered less than 10,000 of the 280,000 registered nurses in the United States in 1940, they represented a valuable resource to the nation. However, the resource could only be used if the discriminating practices could be reversed (Kalisch & Kalisch, 1995).

The crisis of a world war, with its shortage of nursing personnel, led to some changes in discriminatory practices. Educational and employment opportunities for African-American nurses improved. Through the efforts of professional nursing groups, espe-cially the National Association of Colored Graduate Nurses (NACGN), the Cadet Nurse Corps was initiated in the schools that admitted only African-Americans. In addition, some of the traditionally "white-only" schools integrated African-American students in order to meet the necessary quota of students to qualify for Cadet Nurse Corps funding. By 1945 African-American enrollment in the nation's nursing schools had reached a record high of almost 2600 students, a 135% increase from the 1939 figure (Hine, 1989).

Racial barriers were also broken down when restrictive employment practices in hos-pitals and public health agencies were removed. Since many civilian health facilities had lost large numbers of their graduate nurses to the Army and Navy Nurse Corps, they began to meet their staffing needs by employing African-American nurses (Os-borne, 1949).

For African-American nurses, the task of gaining admission to the Army and Navy Nurse Corps proved more difficult than that of being accepted in civilian hospitals. The Army Nurse Corps maintained restricted quotas, and the Navy Nurse Corps ex-cluded all African-Americans. These policies, combined with the willingness of Congress to consider a nurse draft bill in late 1944, turned public opinion against the armed services discriminatory policies. As a result, in January 1945, both military nurse corps lifted their racial barriers and accepted African-American female nurses.

Male nurses faced a different type of discrimination than did African-American fe-male nurses. Tradition and sentiment had long dictated that nursing was uniquely a woman's field, and in establishing the military nurse corps in the 1900s, Congress ruled that only women would be appointed as military nurses. Male nursing students and graduates were subject to the Selective Service draft. Consequently, many of them ei-ther volunteered or were drafted into the armed services. Although their military assignments varied, they possessed no official nursing status and served as enlisted personnel primarily in non-health-related positions (Rose, 1947).

Led by the ANA, several nursing groups appealed to the War Department throughout the war to secure rank and official nurse's designation for male nurses. However, these appeals were consistently opposed by the Army and Navy medical departments. Sentiment among many nurses and the public also endorsed the belief that during the war men should serve on the battlefields while female nurses tended to the sick and wounded. It was not until 1966, when the United States was engaged in the Vietnam War and nurses were in short supply, that Congress authorized the appointment of male nurses to the Army, Navy, and Air Force Nurse Corps.

In a spirit of cooperation and change brought about by the war efforts, there was a steady increase in the integration of African-American and male nurses into the country's nursing schools from 1945 to 1952 (Fig. 1-4). The substantial growth in numbers of African-American graduates stimulated many state nurses' associations to remove their racial barriers to membership. General integration into the ANA was hastened in 1948 when its House of Delegates granted individual membership to African-American nurses barred from state associations and adopted a resolution calling for the establishment of biracial communities at district and state levels. Responding to the fact that by 1950 only two state associations retained discriminatory racial restrictions, the NACGN issued a press release announcing the dissolution of the organization. Recognizing the acceptance of African-American nurses into the ANA, Mabel Staupers, the president of the NACGN, declared that "its program of activities is no longer necessary" (Staupers, 1951).

The end of overt professional discrimination and segregation of both African-American and male nurses did not eradicate more subtle and sophisticated forms of preju-

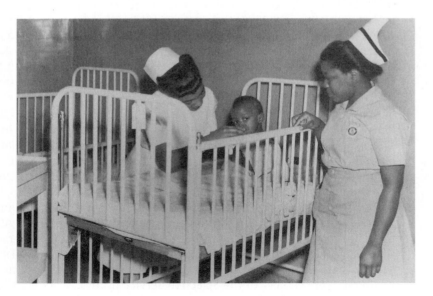

Fig. 1-4   African-American nurses, circa 1950. (Courtesy Hampton University Archives, Hampton, VA.)

dice. It did, however, allow the profession and the health care system to benefit from the contributions of an increased number of minority graduate nurses.

Post–World War II

After World War II, the role of the federal government in health affairs expanded to include not only funding but also policy formation and the establishment of health priorities for the nation. Although funding for nursing education remained modest until 1960, money began to be allocated for nursing research. Under Director Jessie Scott, the restructured U.S. Public Health Division of Nursing assisted Congress in passing the Nurse Training Act of 1964. This act was a response to the nation's demand for more health services. The needs of the country's baby boom population (78 million Americans), the special needs of the elderly, and the availability of private hospitalization insurance had created widespread shortages of nurses. Congress, acknowledging that educated nurses were essential in meeting the public's demand, awarded $242.6 million for scholarships, loans, recruitment, school construction and maintenance, and special projects to improve nursing education (Kalisch & Kalisch, 1982).

The public's growing belief in the power of modern medicine was sustained by advances in pharmacology and surgery. Penicillin, the first of the so-called "miracle drugs," not only successfully treated serious infections, but in preventing postoperative infections, it also promoted new opportunities in surgery. The discovery of new drugs and advances in technology made health professionals and patients optimistic about the conquest of disease. The public, sustained by this optimism, encouraged the government to fund medical research and to subsidize the care of the elderly and the indigent through such programs as Medicare and Medicaid in 1965 (Stevens, 1971).

Nursing, as a key player in the modern health care system, received federal support to expand its role in the provision of care. To fully expand its role, however, the profession needed more than funding. It needed to sever the ties that bound nursing education to hospitals.

NURSING IN HIGHER EDUCATION

After World War II, Congress passed the GI Bill, enabling veterans to acquire a college education (Kiester, 1994). Among those veterans receiving funds to attend college were military nurses who enrolled in collegiate programs, seeking degrees in nursing education and administration. Increased enrollment gave new life to collegiate schools, and by the 1950s many colleges began to develop basic baccalaureate nursing programs. By 1962 there were 178 colleges offering undergraduate degrees in nursing, and the pool of college-educated nurses (Fig. 1-5) began to expand (Brown, 1978).

Community College Nursing

The severity of the nursing shortage in the late 1940s also encouraged the development of experimental programs to educate new and different types of nurses. In 1951

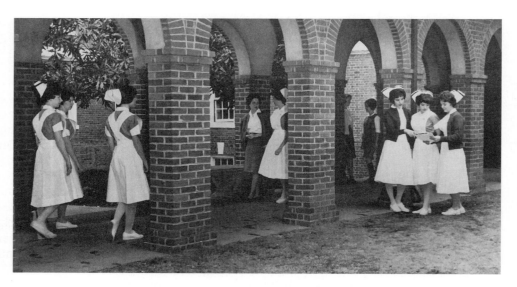

Fig. 1-5   Nursing students at the University of Virginia, circa 1960. (From the collection at the Center for Nursing Historical Inquiry, University of Virginia, Charlottesville, VA.)

Mildred Montag proposed an educational study to prepare nurse technicians in 2-year associate degree (AD) community college programs. After a 5-year study of these AD graduates from seven participating colleges, Montag's program was deemed successful. Success was based on the fact that the AD graduates were able to pass state nursing licensure examinations and demonstrate clinical nursing competency, and all were employed as graduate nurses (Haase, 1990).

Encouraged by these results, the W.K. Kellogg foundation funded similar school projects in four states in 1959. The success of these schools launched the AD nursing education movement across the country. Acquiring funding from the Nurse Training Act of 1964, community colleges opened AD programs at a phenomenal rate. From 1952 to 1974, the number of AD programs in the country doubled every 4 years. During one period, new programs were opening at the rate of one per week (Rines, 1977).

Several important goals were attained by the AD programs' success. A new pool of students, including those who were older than the typical undergraduate, men, and married women with children, were now selecting careers in nursing. These new graduates helped reduce the serious nursing shortages of the 1970s and 1980s. The success of the AD movement also helped move nursing education away from the apprenticeship model of the diploma programs and placed it in community colleges. Although this move enhanced the scope of nursing education, its price was the existence of a confusing mixture of nursing educational programs—diploma, associate degree, and baccalaureate—all leading to registered nurse licensure and entry level positions.

Master's Education in Nursing

The technological and scientific advances continued in the field of medicine during the period 1940 to 1960. As a result, medical care became more complex, and clinical subspecialties and intensive care units developed throughout the nation. The knowledge explosion in medicine, coupled with advances in the social sciences and the results of beginning nursing research, led to the generation of new nursing knowledge and a demand for more nursing research. By the 1970s research courses were incorporated into both baccalaureate and graduate program curricula. Moreover, there was an increased demand for graduate education for nurses, particularly at the master's level.

The scope of nursing's clinical practice had enlarged with the advances in medicine. In addition, society's need for primary care, along with the emphasis on subspecialties within hospitals, shifted the focus of master's programs from administration and teaching to advanced clinical practice and specialization. During the late 1970s and 1980s, nurses sought master's preparation to become nurse practitioners and clinical nurse specialists (Jolly & Hart, 1987). In so doing, nursing took another step toward defining its clinical knowledge, expertise, and identity in the health care system.

Doctoral Education in Nursing

By the 1960s programs leading to doctoral degrees in nursing began to be inaugurated. This logical step in nursing's struggle to attain disciplinary status and independence as a profession had been accelerated by the growing pool of master's prepared nurses in the 1950s. In 1955 the U.S. Public Health Service began to fund doctoral study for nurses through predoctoral research fellowships. The federal government also awarded Nurse Scientist Training Program grants directly to schools of nursing to finance doctoral educational programs (Grace, 1978).

Doctoral education offered the profession a unique opportunity to develop a scientific basis for its caring services. It also provided nurse researchers and scholars opportunities to develop disciplinary knowledge beyond the confines of the medical model of practice. Strongly influenced by the prevalent views of philosophy of science, particularly by empirical methodology and Kuhn's ideas about the nature of science (Kuhn, 1962), early nurse scholars began an attempt to identify theories that would unify nursing's unique body of knowledge. By the 1980s, again influenced by changes in the prevailing views in philosophy of science, the realization of the limitations of "empirical" science guided nurse scholars to expand what they considered phenomena of inquiry to include the subjective nature of human experience. In so doing, they began to use qualitative research methods that emphasized a holistic nursing perspective. In addition, they refocused their work on the development of theories that originated in practice and could be applied to practice. The increased numbers of nurse researchers and the availability of research funding generated not only studies that addressed clinical nursing questions but also multidisciplinary studies that reflected nursing's significant role in the health care system.

•   •   •

Throughout its history, nursing has sought to fulfill its social mandate to provide nursing care. To fulfill its role as a major health care provider, it had to gain professional expertise and autonomy. The development of clinical practice domains and skills, and the movement of nursing education into institutions of higher education were essential to nursing's quest for professional authority.

Nurses of the twenty-first century need to continue to be sensitive to the social and environmental changes that influence clinical practice and the development of nursing knowledge. As the American health care movement broadens, it is reasonable to assume that the new system will demand efficient and cost-effective nursing care. It may require that nurses develop new skills and attitudes. It is also reasonable to assume that much of what is central to the discipline, the concepts of nursing that have survived throughout its development over the last century, will still be of value (Keeling & Ramos, 1995). Understanding the history of the profession offers insight into the social, political, and economic forces that shaped its place in society and its contribution to the health of the nation.

"The ways in which we address the crises and challenges of today have much to do with our understanding and ownership of the past."
Church, 1993, p. 1

 ## Key Points

- The nursing profession is a distillation of over 100 years of development.

- Women have traditionally been expected to care for the ill.

- In 1873 America's first three Nightingale-modeled schools of nursing were established.

- By 1900 there were 432 schools of nursing in the United States.

- In 1983 many superintendents of America's largest nursing schools met to gain control of nursing education and raise its standards.

- In 1903 North Carolina was the first state to require an acceptable program of nursing education, as well as passing an examination, before a person could use the term *registered nurse*.

- By 1923 all states had nurse registration laws.

- Since the beginning of the century, nurses have played a major role in providing health services to the community as public health nurses.

- During World War II, the Cadet Nurse Corps subsidized the education of nursing students who agreed to serve in military or civilian agencies for the duration of the war.

- African-American nurses were first accepted into the military nursing services in 1945.

- From 1952 to 1974, the number of associate degree nursing programs doubled every 4 years.

- Doctoral programs in nursing began in the 1960s and dramatically increased the numbers of nurses prepared to provide leadership and develop nursing research.

Critical Thinking Exercises

1. What do you think might have occurred within the profession of nursing if it had not used an apprenticeship model of education in the early years?

2. Discuss the influences of the growth of hospitals on the profession. How has it changed, and how does this influence the current role of nurses in hospitals?

3. What did public health nursing add to the discipline?

4. How did the federal government influence the nursing profession and its educational preparation? What were the positive and negative implications?

5. In examining the past, how has the nursing profession shaped the current health care system?

6. How does the history of discrimination against men and African-American women in nursing influence current nursing practice?

References

Baer, E. (1992). Aspirations unattained: The story of the Illinois Training School's search for university status. *Nursing Research, 41*(1), 43-48.

Blum, J. (1981). The end of an era. In J. Blum (Ed.), *The national experience* (pp. 652-669). New York: Harcourt Brace Jovanovich.

Brainard, A. (1922). *The evolution of public health nursing.* Philadelphia: W.B. Saunders.

Brodie, B. (1993). Children's Bureau: Guardian of American children. *Nursing Research, 17*(3), 190-191.

Brown, J. (1978). Master's education in nursing, 1945-1969. In M. Louise Fitzpatrick (Ed.), *Historical studies in nursing* (pp. 104-130). New York: Teachers College Press.

Brueggemann, D. (1992). *The United States Cadet Nurse Corps 1943-1948: The Nebraska experience.* Masters thesis, University of Nebraska at Omaha.

Buhler-Wilkerson, K. (1989). *False dawn.* New York: Garland Publishing.

Bullough, B. (1975). The first two phases in nursing licensure. In B. Bullough (Ed.), *The law and the expanding nurse's role* (pp. 7-21). New York: Appleton-Century-Crofts.

Bullough, V., & Bullough, B. (1978). *The care of the sick: The emergence of modern nursing.* New York: Prodist.

Burgess, M. (1928). *Nurses, patients and pocketbooks.* New York: Committee on the Grading of Nursing Schools.

Cannings, K., & Lazonick, W. (1975). The development of the nursing labor force in the United States: A brief analysis. *International Journal of Health Services, 5,* 185-217.

Christy, T. (1969). *Cornerstone for nursing education.* New York: Teachers College Press.

Church, O.M. (1933, September). *In search of nursing's history* (pp. 1-3). A communication service to nursing school deans, administrators, and faculty.

Dock, L. (1900, October). What we might expect from the law. *American Journal of Nursing, 1,* 8-12.

Dock, L. (1907). *A history of nursing* (Vol. 2). New York: G.P. Putnam's Sons.

Dock, L., & Stewart, I. (1931). *A short history of nursing.* New York: G.P. Putnam's Sons.

Faddis, M. (1973). *A school of nursing comes of age: A history of the Frances Payne Bolton School of Nursing.* Cleveland: Alumnae of Frances P. Bolton School of Nursing.

Fitzpatrick, M.L. (1975). Nurses in American History: Nursing and the Great Depression. *American Journal of Nursing, 75,* 2188-2190.

Flood, M. (1981). *The troubling expedient: General staff nursing in United States hospitals in the 1930s: A means to institutional, educational, and personal ends.* Doctoral dissertation, University of California, Berkeley.

Friedman, L. (1965, March-May). Freedom of contract and licensing, 1890-1910. *California Law Review, 53,* 487-534.

Gardner, M. (1936). *Public health nursing* (3rd ed.). New York: Macmillan.

Geister, J. (1926). Hearsay and fact in private duty. *American Journal of Nursing, 26,* 515-528.

Goldmark, J., and the Committee for the Study of Nursing Education. (1923). *Nursing and nursing education in the United States.* New York: Macmillan.

Grace, H.C. (1978). The development of doctoral education in nursing: A historical education perspective. *Journal of Nursing Education, 17,* 17-27.

Haase, P. (1990). *The origins and rise of associate degree nursing education.* Durham: Duke University Press.

Hamilton, D. (1989). The cost of caring: The Metropolitan Life Insurance Company's Visiting Nurse Service, 1909-1953. *Bulletin of the History of Medicine, 63,* 414-434.

Hamilton, D. (1992). Research and reform: Community nursing and the Framingham Tuberculosis project, 1924-1923. *Nursing Research, 41,* 8-13.

Hine, D. (1989). *Black nurses in white.* Bloomington: Indiana University.

Howard, H.B. (1912). The medical superintendent (Section on hospitals). *American Medical Association Transactions,* p. 76.

Johnston, D.F. (1966). *History and trends of practical nursing.* St. Louis: Mosby.

Jolly, M., & Hart, S. (1987). Master's prepared nurses: Societal needs and educational realities. In S.E. Hart (Ed.), *Issues in graduate nursing education* (NLN Publication No. 18-2196, pp. 25-31). New York: National League for Nursing.

Kalisch, B., & Kalisch, P. (1982). *Politics of nursing.* Philadelphia: J.B. Lippincott.

Kalisch, P., & Kalisch, B. (1995). *The advance of American nursing* (3rd ed.). Philadelphia: J.B. Lippincott.

Keeling, A., & Ramos, M. (1995, January-February). The role of nursing history in preparing nursing for the future. *Nursing and Health Care, 16,* 30-34.

Kiester, E. (1994). The GI Bill may be the best deal ever made by Uncle Sam. *Smithsonian, 25*(8), 128-139.

Kimball, J.F. (1934). Prepayment plan of hospital care. *American Hospital Association Bulletin, 8,* 45.

Koch, H. (1951). *Militant angel: Annie W. Goodrich.* New York: Macmillan.

Kuhn, T.S. (1962). *The structure of scientific revolutions.* Chicago: University Press.

Meckel, R. (1990). *Save the babies.* Baltimore: Johns Hopkins University Press.

Numbers, R. (1978). The third party: Health insurance in America. In J. Leavitt & R. Numbers (Eds.), *Sickness and health in America* (pp. 142-145). Madison: University of Wisconsin.

Nutting, A. (1912). *Educational status and nursing* (U.S. Bureau of Education, Bulletin 1912, No. 7). Washington, DC: U.S. Government Printing Office.

Nutting, A. (1926). *A sound economic basis for schools of nursing.* New York: G.P. Putnam's Sons.

Osborne, E. (1949). Status and contributions of the Negro nurse. *Journal of Negro Education, 18,* 364-369.

Reverby, S. (1983). Something besides waiting: The politics of private duty nursing reform in the depression. In E. Lagemann (Ed.), *Nursing history: New perspectives, new possibilities* (pp. 133-156). New York: Teachers College Press.

Reverby, S. (1987). *Ordered to care.* New York: Cambridge University Press.

Rines, A. (1977). Associate degree nursing education: History, development and rationale. *Nursing Outlook, 25,* 496-501.

Roberts, M. (1954). *American nursing: History and interpretation.* New York: Macmillan.

Roren, R. (1930). *The public's investment in hospitals* (Committee on the Costs of Medical Care, Publication No. 7). Chicago: University of Chicago Press.

Rose, J. (1947). Men nurses in military service. *American Journal of Nursing, 47,* 147-148.

Rosenberg, C. (1987). *The care of strangers.* New York: Basic Books.

Sheahan, D. (1979). *The social origins of American nursing and its movement into the university.* Doctoral dissertation, New York University, New York.

Sommers, H., & Sommers, A. (1961). *Patients and health insurance.* Washington, DC: Brooking Institution.

Starr, P. (1982). *The social transformation of American medicine.* New York: Basic Books.

Staupers, M. (1951). Story of the NACGN. *American Journal of Nursing, 51,* 221-222.

Stevens, R. (1971). *American medicine and the public interest.* New Haven, CT: Yale University Press.

Stewart, I. (1943). *The education of nurses.* New York: Macmillan.

Struthers, L. (1917). *The school nurse.* New York: G.P. Putnam's Sons.

Taylor, P. (1971). *The distant magnet.* London: Eyre & Spottiswoode.

Tomes, N. (1983). The silent battle: Nurse registration in New York State, 1903-1920. In E. Lagemann (Ed.), *Nursing history, new perspectives, new possibilities* (pp. 107-132). New York: Teachers College Press.

U.S. Bureau of Census. (1900). *Special reports: Occupation roles, and gender.* Washington, DC: U.S. Government Printing Office.

Vassar preparatory course: A new experiment in nursing education. (1918). *American Journal of Nursing, 18,* 1155.

Wald, L. (1938). *The house on Henry Street.* New York: Henry Holt.

Pathways of Nursing Education 2

Sylvia E. Hart

 Objectives

At the completion of this chapter, the reader will be able to:

- Trace nursing education's history from its inception to the present.

- Compare and contrast nursing education programs for similarities and differences.

- Classify nursing education programs with respect to role preparation, scope of practice, eligibility for LPN or RN licensure, and eligibility for specialty certification.

- Identify and analyze trends in nursing program development, including eligibility for admission, career mobility and advancement opportunities, program accessibility, and modes of program delivery.

- Evaluate the effectiveness of available mechanisms to ensure program quality.

- Discuss and analyze the merits of the current nursing education system.

- Identify effective methodologies for addressing program models needing attention.

Profile in Practice

Joy Tyson, MS, RN
Student, Post-Master's Family Nurse Practitioner Program,
School of Nursing, University of Virginia,
Charlottesville, Virginia

I took the long road into nursing. Even though my mother was a nurse, I didn't think that was what I wanted to do. I went to school and became a medical secretary. I worked in this field for 10 years, primarily working for one physician. I was doing a lot of patient teaching in this position and really enjoyed it. I began to realize, however, that although I enjoyed my current job, as a medical secretary I would always be working for someone else and my job description would be dependent on others. I decided to become a nurse and registered in an associate degree program.

As an associate degree student, the faculty made it clear to us that if we wanted to progress in the profession, we would need at least a baccalaureate degree. So, shortly after graduation from the AD program, I went to the University of Maryland to obtain my bachelor of science degree.

As a student in the BS program, both of my clinical experiences were in the community setting, and I enjoyed both the autonomy and the fact that I could continue to do health teaching. I decided to get a master's in psychiatric nursing, since it seemed to offer the best preparation for learning effective ways to communicate, and I continued to be interested in patient teaching. When I graduated, I took a position as the director of student health in a community college. I loved that position, since I was able to develop a number of innovative health-teaching projects with the students and staff. After a few years, I joined the faculty in the nursing program so that I could work with students to develop their patient-teaching skills. Last year, I decided that I wanted to be a family nurse practitioner in a rural area. I have just started the post-master's family nurse practitioner program at the University of Virginia. I hope to eventually settle in a small community, providing primary care to families.

The proliferation of nursing education programs at all levels provides multiple pathways to the attainment of one or more nursing credentials. For the individual who is planning a career in nursing, entry options into a basic or advanced nursing education program must be examined to facilitate the selection of the most appropriate option to achieve career goals. This chapter presents the various educational opportunities available to students and some considerations for selecting among options. The programs are presented along a historical time line rather than by length or level of program. This method of presentation provides a chronology of events that influenced the development of multiple tracks of nursing education and helps to explain how our current system of nursing education came about.

HISTORY OF NURSING EDUCATION IN THE UNITED STATES

Diploma Programs

The first formal nursing education program in the United States was a 4-month hospital-based diploma program at the New England Hospital for Women and Children in Boston, Massachusetts. That program was established in 1873 and graduated such notables as Linda Richards and Mary Mahoney, the first formally educated African-American nurses in the United States. This program was originally intended to embrace the model put forward by Florence Nightingale when she established collegiate nursing in London, England, in 1860. Anticollegiate forces prevailed, however, and the hospital-based diploma program became the predominant model for nursing education in the United States. The model, in fact, flourished for nearly a century and still exists today.

At their peak in 1958, diploma programs numbered 924. At that time and during the decade that followed, diploma graduates constituted nearly the entire registered nurse (RN) workforce. In 1963 the Surgeon General's Report indicated that 86% of the nursing workforce were diploma graduates. The decline began in earnest in the 1960s and 1970s and continues even today. In 1993 there were 126 diploma programs in 26 states, with over one half of the programs in the three states of Ohio, New Jersey, and Pennsylvania. In 1993 about 6000 nurses graduated from diploma schools.

Diploma programs are typically 2 to 3 years in length plus at least one summer session (National League for Nursing [NLN], 1994a). Graduates of diploma programs are eligible to take the RN licensure examination, now known as the NCLEX-RN. As the length of diploma programs increased over the years from 4 months to 3 years, nursing students increasingly were used to meet hospital staffing needs rather than to function in the student role. The exploitation of nursing students was addressed in several landmark studies of nursing and nursing education, and in good time, student life became more compatible with sound educational practices. Many of these same studies also encouraged the profession to move its programs into collegiate settings (e.g., Goldmark, 1923; Brown, 1948) and to abandon the apprenticeship model. Ultimately, it was the high cost of these programs, both to students and to the hospitals that offered them, coupled with an increasing number of collegiate options, that brought about the closure of many diploma programs.

Some of the programs, rather than closing outright, began to align themselves with academic institutions. Some joined forces with other academic institutions and began to offer joint degrees. Some became freestanding degree-granting institutions in their own right and now grant associate or baccalaureate degrees in nursing. At least 30 diploma programs have made successful transitions to college status, and many of those programs have not only been accredited by the regional accrediting body, but also have achieved specialized accreditation from the NLN.

Baccalaureate Programs

The first baccalaureate nursing program was established in the United States at the University of Minnesota in 1909. The baccalaureate phenomenon caught on slowly and did not gain much momentum until after World War II. Until the mid 1950s many baccalaureate programs were 5 years in length and consisted of 2 years of general education followed by 3 years of nursing. The main difference between the 3 years of nursing in baccalaureate and diploma programs was the inclusion of public health nursing as part of the baccalaureate curriculum. Eventually the nursing content in baccalaureate programs was strengthened and expanded.

Proliferation of baccalaureate programs was slowed by the paucity of faculty members qualified to teach in these programs. While this was an understandable phenomenon, given the relative youth of nursing in academic centers, it created a reluctance on the part of college and university administrators to establish baccalaureate nursing programs. Those that were established were often forced to hire nursing faculty who would not otherwise qualify for university faculty appointments. It has taken several decades for this deficit to correct itself. It is to the lasting credit of the nursing profession and its members that nursing faculty teaching in baccalaureate programs today are, for the most part, bona fide members of their respective academic communities.

Virtually all baccalaureate programs are now 4 academic years in length. The nursing major is concentrated at the upper division level, and a nursing framework or model undergirds the curriculum. Graduates are prepared as generalists to practice nursing in beginning leadership positions in a variety of settings, and unlicensed graduates are eligible to take the NCLEX-RN for licensure. In 1965 the baccalaureate degree was designated by the American Nurses Association (ANA) as the entry point into professional nursing practice. In 1993, 44,000 nurses graduated from the more than 500 baccalaureate programs. It is estimated that by 2005 the shortfall of nurses with baccalaureate degrees will stand at about 400,000 (U.S. Department of Health and Human Services [U.S. DHHS], 1990).

The majority of programs admit both prelicensure students and RNs who are graduates of diploma and associate degree nursing programs, but some programs admit only RNs (NLN, 1994e). The general education requirements are the same for all students. The RN track or option in the baccalaureate program is designed to recognize and reward prior learning and to capitalize on the characteristics of the adult learner (Stecchi et al., 1994). Although some content in the RN track may be configured differently, both RN and prelicensure students meet the same program objectives. Licensed practical nurses (LPNs) also are frequently given credit for prior learning when they enroll in baccalaureate programs. The baccalaureate in nursing degree is the most common requirement for admission to graduate nursing programs (*Peterson's Guide*, 1994).

Vocational Education

Practical nurse programs were begun in 1942 in response to the acute shortage of licensed nurses in the United States created by World War II. Because of the dramatic influx of RNs into the various military branches, U.S. hospitals were largely staffed by nurse's aides, volunteers, and other unlicensed personnel. Practical nurse programs were established to provide some formal training for those who were entering the nursing workforce with little or no knowledge about nursing, and few, if any, nursing skills. The programs were designed to lead to a new kind of licensure for nurses, namely, licensed practical/vocational nurse (LPN/LVN). The license was, and still is, awarded by the state board of nursing, and the examination is now known as the NCLEX-PN.

LPN programs are typically located in technical/vocational education settings. Programs are 9 to 15 months in length and require proof of high school graduation for admission. Programs are designed to prepare LPNs to work with RNs and to be supervised by them. Programs lead to a certificate of completion and to eligibility to take the NCLEX-PN. Currently there are about 1100 such programs in the United States, graduating about 42,000 new practical nurses annually (NLN, 1994c). Since most courses taken by practical nurse students do not carry academic credit, these programs do not always articulate well with collegiate nursing programs. Associate degree programs, however, often have procedures for accommodation of practical nurses into their programs by way of advanced placement.

Associate Degree Programs

In 1952 the associate degree in nursing (ADN) became another program option for those desiring to become RNs. Designed by Mildred Montag, these programs were intended to be a collegiate alternative for the preparation of technical nurses and a reaction to the vocational model for practical nurses.

*"One of the finest contributions of associate degree education to nursing is
its clear delineation of the role of the technical nurse."
Appelgate, 1988, p. 20*

Usually found in community or junior colleges, these 2-year programs consist of a balance between general education and nursing courses, all of which carry academic credit. The programs are designed to prepare technical bedside staff nurses for secondary care settings, such as community hospitals and long-term health care facilities. It was the founder's intent that nurses with associate degrees would work under the direction of registered professional nurses who were prepared at the baccalaureate level. Some confusion arose about roles and relationships, so that by the time the first groups of students had graduated from ADN programs, they were declared eligible for the RN licensure examination, an eligibility that graduates of these programs retain today.

The growth of ADN programs in the United States has been nothing short of phenomenal. Not only did these programs multiply in community colleges, but they also began to appear at 4-year colleges and universities. Currently, there are more than 50 ADN programs in 4-year colleges and universities in 25 states. In all cases, university-based ADN programs are administered by a nursing unit that also offers baccalaureate and sometimes graduate nursing programs. By 1973 there were about 600 ADN programs in the United States. By 1993 there were nearly 900 programs, producing about 57,000 new nurses annually and constituting over 64% of all graduates from programs preparing RNs (NLN, 1994a).

The degree most often awarded on completion of the associate degree program is the ADN. A few institutions award the associate of arts in nursing (AAN) degree.

Master's Degree Education

It is not surprising to note that while the establishment of associate and baccalaureate degree nursing programs was proceeding, a master's program was beginning to emerge on university campuses. The need for nursing faculty to teach in all of the new and developing nursing education programs was apparent. There was also a surge of interest in master's prepared nurses in the service sector as the roles of clinical nurse specialists, nurse practitioners, and nurse administrators became more clearly defined.

Master's education in nursing traces its origins to 1909, when Teacher's College in New York began to offer graduate courses in nursing management. It was not until the late 1950s and early 1960s that program initiatives began to escalate and become nationally visible. The first programs were strong on role preparation and light on advanced nursing content. This was not surprising, since the nurses teaching in these programs did not themselves hold graduate degrees in nursing. As advanced nursing content became more clearly defined, and as increasing numbers of nursing faculty became proficient at teaching it, strong advanced nursing content became the prevailing characteristic of master's programs in nursing. Role preparation received somewhat less attention as clinical emphasis escalated, and by 1990 advanced practice had become the predominant focus for most master's programs.

". . . the expanding authority of APN's [advanced practice nurses] to serve
as autonomous providers of care requires that the education of the
clinicians be sound and that the consumers of APN care be able to have
confidence in the quality of the educational experience."
Booth & Bednash, 1994, p. 2

Master's programs in nursing are typically 1½ to 2 years in length (full-time study) and are built on the baccalaureate nursing major. Program content includes a set of graduate-level foundational (core) courses, a research component, and advanced practice component in a nursing specialty, and appropriate support or role preparation courses. While the bachelor of science in nursing (BSN) degree or its equivalent is usually a requirement for admission to a master's program in nursing, several other interesting models that accommodate other types of students have emerged. Some master's programs admit RNs without a baccalaureate degree or with a baccalaureate degree in another field into a streamlined track that includes both baccalaureate and master's level courses (Creasia, 1994). Other programs admit students who are in fact not nurses at all.

The impetus for opening admissions to other types of students came from noting the kinds of students who were applying in significant numbers to associate degree and baccalaureate nursing programs. Frequently non-nurses with baccalaureate or sometimes graduate degrees in other fields were seeking admission to basic nursing programs. RNs from associate degree and diploma programs who had completed baccalaureate degrees in fields other than nursing were applying for admission to baccalaureate nursing programs so that they could present the appropriate credential for admission to a master's program in nursing. These students brought a rich and diversified background to their educational programs and were highly motivated, self-directed adult learners with a strong and clearly defined career orientation. While some of these students were well served by a "fast track," second baccalaureate degree offered by several institutions, it became clear that master's programs could accommodate them and take them to the master's level in educationally sound and cost-effective ways.

Master's programs in nursing that admit non-nurse college graduates and RNs without a baccalaureate degree in nursing take the necessary steps to ensure that both groups complete whatever undergraduate or graduate prerequisite courses are needed to acquire the equivalent of a baccalaureate nursing major. They then pursue the same graduate-level foundational, specialty, and cognate courses required of master's students; thus they exit the program having met the same program objectives that all graduates of both programs must meet. Non-nurses are eligible to take the NCLEX-RN examination on completion of the generalist or baccalaureate equivalent component of the program or at program completion. There are a number of master's programs in nursing across the United States that have multiple entry options such as those described here, and more are being developed as adult learners with diversified backgrounds migrate toward nursing.

One other item with respect to master's programs in nursing is worthy of note because it represents a relatively new option to nursing students at the master's level: the joint-program concept leading to two master's degrees awarded simultaneously. These programs are especially relevant for nurses seeking administrative positions that require both advanced nursing knowledge and business/management skills. Several joint program models now exist across the country, not only reflecting nursing's responsiveness to documented student need and interest, but also demonstrating nursing's ability to collaborate with other academic disciplines. Available programs in conjunction with the master's in nursing include the master's in business administration (MSN/MBA), master's in public administration (MSN/MPA), and master's in hospital administration (MSN/MHA). Degree candidates must be admitted to both programs and must fulfill requirements for both programs. However, requirements common to both programs may be consolidated. There are at least 15 such programs currently in existence, with several more under development.

Master's programs in nursing have enjoyed phenomenal growth in the past several decades. In 1973 there were 86 such programs; in 1983 the number had increased to 154; and in 1993 there were well over 300 (NLN, 1994b). During the past decade enrollments in master's programs increased from about 18,000 to over 30,000, rising 10.7% in the 1993-1994 academic year alone (Health Professions Report, 1995). Graduations during the past decade increased from nearly 5000 to more than 7500 annually. Despite this steady growth, it is projected that by 2005 the shortage of nurses with advanced nursing degrees will approach 200,000 (U.S. DHHS, 1990). Master's programs currently are offered in all states and territories of the United States.

The degree most often awarded on completion of a master's program is the master of science in nursing degree (MSN). At least 90% of nursing master's degrees are MSN degrees. Other degree designations include master's in nursing (MN), master of science with a major in nursing (MS), and master of arts with a major in nursing (MA). The degree designation is more a matter of institutional policy than it is a reflection of program type or content. There is in fact no substantive distinction among these various degree designations for master's level nursing programs.

Doctoral Programs in Nursing

As might be expected, given nursing's relative youth in academe, the profession has only recently carved out a major doctoral presence in the academic community. Until 1970 there were fewer than a dozen doctoral programs with a major in nursing across the country. Most nurses who earned doctoral degrees did so in related disciplines such as sociology, anthropology, education, and physiology. By 1983 there were 27 doctoral programs in nursing, and by 1990, only 7 years later, there were 50. As of April 1994, there were 56 doctoral programs in nursing in 33 states, and 15 or more were in the planning stages (American Association of Colleges of Nursing, 1995).

The degree most commonly awarded for the doctorate in nursing is the doctor of philosophy (PhD) with a major in nursing. Forty-four of these programs award the PhD. Other degrees awarded include the doctor of nursing science (DNS or DNSc), doctor of science in nursing (DSN), and doctor of education (EdD). These varying degree designations do not necessarily distinguish one program from another with respect to content, rigor, or research emphasis. In most if not all instances, the degree designation is that specified for the discipline by the institution that awards the degree. And, while some are still questioning nursing's readiness for the doctoral community of scholars, the profession is quietly preparing an impressive array of scholars/researchers whose contributions to the health and nursing literature are qualitatively and quantitatively impressive.

Doctoral programs range in length from 3 to 5 years of full-time study or that equivalent in part-time work. All doctoral programs include advanced content in concept and theoretical formulations and testing, theoretical analyses, advanced nursing, supporting cognates, and in-depth research. The culminating degree requirement is the completion and defense of the doctoral dissertation.

Nursing Doctorate Programs

First conceptualized by Rozella Schlotfeldt in the 1970s (Schlotfeldt, 1978), the first nursing doctorate (ND) program was established at the Frances Payne Bolton School of Nursing, Case Western Reserve University in 1979. The ND program, analogous to medical, dental, and legal models of education, is designed to prepare graduates for licensure and professional practice in their field.

"Through completion of the curriculum the student achieves a professional doctorate and receives preparation for professional nursing practice that is truly comparable to the traditional professional preparation of physicians, dentists and lawyers."
Fitzpatrick, 1988, p. 56

Students admitted to the ND program must hold at least a baccalaureate degree in another field and be capable of postbaccalaureate work. The 4-year program prepares a generalist for professional nursing practice who, as part of the program, also acquires an advanced practice specialty. Students are eligible to take the NCLEX-RN on completion of the generalist component of the ND program. Programs are designed to emulate the professional educational model followed by several other distinguished professions without sacrificing the identity of nursing as an academic discipline in its own right. The ND program is not usually listed with the doctoral programs available in nursing, because the focus is on clinical practice rather than research. This program model has not enjoyed much growth since its inception, but it may become more attractive as a direct route to advanced practice now that advanced practice nurses are in such great demand. Currently there are just three programs in three states. However, two more were in the planning stages in early 1995 (American Association of Colleges of Nursing, 1995), and there may be more to come.

To put the various educational programs in perspective, a comparison of their characteristics is presented in Table 2-1.

CONSIDERATIONS IN SELECTING A NURSING EDUCATION PROGRAM

A number of considerations influence a prospective student's choice in selecting either a basic or a graduate-level nursing program. Perhaps among the most important are cost to the student and quality of the program.

Cost

Information available from colleges, national summary documents, and public libraries provide relevant cost information on public and private institutions that offer nursing education programs. From this information some generalizations can be made. First, state-supported community or junior colleges tend to be less expensive than state-supported 4-year colleges and universities. Second, state-supported institutions of higher education usually give a substantial tuition reduction to in-state students. Third, state or government-supported higher education is almost always significantly less expensive than private education, but this fact should not deter investigation of private institutions because of the availability of financial aid.

Financial assistance. Financial aid packages at most institutions are somewhat commensurate with actual costs. Assistance can take the form of scholarships, loans, work-study appointments, employment opportunities within the institution, assistantships, tutoring assignments, or some combination of these or other options. It should also be noted that many of these options are no longer limited to full-time students. Financial assistance awards may be based on scholarships alone, need alone, competitive performance alone, or a combination of two or more of these. Financial support may be, and in most cases should be, sought from more than one source. While most financial assistance awards are administered and awarded by the institution, there are a variety of packages available from community or government-based agencies and organizations. Examples of such agencies include, but are not limited to, state and local governments, Optimist Clubs, chambers of commerce, minority organizations, churches, community clubs, and local or state chapters of health-related organizations (e.g., March of Dimes, American Red Cross, American Heart Association). Local banks frequently have attractive student loan packages. Local hospitals and other health care agencies often sponsor or support nursing students in exchange for a commitment from the student to work for the sponsoring agency for a specified period of time after graduation. It is clear, therefore, that some form of nursing education is fiscally and geographically within reach of all interested and qualified individuals.

Quality

Issues of program quality relate to the quality of the educational program itself, as well as the eligibility of its graduates to become licensed and/or certified. With regard to program quality, how are prospective students protected from program mediocrity or less? And how is the public protected from low-quality nursing practice that can frequently be traced to low-quality programs?

The public is protected by licensure and certification procedures that ensure a standardized level of competence. The student is protected from marginal programs by institutional accreditation through regional accrediting bodies, by specialized accreditation of the nursing program(s) by the NLN, and by approval of the legal regulatory body for programs preparing for licensure, specifically the respective state boards of nursing.

Accreditation. Appropriate questions to ask about the quality of nursing programs include the following:

- Is the parent institution accredited by the appropriate regional accrediting body?
- Is the nursing program unconditionally approved by the state board of nursing and fully accredited by the NLN (if eligible)?
- What is the usual pass rate for first-time writers of the licensure examination from the school or program of interest?
- Are the faculty appropriately credentialed for their area of responsibility?
- Are they certified in their clinical specialty, if appropriate?
- Are graduates of the program eligible for the appropriate certification examination for the program being pursued?
- Does the program have a troubled history with respect to licensure examination performance, accreditation, or state approval?

Specialized accreditation. Some new developments are occurring with respect to specialized accreditation of nursing programs that need to be factored into assessment of program quality, especially at the master's level. The NLN is, and has been, the specialized accrediting body for nursing programs, LPN through master's. In times past, when a master's program was accredited by the NLN, the accreditation covered all specialties that were offered within the master's program. However, when a nurse-midwifery program was one of the options in the master's program, even though it was covered by NLN accreditation, separate specialized accreditation for the nurse-midwifery program was sought from the American College of Nurse Midwives. This was done so that graduates of that program could take the midwifery license/certification examination and therefore practice as nurse midwives. Now nurse anesthesia programs are being upgraded from diploma or certificate programs (which most of them were) to master's level programs. Although several of these nurse anesthesia programs at the master's level are now accredited by the NLN as one of the offerings within the master's program, these programs are continuing to seek and receive specialized accreditation from their specialty organization, the American Association of Nurse Anesthetists. This practice will continue so that nurse anesthetists are eligible for the credentials that en-

Table 2-1 **Characteristics of Different Nursing Programs**

	Diploma	Baccalaureate	Practical Nurse Programs
Year established	1873	1909	1942
Location	Hospitals	4-year colleges and universities	Vocational/technical schools
Accessibility	Limited to 126 programs in 26 states with over half of the programs in 3 states: Ohio, New Jersey, and Pennsylvania	Universal: all states, most cities; more than 500 programs	Universal: all states, most cities; more than 1200 programs
Length	2-3 years	4 academic years	9-15 months
Cost	A few hundred dollars per term	Highly variable; a few thousand to several thousand dollars per year	Minimal: mostly books and cost of living
Purpose	Prepare clinically competent bedside nurses	Prepare professional nurse generalists for acute care settings, community-based practice, and beginning leadership/management positions	Prepare assistive licensed nurse workers
Advanced placement or acceleration opportunities	For LPNs	For LPNs or RNs from diploma and associate degree nursing programs	None
Degree/certificate	Diploma	BSN	Certificate of completion
License eligibility	RN	RN (if not already licensed)	LPN/LVN
Certificate eligibility	None	Limited	None
Program growth pattern	Significant decline: from 944 programs in 1958 to 126 in 1993	Slight increase: 420 programs in 1983; 507 programs in 1993	Very slight decline: reduction by approximately 100 programs in 1991-1994 (from 1300 to 1200)
Graduates in 1993	6000	44,000	42,000

NOTE: This table contains 1993 data published by the National League for Nursing in 1994 (NLN, 1994a, 1994b, 1994c, 1994d, 1994e).

Associate Degree Nursing Programs	Master's Programs	Doctoral Programs in Nursing	Nurse Doctorate Programs
1952	Late 1950s	1960s	1979
Community, junior, or 4-year colleges and universities	Universities and colleges	Universities and colleges	Universities and colleges
Universal: all states, almost all cities; nearly 900 programs	Very good: more than 300 programs with at least 1 in every state; also available through distance learning	56 programs in 33 states	3 programs in 3 states: Ohio, Illinois, and Colorado
2 years	3 to 4 semesters or their equivalent for postbaccalaureate BSN-prepared nurses; additional work for other types of students	3 to 5 years post master's	4 years post baccalaureate
Reasonable in state or other public colleges; a few hundred to a few thousand dollars per year	Variable: several hundred to several thousand dollars per term	Several thousand dollars per term	Several thousand dollars per term
Prepare competent technical bedside nurses for secondary care settings	Prepare advanced practice nurses in a specialty	Prepare leaders for education, administration, clinical practice, and research	Prepare clinically adept, advanced practice nurses for leadership positions in clinical settings
For LPNs	For non-nurse college graduates; RNs with degrees in other fields; some RNs without degrees	For BSNs (limited number of programs)	Not applicable; all students are non-nurse college graduates
ADN (usually); AAN	MSN (most common) or MN, MS, MA	PhD (most common), DSN, DNS, DNSc, EdD	ND
RN	RN if unlicensed at entry	Not applicable	RN
None	Multiple	None	Multiple
Significant increase: from 600 programs in 1973 to nearly 900 in 1993; approaching plateau	Strong increase in past decade: 150 programs in 1983; more than 300 in 1993	Upward: 27 programs in 1983; 56 programs in 1993	Flat: three programs in 15 years
57,000	7500	400+	Very few

able them to practice their specialty. It is entirely possible that some other nursing specialties may seek programmatic accreditation that goes beyond the broader accreditation that the NLN makes available. This movement is closely tied to the increasing emphasis on specialty certification and the organizations in the best position to provide it. It is an issue that persons pursuing advanced specialty preparation need to monitor with vigilance.

Certification. Certification of individual nurses is a growing quality control activity being implemented by a variety of nursing and nursing-related organizations. This effort is directed toward attesting to or endorsing the demonstrated knowledge base and clinical practice behaviors associated with high-quality performance in an area of specialization. This movement is a very important one for the profession. Initiatives are now in place to make eligibility and certification requirements more uniform, to reduce duplicate or similar certification requirements across organizations, and to match certification programs with the specialties being practiced.

"Certification is the process by which the AACC Boards on certification validate, based upon predetermined standards, an individual registered nurse's qualifications, knowledge, and practice in a defined . . . area of nursing."
American Nurses' Credentialing Center, 1994, inside front cover

Currently, the American Nurses' Credentialing Center, an arm of the ANA, offers 24 certification examinations, among which are four for generalist areas of practice, five for nurse practitioner specialties, five for clinical specialists, and two for nurse administrators. A certification examination in nursing informatics, an emerging master's level specialty of increasing importance, became available in 1995.

Many nursing specialty organizations are members of the American Board of Nursing Specialties. As of October 1993, 15 nursing certification boards were members of this board. An organization called National Specialty Nursing Certifying Organizations includes some additional specialty-certifying bodies among its members. More than 40 associations are members of this organization. Some are rather highly specialized and offer certification in such specialty areas as addiction, neuroscience, nephrology, ophthalmology, and perioperative nursing. All certification efforts are designed to recognize competence of nurses in specific areas and to protect the public from unsafe or uninformed nursing practice.

IMPACT OF STUDIES OF THE PROFESSION

Throughout this chapter the history of nursing education has been traced from professional, organizational, regulatory, and institutional perspectives. The system has been described, analyzed, compared and contrasted within itself, and presented for what it is and what it is becoming. One frame of reference that has not been formally considered from the standpoint of impact or programmatic direction is that provided by the multiple studies that have been published about nursing and nurses. Many such studies have been conducted—some by nurses, some by the federal government, and some by human behavior experts from other disciplines (e.g., sociology, anthropology). The findings and recommendations from these studies were not ignored by the profession. The best of them were used to bring about improvements and needed change.

To analyze these studies and their impact on the developments that have occurred would constitute a book in its own right. The analysis of nursing education that completes this chapter is presented without direct reference to these studies, while recognizing fully that the studies are quite directly related to what *is* and what *will be* in nursing education. The five studies that are recommended to the reader for serious review are The Goldmark report, *Nursing and Nursing Education in the United States* (1923); The Brown report, *Nursing for the Future* (1948); The Lysaught report, *An Abstract for Action* (1970); The Institute of Medicine report, *Nursing and Nursing Education: Public Policy and Private Actions* (1983); and The Pew Commission report, *Health America: Practitioners for 2005* (Sugars, O'Neil, & Bader, 1991).

OBSERVATIONS AND ANALYSIS

One may argue, and many have, that regardless of the reasons, the system of nursing education that has been created is chaotic, confusing, and redundant. There are those who are holding out for the day when there will be only one way to become a nurse, only one degree to be obtained, only one license to be acquired, and only one way to be approved and recognized as a specialist. That, after all, is the way medicine, dentistry, and law do it. Can there possibly be any more likely professions to which nursing might look for modeling and emulation? Probably not.

But consider for a moment how different medicine's evolution has been. Consider the venerable age of the profession. Consider how readily and completely the European model for medical education was transplanted unchanged to the United States. Consider the unquestioned dominance of the medical profession in the United States from the time the health care "system" was first defined until it began to crumble. And now that it is crumbling, consider the serious criticism being leveled at the medical profession—criticism about education, practice, costs, and societal insensitivities. Medical reform is being demanded by the federal and state governments, by consumers, and by the profession itself. And this reform must be conducted and completed by those who entered that profession in good faith and with a set of information-based expectations that they thought would last a lifetime. This state of affairs is by no means an indictment of the medical profession or the vast majority of its members. It is, instead, an example of what can happen when the status quo is unquestioned, when a service profession loses touch with its constituencies, and when hard questions are not answered because they are not asked.

Wherever the nursing education system is right now, it is clearly in a better place than many of its other health profession counterparts. Nursing does not necessarily need to look to other health professions to take the right cues or develop the right models. Rather, it needs to look within itself to examine what has been created; to retain, build on and reconfigure as needed that which is good; to abandon or revamp that which is no longer germane; to clarify ambiguities; to underline uniqueness; to stay in touch with our consumers; and to continue the marvelous and now undeniable trend of the profession to embrace and participate fully in the higher education academic community, enjoying and benefitting from all of the collegial and professional relationships that accrue from that participation. Those, after all, are relationships that can only get better.

With those observations as a backdrop, an analysis of strengths, weaknesses, and areas needing attention is presented. The information is organized around program types and follows the historical evolution presented earlier.

Diploma Programs

Strength. Programs prepare competent bedside nurses who are eligible to take the NCLEX-RN.

Weaknesses. Programs, for the most part, are not collegiate based and are expensive, and nursing courses are not readily transferable for career advancement purposes.

Recommendation. Continue admirable and effective efforts to align with degree-granting institutions or become degree-granting as newly established academic institutions.

Baccalaureate Programs

Strengths. Programs provide a solid liberal education and are a substantive upper-division nursing major. Both components are combined in ways that prepare a nurse generalist who is able to provide professional nursing services in beginning leadership positions in a variety of settings and who is eligible to take the NCLEX-RN. Programs are accessible. Programs accommodate RNs who are graduates of associate degree and diploma programs. Baccalaureate programs in nursing have been designated by the ANA as the entry point for professional practice.

Weaknesses. The legal scope of practice for associate degree and baccalaureate-prepared nurses is undifferentiated because both groups are awarded the same license. This limits differentiated roles in work settings and hinders the reward system for leadership responsibilities.

Recommendations. Develop a different or additional license for baccalaureate-prepared nurses. Expand community focus and give additional emphasis to managed care in the curriculum.

Practical Nurse Programs

Strengths. Programs are short, economical, and accessible. Programs prepare licensed assistive nurse workers.

Weaknesses. Programs are not collegiate based. Graduates are not prepared to do what they are called on to do in the workplace. Practical nurses are exploited and are frequently called on to perform functions beyond their legally defined scope of practice.

Recommendations. Elevate these programs to the community college level and award the ADN. Adjust enrollments downward to reflect market demands.

Associate Degree Programs

Strengths. Programs are offered in academic/collegiate settings and are affordable, accessible, and reasonably brief. Programs prepare competent technical bedside nurses who are eligible to take the NCLEX-RN.

Weaknesses. Programs and their graduates go beyond the purposes and scope of the practice envisioned by the program founder. When combined with practical nurses, the total number of technical nurse types being produced is excessive, given current and future market demands (Fagin & Lynaugh, 1992).

Recommendations. Collaborate with the LPN leadership to develop one program type that prepares the technical nurse, using that which is most effective from both programs to bring this outcome about. Once the two programs have become one, assess the marketplace and consumer needs for this type of nurse and adjust the program output accordingly. Seek guidance from North Dakota, where successful program unification (LPN and ADN) has already occurred.

Master's Programs

Strengths. Programs are accessible. Programs prepare graduates for advanced practice in a nursing specialty. Some of the programs admit non-nurse college graduates, RNs with baccalaureate degrees in other fields, and some RNs without baccalaureate degrees. Graduates of these programs are prepared to engage in advanced practice nursing as nurse practitioners, clinical nurse specialists, nurse anesthetists, or nurse midwives and in other specialty practices.

Weaknesses. Non-nurses take the same licensure examination as associate degree graduates. Certificate programs for master's prepared nurses are not uniformly consistent in terms of eligibility requirements and examination rigor.

Recommendations. Collaborate with baccalaureate nurse educators and other interested professionals in bringing to fruition the second or different examination for professional nurses. Bring greater uniformity and meaning to certification programs.

Doctoral Programs in Nursing

Strengths. Programs prepare leaders for responsible advanced positions in nursing education, nursing administration, nursing research, nursing practice, or some combination of these roles. Programs are fairly accessible, as doctoral programs go.

Weakness. Program proliferation has resulted in the use of some unqualified faculty members for program delivery

Recommendation. Stabilize program growth at the current level so that faculty can fine-tune their qualifications and participate more fully in the life of scholarship.

Nursing Doctorate Program

Strength. Programs prepare clinically adroit, theoretically strong, advanced practice nurses.

Weaknesses. Programs are not widely accessible (only three programs in three states) and are expensive.

Recommendation. Market the program as an effective alternative route to preparation for advanced practice nursing.

•   •   •

However nursing education programs are configured for the future, we must retain those facets of the system that ensure continued and growing representation of the gender and cultural diversity that exists in the society that the profession serves. This means that we must intensify efforts to attract ethnic and racial minorities and men into nursing.

*"Male nurses are still a minority but their ranks are increasing. Last year
(1993), more than 8% of the U.S. RN graduates were men . . . up from
0.8% in 1949. Besides the increasing number of males in nursing there is
also an increasing number of nurses who represent a wide variety of
ethnic and cultural backgrounds."*
Peterson's Guide to Nursing Programs, 1994, p. 19

We must retain a system that maximizes career development and advancement. We must bring greater clarity and meaning to our licensure and certification programs. And we must monitor and control the kinds and numbers of nurses we educate to meet societal and professional needs (Aiken & Salmon, 1994). As we do so, we must bear in mind that to the extent that the profession attracts and uses the people who earn the most respected advanced degrees and then gives them the opportunity to be role models and spokespersons for nursing, the profession will grow in viability, usefulness, and esteem.

If this chapter conveys a message of endorsement of and enthusiasm for the nursing profession and most components of its educational enterprise, a major outcome has been realized. There is every reason to believe that our successes will continue and that our problems can be solved. Nursing is a profession where exciting things are happening and where the best is yet to come.

 ## *Key Points*

- Health care needs in our society, along with certain historical events, influenced the development of multiple tracks of nursing education.

- Hospital-based diploma programs became the predominant model of nursing education in the United States for nearly 100 years.

- Although the first baccalaureate program in nursing was established in 1909, the development of significant numbers of these programs progressed slowly.

- Practical nursing programs were established to provide formal training for unlicensed personnel who, in large numbers, staffed U.S. hospitals during World War II.

- As a reaction to the vocational model of practical nursing, associate degree programs were established to educate technical nurses in collegiate programs.

- Master's programs prepare advanced practice nurses and other nurse specialists to assume significant roles in a variety of health care settings.

- The nursing doctorate program, similar in design to medical, dental, and legal models of education, prepares graduates for licensure and professional practice.

- Doctoral programs in nursing are designed to prepare scholars and researchers to expand the body of nursing knowledge.

- Cost and quality are two major considerations in selecting educational programs in nursing.

- Indicators of academic program quality include the status of program accreditation and approval, pass rates on licensure examinations, and pass rates on certification examinations.

- While each nursing education program has unique strengths, each also has weaknesses to which attention must be given.

 ## *Critical Thinking Exercises*

1. Defend or refute the following statement: There should be a separate licensing examination for nurses with baccalaureate degrees.

2. What is your career goal in nursing? What, if any, further education will you need to fully achieve your goal?

3. How does certification of advanced practice nurses and nurse specialists protect the public?

4. Consult your state nurse practice act to determine the scope of practice of advanced practice nurses and other nurse specialists. What are the constraints on advanced practice nursing in your state?

5. Clarify the differences between nursing doctorate programs and doctoral programs in nursing.

6. Discuss the validity of state board pass rates, regional and specialized accreditation status, and pass rates on certification examinations as indicators of the quality of a nursing education program.

7. What changes must be made in nursing education to ensure a culturally diverse nursing profession, nonpunitive career advancement opportunities, and credibility in the higher-education community?

References

Aiken, L.H., & Salmon, M.E. (1994). Health care workforce priorities: What nursing should do now. *Inquiry, 31,* 318-329.

American Association of Colleges of Nursing. (1995). *Schools planning doctoral programs* [List compiled by AACN]. Washington, DC: The Association.

American Board of Nursing Specialties Governing Council—revised October, 1993. Uncopyrighted list.

American Nurses' Association. (1991). *Nursing's agenda for health care reform.* Washington, DC: The Association.

American Nurses' Credentialing Center. (1994). *Certification catalog.* Washington, DC: The Center.

Appelgate, M.H. (1988). Associate degree nursing and health care. In *Perspectives in nursing—1987-1989* (NLN Publication No. 41-2199, pp. 207-219). New York: National League for Nursing.

Booth, R.Z., & Bednash, G. (1994). *Syllabus: The newsletter of the American Association of Colleges of Nursing, 20* (5).

Brown, E.L. (1948). *Nursing for the future.* New York: Russell Sage Foundation.

Creasia, J.L. (1994). Issues in designing an RN-MS track. *Nurse Educator, 19*(1), 27-32.

Diploma programs in nursing accredited by the NLN 1994-95 and practical nursing programs accredited by the NLN 1994-95. (1994). *Nursing and Health Care, 15*(7), 386-389.

Fagin, C.M., & Lynaugh, J.E. (1992). Reaping the rewards of radical change: A new agenda for nursing education. *Nursing Outlook, 40,* 213-220.

Fitzpatrick, J.J. (1988). The professional doctorate as an entry level into clinical practice. In *Perspectives in nursing—*

1987-1989 (NLN Publication No. 41-2199, pp. 53-56). New York: National League for Nursing.

Goldmark, J., and the Committee for the Study of Nursing Education. (1923). *Nursing and nursing education in the United States.* New York: Macmillan.

Health Professions Report. (1995). *More nurses pursuing master's degrees: More schools plan NP programs in 1994.* Fanwood, NJ: Whitaker Newsletters.

Institute of Medicine. (1983). *Nursing and nursing education: Public policies and private actions.* Washington, DC: National Academy Press.

Lysaught, J. (1970). *An abstract for action.* New York: McGraw-Hill.

National League for Nursing. (1994a). *Nursing data source 1994: Vol. 1. Trends in contemporary nursing education* (NLN Publication No. 19-2642). New York: NLN Division of Research.

National League for Nursing. (1994b). *Nursing data source 1994: Vol. 2. Graduate education in nursing: Advanced practice nursing* (NLN Publication No. 19-2643). New York: NLN Division of Research.

National League for Nursing. (1994c). *Nursing data source 1994: Vol. 3. Focus on practical/vocational nursing* (NLN Publication No. 19-2644). New York: NLN Division of Research.

National League for Nursing. (1994d). *State approved schools of nursing LPN/LVN 1994* (NLN Publication No. 19-2623). New York: NLN Division of Research.

National League for Nursing. (1994e). *State approved schools of nursing RN 1994* (NLN Publication No. 19-2622). New York: NLN Division of Research.

National Specialty Nursing Certifying Organizations—updated August 1, 1994. Uncopyrighted list.

Peterson's guide to nursing programs: Baccalaureate and graduate nursing education in the U.S. and Canada. (1994). Princeton, NJ: In cooperation with the American Association of Colleges of Nursing.

Schlotfeldt, R.M. (1978). The professional doctorate: Rationale and characteristics. *Nursing Outlook, 26*(5), 302-311.

Stecchi, J.M., Pearce, C., Tyra, P.A., Gelser, L., Durkin, M.A., & Rogers, H. (1994). RN to BSN in nursing: Historical re-view leads to articulation agreement. *Journal of Continuing Education in Nursing, 25*(5), 219-223.

Sugars, D.A., O'Neil, E.H., & Bader, J.D. (Eds.) (1991). *Healthy America: Practitioners for 2005: An agenda for action for U.S. health professional schools: A report of the Pew Health Professions Commission.* Durham, NC: Pew Health Professions Commission, Duke University Medical Center.

U.S. Department of Health and Human Services. (1990). *Eighth report to the President and Congress on the status of health personnel in the United States.* Bethesda, MD: The Department.

Socialization to Professional Nursing

3

Marian M. Larisey

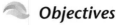

Objectives

At the completion of this chapter, the reader will be able to:

- Identify characteristics of a profession.
- Evaluate nursing's current status as a profession.
- Describe models of professional socialization.
- Discuss factors that influence professional socialization.
- Differentiate between accountability, autonomy, and shared governance as characteristics of professional practice.
- Discuss the importance of actively participating in professional nursing associations.

Profile in Practice

Shari Janes Knowles, BSN, RN
Master's Degree Student,
School of Nursing, University of Virginia,
Charlottesville, Virginia

When I first graduated from a diploma nursing program, I knew that I had excellent clinical skills. I worked nights in Labor and Delivery and always felt confident, even though I was sometimes the only nurse working in L&D. Even as a student in the diploma program, I knew I would eventually go for my baccalaureate degree. I finished my diploma program on a Friday, and on Monday I was in the baccalaureate program. Because I was a registered nurse, I was able to work while in school to support myself financially.

I am now enrolled in a master's program. I tell my son that I'm still in school because I'm still alive! I want to always keep learning and growing. I believe that the diploma program provided me with strong clinical skills. The baccalaureate and master's courses have given me a broader perspective of nursing and health care. For example, I now look at systems and analyze the efficiency of health care delivery systems. Another difference is the use of theories. Nursing theorists were not discussed in my diploma program. Of course, I was in a diploma program many years ago, and I don't know if they have changed or not.

I think the biggest challenge facing professional nurses today is to remember the person receiving our nursing care. This is why I first went into nursing, and my interest and commitment have not changed. I think my continuing in school has made me a better nurse, as well as a more thoughtful person and informed parent.

Socialization to professional nursing is a lifelong process that begins in the educational setting and continues throughout one's nursing career. After being initially socialized in a basic nursing program, a nurse must be resocialized at each of the following junctures: (1) when the new graduate leaves the educational setting and enters the work world; (2) when the experienced nurse changes work settings, either in a new organization or within the same organization; and (3) when the nurse undertakes new roles, such as assuming a leadership role or returning to school. Both initial socialization and resocialization involve changes within the individual as a new self-identity emerges. Often, these changes are stressful, evoking strong emotional reactions and inner conflict.

Embedded in the idea of socialization to professional nursing are two concepts: professionalism and socialization. An exploration of these concepts will facilitate an understanding of the professional status of nursing and the process of professional socialization.

NURSING AS A PROFESSION

Professional nursing practice embodies the social service ideal whereby the client rather than the task takes on the highest level of importance (Whitman et al., 1992). Since the days of Florence Nightingale, nurses often have commented that they entered nursing to help people and serve the needs of society in the area of health care. The Nightingale Pledge, which has been spoken by millions of nurses since the late 1800s, concludes "...devote myself to the welfare of those committed to my care." But are devotion and caring sufficient for nursing to call itself a profession? This question has stimulated discussion, debate, and controversy within health care disciplines and related disciplines. As scholars and researchers attempted to describe a profession, several sets of characteristics emerged. Taken as a whole, these characteristics address the level of knowledge, attitudes, and values that symbolize a profession.

Characteristics of a Profession

In the early 1900s the Carnegie Foundation issued a series of papers on professional schools. A classic piece of literature by Abraham Flexner (1910) was the catalyst for the reform of medical education in the United States and Canada. Flexner also studied other disciplines, and in 1915 he published a list of criteria he believed were characteristics of all true professions. According to Flexner, a true profession:

- Is basically intellectual (as opposed to physical)
- Is based on a body of knowledge that can be learned
- Is practical, rather than theoretical
- Can be taught through the process of professional education
- Has a strong internal organization of members
- Has practitioners who are motivated by altruism (the desire to help others)

Since Flexner's work in 1915, additional characteristics of a profession have been identified. In 1959 Bixler and Bixler presented the following criteria against which to evaluate nursing's status as a profession. According to them, a profession:

- Uses a well-defined and well-organized body of specialized knowledge on the intellectual level of higher learning
- Continuously enlarges its body of knowledge and uses the scientific method to improve its techniques of education and service
- Prepares its practitioners in institutions of higher education
- Applies its body of knowledge through practical services that are vital to human and social welfare
- Functions autonomously in formulating professional policy and controlling professional activity
- Attracts individuals who exalt service above personal gain and who recognize their chosen occupation as their life's work
- Compensates its practitioners by providing freedom of action, opportunity for continuous professional growth, and economic security

The works of Greenwood (1957), Houle (1980), and Kelly (1981) extend that of Flexner, and Bixler and Bixler and are summarized in Table 3-1.

At the time these criteria were being developed, nursing fell short of professional status in a number of areas. For example, most nursing education programs were based in hospitals rather than in institutions of higher education. Nursing research was in its infancy, thereby offering little toward the improvement of education and service. In addition, autonomous nursing practice was relatively uncommon, and there was no formalized code of ethics. Today, most nursing education programs are based in institutions of higher education. There is an expanding body of knowledge derived from a basis of scientific research. Opportunities for autonomous practice are increasing (although nurses do not universally desire autonomy), and there is a well-defined code of ethics. Areas still needing attention are control by nursing over policies and activities, commitment to nursing as a profession rather than a job, and viewing the professional association as an important component of the professional culture.

PROFESSIONALIZATION OF NURSING

Professionalization is the process by which an occupation achieves professional status. The status of nursing as a profession is important because it reflects the value society places on the work of nurses and the centrality of this work to the good of society (Strader & Decker, 1995). Although the terms *occupation* and *profession* are often used interchangeably, it is important to understand the critical differences between the two concepts. A *profession* is characterized by prolonged education that takes place in a college or university. Values, beliefs, and ethics relating to the profession are an integral part of the educational preparation. By definition, a professional is autonomous in decision making and is accountable for his or her own actions. Personal identification and commitment to the profession are strong, and individuals are unlikely to change professions. In contrast, an *occupation* is characterized by training that may occur on the job for varying lengths of time. The training does not incorporate, as a prominent feature, the values, beliefs, and ethics of the occupation. The workers are supervised, and ultimate accountability rests with the employer. Thus the commitment

Table 3-1   **Characteristics of a Profession**

Greenwood (1957)	Houle (1980)	Kelly (1981)
Systematic body of knowledge	Concept of mission open to change	Services are vital to humanity and the welfare of society
Professional authority	Mastery of theoretical knowledge	Special body of knowledge that is continually enlarged through research
Sanctions of community	Capacity to solve problems	
Ethical codes	Use of theoretical knowledge	
Professional culture	Continued seeking of self-enhancement by its members	Services involve intellectual activities where accountability is strong feature
	Formal training	
	Credentialing system to certify competence	Practitioners educated in institutions of higher learning
	Creation of subculture	Practitioners relatively independent and control own policies and activities
	Legal reinforcement of professional standards	
	Ethical practice	Practitioners motivated by service, and work is important component of their lives
	Penalties against incompetent or unethical practice	
	Public acceptance	Code of ethics to guide decisions and conduct of practitioners
	Role distinctions that differentiate professional work from that of other vocations and permit autonomous practice	
	Service to society	Association that encourages and supports high standards of practice

is not always strong, and individuals often change jobs (Chitty, 1993). Styles (1982), taking a different approach to professionalization, proposed that instead of applying a list of external criteria to determine nursing's professional status, nursing and nurses should focus on the "characteristics of the individual as a member of the profession" (p. 8). She defined this as *professionhood.*

Development of nursing knowledge is fundamental to the professionalization of nursing. The science of nursing is concerned with a unified body of knowledge and includes the skills and methodologies to apply that knowledge (Keck, 1994). Until the 1980s, knowledge by definition was empirically-based, focusing on objective and observable data with an analytical and linear line of reasoning. Since that time, there has been a growing awareness that total reliance on empirical data provides a distorted view of the world (Christensen & Kenney, 1995). Thus nursing knowledge is derived not only from theoretical formulations and scientific research, but also from personal experience that leads to clinical expertise. This distinct body of knowledge can differentiate nursing from other health professionals by providing a basis for practice.

Professional Nursing Practice

Professional nursing practice involves "specialized skills essential to the performance of a unique, professional role" (ANA, 1975, p. 3). Although skills change and evolve with time, a basic value of nursing that has persisted over the years is service to society. The service component of nursing requires integrity and a lifelong commitment. Two concepts that are in the forefront of professional nursing and its service ideal are accountability and autonomy.

Accountability. *Accountability* is the state of being responsible and answerable for one's own behavior. According to the American Nurses' Association (ANA) *Code for Nurses* (1985), the nurse assumes responsibility and is accountable for individual nursing judgments and actions. The spheres of a nurse's accountability are to self, the client, the employing agency, and the profession. The *Standards of Clinical Nursing Practice* (ANA, 1991) presented in Table 3-2 and standards of the various specialty nursing practices document the professional nurse's scope and limits of accountability.

By virtue of these standards, society holds nurses and those under their supervision accountable for their actions. The nurse has a responsibility to demonstrate sound judgment, critical thinking, and competence in the caregiver role. In the supervisory role, the nurse must ensure that only competent health care workers be allowed to care for clients and must take action against those whose knowledge and skill are questionable. Clients have a right to receive high-quality care that is grounded in a scientific knowledge base, performed by those who make good judgments, and based on an appropriate value system.

The nursing profession exercises accountability to itself by controlling its activities, formulating policies, and advocating for professional issues in the political system. The standards of practice for general and specialty nursing care have been developed by nursing organizations and contain the terms of professional accountability. The terms

---

Table 3-2 **Standards of Clinical Nursing Practice**

Standard	Responsibilities of the Nurse
I. Quality of care	The nurse systematically evaluates the quality and effectiveness of nursing practice.
II. Performance appraisal	The nurse evaluates his/her own nursing practice in relation to professional practice standards and relevant statutes and regulation.
III. Education	The nurse acquires and maintains current knowledge in nursing practice.
IV. Collegiality	The nurse contributes to the professional development of peers, colleagues, and others.
V. Ethics	The nurse's decisions and actions on behalf of clients are determined in an ethical manner.
VI. Collaboration	The nurse collaborates with the client, significant others, and health care providers in providing client care.
VII. Research	The nurse uses research findings in practice.
VIII. Resource utilization	The nurse considers factors related to safety, effectiveness, and cost in planning and delivering client care.

From American Nurses' Association. (1991). *Standards of clinical nursing practice.* Kansas City, MO: The Association.

of legal accountability are contained in the licensing procedures, certification, and disciplinary actions that are established and controlled by nursing. In the political arena, nurses are becoming more involved in advocating for health care legislation that strengthens nursing practice, protects the public, and offers choice to the consumer.

Autonomy. *Autonomy* in nursing is the freedom and the authority to act independently. It implies control over one's practice, and it applies to both decisions and actions. Autonomy involves independence on the part of the nurse, a willingness to take risks, and accountability for actions. The notion of autonomy in nursing practice must be balanced with interdependence, however, since health care is a multidisciplinary endeavor and several disciplines contribute to total client care. In addition, freedom to act or not act is a human right, and therefore autonomy of the client must also be respected.

Lack of autonomy has been cited as one of nursing's shortcomings in its efforts to achieve professional status. One reason given for the lack of autonomy in nursing practice is that nurses, being predominantly female, are an oppressed group (Roberts, 1983; Stein, Watts, & Howell, 1990). Women in our society have been socialized to shy away from power and assume more subservient roles. A second reason is that many nurses have a job orientation instead of a professional orientation (Gardner, 1992) and therefore do not have a commitment to advance nursing to a full professional status through autonomous practice. A third reason is that nurses are fragmented by subgroups, internal dissension, and rivalry. Other groups that attempt to control nursing, such as organized medicine and health services administration, are well organized and have effective lobbies.

The Climate for Professional Practice

To practice as professionals, nurses must have control over the practice environment so that clinical judgments and interventions can reflect the uniqueness of each client. Lateral communication and dialogue among peers allow nurses to validate clinical judgments according to standards of professional practice. Through peer-based quality evaluation and assurance, nurses can maintain high standards of client care. When nurses have a defined role in governance, policies that could have a negative impact on high-quality care can be averted.

According to Porter-O'Grady (1986), there are five key issues involved in creating a professional practice climate. The nurse must have:

- The freedom to function effectively
- A sense of support from peers and leaders
- Clear expectations of the work environment
- Appropriate resources to practice effectively
- An open organizational climate

A number of contemporary client care delivery models were developed to facilitate the practice of nursing as a professional discipline. Many of the models address the issues cited by Porter-O'Grady with systems such as shared governance or self-governance. While specific organizational designs may vary, all can be classified as professional governance models because they focus on autonomy over, and accountability for, nursing practice.

Overview of professional governance models. An accountability-based governance system is a predominant feature of professional practice models. Responsibility and authority are established in specified processes rather than in particular individuals who, in turn, determine the placement of accountability. The nurse is central to the organization and is supported by major service components such as standards, quality assurance, continuing education, and peer process. Nursing management has no legitimate role in practice-related decisions; rather, management facilitates, integrates, and coordinates nursing operations to support the practitioner. Organizational administration is concerned with system-wide operations and serves as a link to the external environment (i.e., consumers). These elements, which constitute a framework for professional governance, are illustrated in Fig. 3-1.

There are three prevailing models of professional governance (Porter-O'Grady, 1987). The *councilor model* uses elected councils to structure the governance processes of staff and management. Councils on practice, quality assurance, and education are composed primarily of practicing nurses, with management having minority representation. These councils make decisions related to clinical practice. The management team has a management council, with clinical staff having minority representation. It is in this council that decisions regarding system operations are made. A second model,

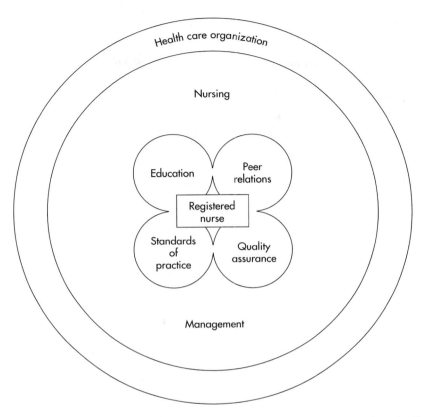

Fig. 3-1 Model for professional governance. (Modified from Porter-O'Grady, T. [1987]. Shared governance and new organization models. *Nursing Economics, 5*[6], 284.)

the *congressional format,* consists of a president and cabinet of officers who are elected from the staff of the organization and who oversee the operations. Cabinet members are a mixture of clinical and management representatives. There may be equal representation from each group or, consistent with the belief that the organization is a clinical service, it may be weighted with more clinical representatives. Committees, often chaired by cabinet officers, are empowered with certain responsibilities and accountabilities and report back to the cabinet. The third model, the *administrative model,* is perhaps the least professionally structured. Although a management and clinical forum are the basic structural units, each forum is more typically aligned in a hierarchical fashion, and the nurse executive often has a mechanism for vetoing considerations of the various decision-making groups.

SOCIALIZATION

Socialization is the process of acquiring knowledge and skills and internalizing attitudes and values specific to a given social group. Much of the literature on socialization has focused on child development and the influence of the family on the child's socialization. This process occurs through role modeling and reinforcement of socially relevant behaviors. Increased attention is now being given to *adult socialization,* the process by which individuals develop new behaviors and values associated with roles they assume as an adult. Brimm (1966) identified six major differences between socialization of the child and of the adult as presented in Table 3-3.

When an adult assumes a new role, such as parent, nurse, or student, socialization to that new role occurs. With the assistance of others, the individual learns the necessary behaviors, values, skills, and identity to successfully assume the new role.

Socialization to Professional Nursing

Socialization to professional nursing is the process of learning the skills, roles, and values of the profession. It represents the process by which a student or practicing nurse acquires the knowledge and skills needed to practice nursing and internalizes the attitudes, beliefs, norms, values, and ethical standards of the profession into his or her own behavior pattern. The development of an occupational and professional identity occurs initially through education and is extended in the work setting.

Socialization through education. Learning any new role can be a difficult and anxiety-producing task. Professional socialization through education is one pathway to learning new roles and the culture of nursing. A number of models have been developed to describe this process. Malcolm Knowles (1970), through his classic work in adult education, used the term *andragogy* to describe the "art and science of how adults learn." Knowles believed that adult learners, motivated by the desire for self-growth and self-direction, have four unique characteristics:

1. They shift from dependent learners to self-directed learners.
2. They have acquired experience that serves as a resource for learning.

Table 3-3   Comparison of Childhood and Adult Socialization

Childhood Socialization	Adult Socialization
Learns values and motives of society	Learns new overt role behaviors
Acquires new materials	Synthesizes previously learned material
Concerned with idealism	Concerned with realism
Learns general demands of society	Learns role-specific expectations
Learns basic role expectations	Develops methods of role conflict resolution
Focuses on self as identity	Involves others in maturing identity

From Brimm, O.G., Jr. (1966). Socialization through the life cycle. In O.G. Brimm, Jr., & S. Wheeler (Eds.), *Socialization after childhood: two essays.* New York: John Wiley & Sons.

3. They have a readiness to learn that is oriented toward the developmental tasks of their social roles.
4. Their orientation to learning shifts from a postponed application of learning toward an immediate application. This model is particularly applicable to the nurse who returns to school for an advanced degree.

Initial socialization. Initial socialization to nursing occurs in the educational setting and is subsequently transferred to the practice setting. Wilson (1994) conducted a study to determine nursing students' perspectives of learning in the clinical setting. The students defined roles for themselves, their instructors, and the staff nurses. The configuration and interaction of these roles may provide some insight to the socialization of nurses in educational programs.

Two models that describe socialization through education are proposed by Hinshaw (1976) and Cohen (1981). Based on the classical doctrinal conversion model, Hinshaw's model is marked by six stages, and corresponding behaviors of the nurse are identified:

Initial innocence. The initial image of nursing is based on what "should" be.
Incongruities labeled. Initial expectations and reality collide.
Identification. Behaviors of experienced nurses are observed.
Role simulation. Observed behaviors are practiced, but feelings of being uncomfortable in the role occur.
Vacillation/provisional internalization. Old images conflict with a new professional image.
Internalization. The new role is accepted with feelings of comfort.

Cohen drew on theories of cognitive development to propose a model of professional nursing socialization through education. The model consists of four states that students must experience as they become professionals:

Unilateral dependence. Students rely on external limits and controls and are unlikely to question the concepts presented.
Negativity/independence. Students' critical thinking abilities are expanded. Students begin to question the instructor and rely more on their own judgment.
Dependence/mutuality. Students evaluate the ideas of others and are more impartial in accepting some ideas and rejecting others.
Interdependence. Students make independent judgments while working in collaboration with others. Students become professionals.

Resocialization. Returning to school represents a period of resocialization in nursing during which new role expectations are synthesized. Larisey (1985) found that registered nurses returning to school came from diverse backgrounds and were motivated by advancement of career goals, program availability, future job security, and financial security. If resocialization through education is fully effective, the student leaves the educational program with changes in behavior that reflect an integration of the values and norms of a professional practitioner. Lawler and Rose (1987) documented the effectiveness of resocialization of registered nurses (RNs) in a baccalaureate program.

Shane (1983) proposed that RNs who return to school experience a "returning-to-school syndrome" that is marked by three phases. The first phase, the *honeymoon,* is very positive, and the student is excited about returning to school to increase knowledge and skills. The student relates the present educational experience to earlier education. The honeymoon phase typically ends when the student takes the first nursing theory or practice course. Thus the first phase may be short-lived. The second phase, *conflict,* is characterized by a plethora of negative emotions, such as anger, depression, and feelings of helplessness. The old rules are no longer valid, and the new rules are not accepted. Feelings of inadequacy may lead to academic difficulties. A conflict response may be intensified if the RN is trying to integrate multiple roles, such as student, practitioner, and significant other. The beginning of the next phase, *reintegration,* is characterized by hostility and a strong rejection of the educational program. The conflict response is ongoing. Some students may leave the program if the hostility is severe, whereas others are able to resolve this conflict. The ability to integrate the original culture of work with the new culture of school is the positive resolution of the "returning-to-school syndrome." Students who remain in school but are not successful in moving through this phase resist growth and change.

Throwe and Fought (1987) believe that the stages RN students must master during the resocialization process can be assessed according to the eight stages of Erikson's (1950) developmental theory. For each of the eight stages, there are examples of role-resisting and role-accepting behaviors that can be observed as the RN student progresses through the socialization process. These can be regarded as developmental tasks associated with role identification. The final stage reveals an RN learner who achieves consistent role enactment. The student's knowledge base is strengthened, new options are explored, and problem solving is more creative. The student is ready to try out new roles.

Socialization to the Work Setting

Education is only the initial process in socialization. The professional nursing role learned in the educational setting must now be transferred and modified to fit the workplace. Thus the continuum of socialization extends as resocialization begins.

The phenomenon of socialization is built around role theory (see Chapter 4). Individuals learn behaviors that accompany each role by two simultaneously occurring processes: (1) interaction involving groups and significant others in a social context and (2) learning through role-playing, identification, modeling, instruction, observation, trial and error, and role negotiation (Hardy & Conway, 1988). Early research on the socialization of nurses in the work setting was conducted by Brimm (1966), who concluded that socialization or resocialization produces difficulty in three areas: (1) ignorance of the particular role prescription and expectations, (2) inability to meet role demands, and (3) deficiencies in motivation.

Kramer's resocialization model. One of the best-known models of resocialization in nursing is that proposed by Kramer (1974). She described special fears and difficulties of new graduate nurses in adapting to the work setting and referred to these feelings of powerlessness and ineffectiveness as *reality shock*. Reality shock is a result of conflict between a new graduate's knowledge and skills acquired in the educational program and the reality of the behaviors required in the actual work setting. Kramer's model consists of four stages through which new graduates progress before feeling comfortable in the professional role.

Stage one is *mastery of skills and routines*. New graduates feel inadequate and frustrated and as a result tend to focus on the mastery of essential skills. A potential problem here is that the nurse may become fixated on technical skills and fail to see other important aspects of client care, such as emotional needs.

Stage two is *social integration*. The new nurse's major concern is getting along with co-workers and fitting into the work group. Conflict occurs when the new nurse strives to maintain high ideals and standards learned in the educational setting and at the same time avoid alienating co-workers.

Stage three is *moral outrage*. During this stage incongruities among roles in the work setting cause the new nurse to feel angry, frustrated, and inadequately prepared. Determining priorities is a challenge.

In stage four, *conflict resolution,* nurses either give up their values or successfully integrate them into the professional and bureaucratic systems. There are four possible resolutions for the conflict stage:

- Behavior capitulation, wherein the new nurse changes the behaviors but retains the values. Nurses who choose this solution either find work situations that are more compatible with their beliefs or leave nursing altogether.
- Values capitulation, wherein the new nurse accepts the values of the bureaucracy and gives up the values gained in the educational program. The nurse just tries to fit into the organization.
- Capitulation of both behaviors and values for the purpose of conforming, and thereby retaining the position. Survival is the goal.
- Biculturalism, wherein the new nurse learns to use the values of both the profession and the bureaucracy to influence positive change in the system.

According to Kramer, biculturalism is the healthiest and most successful resolution. The nurse balances the cultures of the educational setting and the work setting and recognizes the ability to influence others. Values and behaviors of both the professional and bureaucratic systems are identified, and they are used appropriately.

Following publication of Kramer's work, educational programs and work settings, primarily hospitals, began to look at methods that could be used to reduce reality shock in the transition from student to professional. For example, educational programs encouraged students to gain practical experience outside of school settings, such as during the summer, school breaks, and weekends. In addition, some educational programs began to pair students with preceptors so that they could work closely with a practicing registered nurse. In the work setting, longer orientation programs provided an opportunity for smoother transition. Preceptor programs were also offered to allow the new nurse to work alongside an experienced nurse. These are but a few examples of measures that can be taken to minimize reality shock. Creativity and commitment by educational programs and work settings are two key factors in helping the new graduate to successfully assume the professional role.

Socializing agents. Both educational programs and practice settings can assist in clarifying role expectations and decreasing conflict through the use of role models, preceptors, mentors, and sponsors. Historically, the functions and purposes of these roles have been compartmentalized, but the model of "learning partners" proposed by Crim and Hood (1995) suggests that nurses must move back and forth between roles to function competently in the changing health care system. Despite the somewhat blurred boundaries and functions of these roles, each has an important part to play in the nurse's socialization process.

Role models are experienced, competent nurses who exemplify excellence in practice. They provide inspiration, intellectual stimulation, and psychological support, and may serve as teacher and advisor (Fields, 1991). Although the relationship may be a passive one, research on excellence in hospitals has found that the greater the number of excellent role models available, the greater the possibility for the nurse to perform well (Kramer & Schmalenberg, 1988).

Preceptors usually serve in a short-term role that is active and purposeful. Specifically, the *preceptor* models behavior and supports the development of functional and technical competence (Carey & Campbell, 1994), and socializes the novice to the work environment. As a result, the inexperienced person learns a set of skills from observing, working with, and relating to the preceptor (Douglas, 1992). To be effective, preceptors must have some knowledge of adult learning theory and strong clinical skills. A sample of nurses identified the five most important preceptor characteristics as clinical competence, positive attitude, effective teacher, effective communicator, and role model (Scherwin et al., 1994).

Mentors take on an even more powerful role in the socialization process. *Mentoring* is defined as an "intense relationship calling for a high degree of involvement between a novice in a discipline and a person who is knowledgeable and wise in that area" (May, Meleis, & Winstead-Fry, 1982). The mentor takes a personal interest in helping an individual over a period of time to develop the knowledge and skills needed to realize the protégé's full potential and major life goals (Fuszard & Taylor, 1995). The mentor role involves listening, affirming, counseling, encouraging, seeking input, helping the protégé gain expert status, and developing a career direction (Carey & Campbell, 1994; Haynor, 1994). The mentor and the protégé often develop a long-term, close working relationship. Mentors serve a particularly helpful role in assisting nurses who are expanding their career opportunities. Unfortunately, not every nurse has the benefit of having a mentor during each career change. Specific roles of the mentor are presented in the box on p. 59.

Sponsors contribute to the socialization process by teaching strategies for dealing with the politics of career advancement and introducing the protégé to the right peo-

---

Roles of the Mentor

Challenger—encourages the critical look at issues
Counselor—helps to make short- and long-term goals
Door-opener—by virtue of position provides new experience or opportunities
Energizer—stimulates action
Envisioner—communicates the meaning and potential of professional nursing
Eye-opener—broadens perspective
Feedback-giver—gives honest positive and negative feedback
Idea bouncer—listens and discusses ideas
Model—someone to emulate
Problem solver—assists in looking at problems and possible solutions
Supporter—offers emotional support and builds self-confidence
Standard-prodder—accepts nothing less than excellence
Teacher—teaches skills essential for career advancement

From Darling, L.A. (1984). What do nurses want in a mentor? *Journal of Nursing Administration, 14*(10), 42-44.

---

ple (Carey & Campbell, 1994). For example, Beth Israel Hospital in Boston uses clinical nurse sponsors to guide the novice beyond mere skill acquisition to become socialized to professional roles and values, such as how to work on interdisciplinary teams and follow a client's illness throughout its course, both in the hospital and in other settings (American Association of Colleges of Nursing, 1995).

Socialization as Career Development

Career development is a longitudinal process beginning when the new graduate enters the work setting and proceeding at varied rates along a career path. Two models of career development in nursing are presented here. The stages of one model lead to an increased level of responsibility (Dalton, Thompson, & Price, 1977); the stages of the other lead to a high level of clinical proficiency (Benner, 1984).

Dalton's longitudinal model. Dalton described a four-stage model of career development that builds on prior knowledge and experience. In stage 1 the nurse learns to perform routine duties competently and to use both formal and informal channels of communication. Ideally, the nurse works with an experienced preceptor who also serves as a role model. A problem occurs when the organization does not permit enough time to master this stage. In stage 2 the individual develops a reputation as a competent nurse, often in an area of clinical specialty. Again, adequate time is needed in this stage to master this level of expertise. In stage 3 the nurse assumes responsibility for others. The nurse may take on multiple roles, such as informal mentor, manager, supervisor, or coordinator. In stage 4 the nurse assumes the roles of manager and innovator of ideas to influence the direction of the organization. Relationships are developed inside and outside the organization. Individuals in stage 4 think more broadly about the organization and feel comfortable in exercising power and taking a position with which others may disagree. Only a small percentage of nurses achieve this level of career development, either by choice or because of the limited number of positions.

Benner's novice-to-expert model. Benner (1984) described five stages in the acquisition of skill and knowledge that result in clinical proficiency. The model illustrates how the inexperienced nurse moves from the novice stage (stage 1) into the role of the advanced beginner (stage 2), where performance as a new graduate is marginally acceptable. While recognizing overall global aspects that are meaningful, the advanced beginner needs help in setting priorities. The competent practitioner in stage 3 has typically worked in the same setting for 2 to 3 years and has a feeling of mastery and efficiency. This practitioner is aware of long-range goals, engages in deliberate planning, and feels efficient and organized. By stage 4 the practitioner is proficient and does not need to think about individual actions. This nurse typically has 3 to 5 years of experience. Situations are perceived as wholes, and significant aspects of the situation are recognized with ease. The fifth stage of expert practitioner is achieved only after extensive experience. Because of a vast array of previous clinical experiences, the expert does not need to analytically think through familiar situations but uses intuition to deal with them. Analytical reasoning is used when new situations are encountered.

Benner identified 31 different competencies that are evident in clinical practice. These are organized into seven domains of nursing practice:

1. The helping role
2. The teaching-coaching function
3. The diagnostic and patient-monitoring function
4. Effective management of rapidly changing situations
5. Administration and monitoring of therapeutic interventions and regimens
6. Monitoring of (and ensuring the quality of) health care practices
7. Organizational and work role competencies

ISSUES IN SOCIALIZATION

Socialization is the adaption to changing roles and is a continuing, interactive, life-long process (Conway, 1984). Each role change may produce stress and conflict whether or not the nurse is experienced. For successful socialization to nursing roles, an awareness and understanding of factors in the work environment that may enhance or restrain professional nursing practice is helpful.

Professionals in a Bureaucratic Environment

Nursing education focuses on the skills, behaviors, and values of the profession. Once in the work setting, the nurse may have difficulty putting the profession's values into operation if the setting is highly bureaucratic and not supportive of professional practice. In a bureaucratic organization, decision making takes place above the level of the practitioner. Under these circumstances, conflict between the practitioner and the bureaucracy is inevitable. In an organization where decision making occurs at the level of the practitioner, conflict is reduced. Characteristics of professional and bureaucratic organizations are summarized in Table 3-4.

Three role conceptions that all nurses hold to some degree were identified by Corwin (1961):

1. *Bureaucratic role conception* is associated with rules and regulations of the organization. Primary loyalty is to hospital administration.
2. *Professional role conception* is associated with principles and standards. Primary loyalty is to the profession.
3. *Service role conception* is associated with values such as compassion, dedication, and understanding. Primary loyalty is to the patient as an individual.

Successful blending of these role conceptions will facilitate the socialization process and decrease the amount of perceived stress and conflict. The nurse must learn how to balance the values of both the profession and the organization. The strong service ideal inherent in nursing sometimes helps to mediate the effects of clashes between professional and bureaucratic values.

Research on Socialization

Published literature and research suggest that interest in professional socialization of entry-level nurses has been replaced by interest in socialization through the educational process. Several recent studies have focused on the clinical educational preceptorship as a mechanism for preparing the student for the role of beginning professional nurse. The preceptorship is based on the assumption that a one-to-one relationship facilitates learning and socialization to the professional role. Increased self-esteem and

Table 3-4   Characteristics of Professional and Bureaucratic Organizations

Bureaucratic	Professional
Hierarchical power with centralized decision making	Knowledge-based power with decentralized decision making
High formalization	Low formalization
Work performed according to division of labor	Work performed according to professional norms
Uniformity of product emphasized; work standardized	Uniqueness of client emphasized; work unstandardized
Routine tasks	Nonroutine tasks
Service to organization	Service to client and profession
Achievement of organizational goals	Loyalty to profession

confidence are demonstrated benefits of the preceptorship experience (Collins, Hilde, & Shriver, 1993). Preceptored experiences have also enhanced the collaboration between faculty and practitioners and serve to create alliances between nursing education and practice (Clayton, Broome, & Ellis, 1989; Coudret et al., 1994). Students report satisfaction with the preceptored experience and are grateful for the early sensitization to reality shock. They are challenged to work up to the RN level and, as a result, their clinical competencies improve (Haddock, 1994).

Additional research about factors related to socialization of nurses in today's health care environment is needed. Diverse needs of the learner, multiple roles of students, processes and strategies that best facilitate role transition, effectiveness of role models in the socialization process, and effectiveness of resocialization for RNs returning to school are some of the issues that must be addressed.

PROFESSIONAL ASSOCIATIONS

Merton (1958) defined a *professional association* as "an organization of practitioners who judge one another as professionally competent and have banded together to perform social functions which they cannot perform in their separate capacity as individuals" (p. 50). Professional associations exist to assure the public that high-quality services are provided. Nursing associations provide a way for nurses to meet the needs of the present and prepare for the challenges of the future.

Associations can be classified as one of three main types: broad-purpose associations, specialty practice associations, and special-interest associations. The National League for Nursing (NLN) and the ANA are two broad-purpose associations. They were both founded around the turn of the century. In 1894 the Society of Superintendents of Training Schools for Nurses of the United States and Canada gathered. This organization became the National League of Nursing Education (NLNE) in 1912 and the NLN in 1952. In 1896 a group of representatives from nursing school alumnae associations met and founded the Nurses' Associated Alumnae of the United States and Canada, which became the ANA in 1912. From the beginning, nurses were separated into two national nursing organizations with different purposes. However, all nurses are eligible for membership in both organizations, and some nurses belong to both. The NLN is composed of nurses, other health professionals, and consumers working to improve the quality of health care through accreditation of nursing education programs. This organization is also involved in continuing education programs, testing services, research, publications, videos, and lobbying efforts. The NLN is recognized as the national professional accrediting body for all basic nursing programs and master's degree nursing programs. The NLN also provides a voluntary peer-review accreditation program for home health agencies and community nursing services. The NLN continues to promote the original mission of the Superintendent's Society of improving education.

The ANA is the professional association for RNs in the United States, with constituent nursing associations in each of the 50 states and in the District of Columbia,

Guam, and the Virgin Islands. The purposes of the ANA are to "work for the improvement of health standards and the availability of health services for all people, to foster high standards of nursing, and to stimulate and promote the professional development of nurses and advance their economic and general welfare" (ANA, 1987, p. 366). The ANA is involved in many activities, including specialty certification of RNs; accreditation of continuing education programs; maintenance of government relation activities; development of standards for nursing practice; and programs to promote economic and general welfare, research, and priorities for human rights. Unfortunately, only about 10% of all RNs belong to the ANA. Because the ANA represents every RN, it is critical that all nurses become active, contributing members.

Sigma Theta Tau International is the nursing honor society. Although not a clinical specialty organization, Sigma Theta Tau, as a specialty purpose organization, encourages and recognizes superior scholarship and leadership. It was founded in 1922 by students at the Indiana University Training School for Nurses. From a beginning of 6 members and 1 chapter, the organization has grown to more than 120,000 members and over 300 chapters, including international chapters. Membership is by invitation and is based on superior scholastic achievement, professional leadership potential, or achievement in the field of nursing. Students in baccalaureate or higher-degree programs in nursing and nurse leaders in the community with a minimum of a baccalaureate degree are eligible for membership. The organization contributes to the advancement of nursing through its support of research, conferences, and publication of research in its professional journal, *Image: The Journal of Nursing Scholarship*. In 1989 the Center for Nursing Scholarship and International Nursing Library were dedicated in Indianapolis.

As nursing continues to grow, many nurses have chosen to join the specialty practice nursing organization that represents their area of clinical practice. These include organizations representing maternal-child, community, medical-surgical, and mental health nursing specialties and many areas where nurses work, such as the emergency department, operating room, and critical care units.

What are the benefits of belonging to a professional association? In other words, what is the return on the investment of money? Membership in professional associations benefits both the individual and the profession of nursing. Recognition of expertise through certification, collective bargaining to improve salary and working conditions, lobbying to influence laws affecting nursing, and promoting state laws that will assure the public of quality care are some of the initiatives undertaken by these organizations. These initiatives benefit all nurses, whether or not they are members of the professional association. To increase their effectiveness as official representatives of nursing, more nurses must become active participants in professional associations by becoming members, attending meetings, and participating in the organization's activities. Through active participation, nurses become a powerful collective of professionals. They can view nursing and health care beyond their present employment situation, and they can work to make the profession stronger. It is through participation and support of professional associations that nurses can make a difference.

Key Points

- Socialization to professional nursing is a dynamic and lifelong process.

- The status of nursing as a profession can be assessed using the criteria for professions as benchmarks.

- Accountability, autonomy, and self-governance are concepts embedded in professional practice.

- Socialization to professional nursing involves initial socialization in an educational setting followed by resocialization in the workplace.

- Several models of socialization identify stages of progression that occur as one is socialized into the professional role.

- Role models, preceptors, mentors, and sponsors play an important part in socializing nurses to specific roles or in helping them develop their career paths.

- Nurses who work in highly bureaucratic settings must integrate that value system with their own professional values.

- Professional associations are the vehicles that promote high standards of practice and advance the profession of nursing.

 ## Critical Thinking Exercises

1. Select one set of criteria of a profession and use it to analyze nursing's status as a profession.

2. Select a model of socialization and evaluate your current status in progressing through the stages of the model.

3. Who or what has been the greatest influence on your socialization to the professional nursing role?

4. Talk with five nursing graduates who have been working from 3 months to 3 years about the process of their professional socialization after graduation. Was reality shock experienced? If so, how long did it last? How was it resolved? If you were their preceptor, what measures would you take to make their socialization more meaningful and less stressful?

5. What are the advantages of being actively involved in a professional association? Contact at least one professional association to discover what the organization offers its members.

6. Defend or refute this statement: "All nurses should belong to the same professional association."

References

American Association of Colleges of Nursing. (1995, July). *Issue bulletin.*

American Nurses' Association. (1975). *Standards for nursing education.* Kansas City, MO: The Association.

American Nurses' Association. (1985). *Code for nurses with interpretive statements.* Kansas City, MO: The Association.

American Nurses' Association. (1987). *Facts about nursing.* Kansas City, MO: The Association.

American Nurses' Association. (1991). *Standards of clinical nursing practice.* Kansas City, MO: The Association.

Benner, P. (1984). *From novice to expert.* Menlo Park, CA: Addison-Wesley.

Bixler, G.K., & Bixler, R.W. (1959). The professional status of nursing. *American Journal of Nursing, 59*(8), 1142-1147.

Brimm, O.G., Jr. (1966). Socialization through the life cycle. In O.G. Brimm, Jr., and S. Wheeler (Eds.), *Socialization after childhood: Two essays* (pp. 24-33). New York: John Wiley & Sons.

Carey, S.J., & Campbell, S.T. (1994). Preceptor, mentor, and sponsor roles: Creative strategies for nursing retention. *Journal of Nursing Administration, 24*(12), 39-48.

Chitty, K. (1993). *Professional nursing: concepts and challenges.* Philadelphia: W.B. Saunders.

Christensen, P.J., & Kenney, J.W. (1995). *Nursing process: Application of conceptual models,* (4th ed) St Louis: Mosby.

Clayton, G., Broome, M., & Ellis, L. (1989). Relationship between a preceptorship experience and role socialization of graduate nurses. *Journal of Nursing Education, 28*(2), 72-75.

Cohen, H.A. (1981). *The nurse's quest for professional identity.* Menlo Park, CA: Addison-Wesley.

Collins, P., Hilde, E., & Shriver, C. (1993). A five-year evaluation of BSN students in a nursing management preceptorship. *Journal of Nursing Education, 32*(7), 330-332.

Conway, M.E. (1984). Socialization and roles in nursing. In H. Werley and J. Fitzpatrick (Eds.), *Annual review of nursing research* (Vol. 1, pp. 183-208). New York: Springer.

Corwin, R.G. (1961). The professional employee: A study of conflict in nursing roles. *American Journal of Sociology, 66*(6), 604-615.

Coudret, N., Fuchs, P., Roberts, C., Suhrheinrich, J., & White, A. (1994). Role socialization of graduating student nurses: Impact of a nursing practicum on professional role conception. *Journal of Professional Nursing, 10*(6), 342-349.

Crim, B.J., & Hood, A.W. (1995). Learning partners: Preceptor, mentor, facilitator, learner. *Seminars in Perioperative Nursing, 4*(1), 67-72.

Dalton, G.W., Thompson, P.H., & Price, R.L. (1977, summer). The four stages of professional careers: A new look at performance by professionals. *Organizational Dynamics, 6,* 19-42.

Darling, L.A. (1984). What do nurses want in a mentor? *Journal of Nursing Administration, 14*(10), 42-44.

Douglas, L.M. (1992). *The effective nurse: Leader and manager* (4th ed). St Louis: Mosby.

Erikson, E. (1950). *Childhood and society.* New York: W.W. Norton.

Fields, W.L. (1991). Mentoring in nursing: A historical approach. *Nursing Outlook, 39,* 257-261.

Flexner, A. (1910). *Medical education in the United States and Canada.* New York: Carnegie Foundation for the Advancement of Teaching.

Flexner, A. (1915). Is social work a profession? *School Society, 1*(26), 901.

Fuszard, B., & Taylor, L.J. (1995). Mentorship. In B. Fuszard, *Innovative teaching strategies in nursing* (2nd ed., pp. 200-208). Gaithersburg, MD: Aspen.

Gardner, D.L. (1992). Career commitment in nursing. *Journal of Professional Nursing, 8,* 155-160.

Greenwood, E. (1957). Attributes of a profession. *Social Work, 2*(3), 45-54.

Haddock, S. (1994). A precepted leadership course based on Bandura's social learning theory. *Nursing Connections, 7*(3), 55-61.

Hardy, M.E., & Conway, M.E. (1988). *Role theory: Perspectives for health professionals.* New York: Appleton-Century-Crofts.

Haynor, P.M. (1994). The coaching, precepting, and mentoring roles of the leader within an organizational setting. *Holistic Nursing Practice, 9*(1), 31-40.

Hinshaw, A.S. (1976). *Socialization and resocialization of nurses for professional nursing practice* (NLN Publication No. 15-1659). New York: National League for Nursing.

Houle, C.O. (1980). *Continued learning in the professions.* San Francisco: Jossey-Bass.

Keck, J.F. (1994). Terminology of theory development. In A. Mariner-Tomey, *Nursing theorists and their work* (pp. 17-26). St. Louis: Mosby.

Kelly, L. (1981). *Dimensions of professional nursing* (4th ed). New York: Macmillan.

Knowles, M. (1970). *The modern practice of adult education: From pedagogy to andragogy.* Chicago: Follett.

Kramer, M. (1974). *Reality shock: Why nurses leave nursing.* St. Louis: Mosby.

Kramer, M., & Schmalenberg, C. (1988). Magnet hospitals. *Journal of Nursing Administration, 18*(2), 13-24.

Larisey, M. (1985). Characteristics and motivators of non-BSN nurses returning to school. In *Proceedings of RN to BSN: Alternative approaches,* Buffalo: State University of New York.

Lawler, T., & Rose, M. (1987). Professionalization: A comparison among generic baccalaureate, and RN/BSN nurses. *Nurse Educator, 12*(6), 19-22.

May, K., Meleis, A., & Winstead-Fry, P. (1982). Mentorship for scholarliness: Opportunities and dilemmas. *Nursing Outlook, 30*(1), 22-28.

Merton, R. (1958). The functions of the professional association. *American Journal of Nursing, 58*(1), 50-54.

Porter-O'Grady, T. (1986). *Creative nursing administration: Participative management into the 21st century.* Rockville, MD: Aspen.

Porter-O'Grady, T. (1987). Shared governance and new organizational models. *Nursing Economics, 5*(6), 281-287.

Roberts, S.J. (1983). Oppressed group behavior: Implications for nurses. *Advances in Nursing Science, 5*(4), 21-30.

Scherwin, J., Gaster, K., Krolikowski, J., & Sherman-Justice, D. (1994). Staff nurse leadership and professional growth in the mentor role. *Journal of Nursing Staff Development, 10*(3), 139-144.

Shane, D. (1983). *Returning to school: A guide for nurses.* Englewood Cliffs, NJ: Prentice Hall.

Stein, L.I., Watts, D.R., & Howell, T. (1990). The doctor-nurse game revisited. *New England Journal of Medicine, 322,* 546-549.

Strader, M.K., & Decker, P.J. (1995). *Role transition to patient care management.* Norwalk, CT: Appleton & Lange.

Styles, M. (1982). *On nursing: Toward a new endowment.* St. Louis: Mosby.

Throwe, A., & Fought, S. (1987). Landmarks in the socialization process from RN to BSN. *Nurse Educator, 12*(6), 15-18.

Wilson, E. (1994). Nursing student perspective of learning in clinical setting. *Journal of Nursing Education, 33*(2), 81-86.

Whitman, N.I., Graham, B.A., Gleit, C.J., & Boyd, M.D. (1992). *Teaching in nursing practice* (2nd ed.). Norwalk, CT: Appleton & Lange.

Professional Nursing Roles

4

Joan L. Creasia

 Objectives

At the completion of this chapter, the reader will be able to:

- Discuss the theoretical foundations of personal and professional roles.

- Differentiate between the structural-functional and symbolic interaction perspectives of nursing roles.

- Discuss the impact of the multiple roles experienced by the professional nurse.

- Analyze common role stressors as they relate to the role of the nurse.

- Describe selected roles commonly assumed by the professional nurse and the responsibilities associated with each.

Profile in Practice

Deborah Williamson, MSN, RN, CNM
College of Nursing Midwifery Faculty Practice,
Medical University of South Carolina,
Charleston, South Carolina

After graduating from nursing school in 1972, I worked as a community health nurse at an inner-city neighborhood health center in Rochester, New York. All of the OB-GYN care for the health center was provided by a group of obstetricians and a nurse midwife. This was the first opportunity I had to work with a nurse midwife. I was impressed by her knowledge, her clinical skills, and her independent mode of practice. My primary area of interest, even then, was in the health care of women. Nurse midwifery provided an avenue for specialization in my area of interest. I also saw nurse midwifery as a way to become a primary care provider. I wanted to be the person responsible for managing the care of the women in my practice. I wanted to do the clinical exams and necessary procedures. I enjoyed the mental challenge of problem solving that exists in clinical nurse midwifery. Most important, I wanted to provide health care that was sensitive to the needs of women.

My first practice after completion of nurse midwifery school was a major influence on the rest of my career. I practiced in a rural community with three family physicians. The similar philosophy of care made the practitioners cohesive and enhanced the community's sense of being cared for by the practice. I learned about continuity of care, the importance of recognizing your own limits, and the importance of follow-up. On a personal level, I felt the intense relationships that comes from living and providing health care in a small town. The sense of connectedness that comes from sharing the joy of birth is powerful, and the bond established is forever.

Being a midwife means being part of the community whether you practice in a small town or in the city. Birth is a family affair—it's not unusual to know the mother and several generations of her family by the end of the postpartum period. After practicing almost 20 years, I can honestly say there is nothing I would rather do than practice midwifery. I feel lucky to have chosen a career that I have loved and have always felt was challenging.

I enjoy the challenge of clinical practice. But there are other challenges in the practice of midwifery. The ongoing political struggles to have nurse midwifery recognized as part of the mainstream of the American health care system is exhausting. Midwifery attracts ardent supporters and fanatical opposition. The players are physicians, nurses, and administrators. The role of supporter or oppressor is different from practice to practice. However, uniformly, women and their families are the ardent supporters of nurse midwifery care.

Another major challenge of practice is the blending of one's personal and professional life. The irregular hours and the physical and emotional fatigue take their toll on family members. To be a midwife requires a family that is supportive of the career. But I can also say that I can sense the pride my children and my husband feel when we're out and a parent shows me the child that I helped deliver. The radiance of this interaction is a mixture of the loving parent-child relationship and a special bond that formed between the parents and myself at the time of childbirth.

In today's rapidly changing health care environment, the nursing role is becoming less traditional and increasingly diverse. As the professional disciplines are called on to provide expanded and more diverse health care services in a wide variety of settings, the traditional structure of provider roles is being challenged. Nursing is responding to this challenge by examining the nature of the professional role, identifying its component parts, and adapting it to better meet the needs and changes of a dynamic health care system.

This chapter focuses on role taking in nursing by examining theoretical foundations of roles, the types of roles nurses commonly assume, the impact of multiple roles, and common role stressors. Finally, selected nursing roles and associated responsibilities are discussed.

THEORETICAL FOUNDATIONS OF ROLES

Individuals assume roles that define their position in society. Although the concepts of role and position are often used interchangeably, it is important to differentiate between the two. *Roles* are sets of patterned behaviors unique to a given position and may be reflective of personal, social, or occupational domains. The behavior patterns are manifested in the performance of duties and tasks and the assumption of certain responsibilities. *Position,* on the other hand, denotes status or a place within a specified context, such as a health care organization. An organizational chart is used to illustrate the placement of positions within the organization and to depict vertical and horizontal relationships. Thus roles are classifications of behavior, whereas positions are classifications of people (Biddle, 1979).

The expected behaviors of those who occupy a social position determine how a person in a given role should act. A *social position* refers to an identity that is widely known and held by persons who behave in a characteristic way. Roles, then, are associated with social positions and are shaped by the expectations of others in an individual's social network, often referred to as *socializing agents* (Biddle, 1979). Either explicitly or implicitly, socializing agents communicate the values and norms that are associated with a given role. Over time, the values and norms are assimilated by the person assuming that role and develop into a behavior pattern.

The context in which the social position exists also contributes to role expectations. *Context* refers to the environment in which the role is enacted and may be defined as a setting (e.g., community), an organization (e.g., hospital), or a social situation (e.g., discussion group). Although a person could theoretically hold an identical position in all three contexts (e.g., a nurse), it is clear that the expected behavior patterns would vary markedly. Thus role behaviors are limited by the physical, environmental, or temporal boundaries of the context. These concepts of role theory can be applied to professional nursing roles; the expected behaviors or roles of the nurse are determined by the nurse's social position and the context in which nursing care is delivered.

"Individuals enact roles mainly according to their personal knowledge of the role, the behavior modeling they have witnessed, the sets of expectations of others interacting with the role, and the social structure in which the role is being expressed."
Christman, 1991, p. 210.

Role Theories and Paradigms

There are two competing theoretical perspectives that may be used to analyze roles. The first perspective is the *structural-functional* paradigm, which links the individual to the social structure and focuses on the division of labor within that context (Hardy & Conway, 1988). There are formal prescriptions for actions that result in appropriate behavior. For example, this perspective might focus on the "formal prescription for action" found in the job description of a nurse who holds a staff nurse position in a large teaching hospital. An additional assumption of the structural-functional perspective is that norms and values attached to the position are handed down from generation to generation (Berger & Luckman, 1966), but as the social structure changes over the years, the values and norms of a given position adapt to that change. For example, when the length of stay in hospitals was much longer than it is today, it was the norm for nurses to implement the teaching plan after the client had sufficiently recovered from the acute stage of illness. Nurses valued client teaching and viewed it as an important dimension of the nursing role. As resource-driven care resulted in shortened lengths of stay, the norm was altered. Teaching plans and strategies were adapted to accommodate early discharge, and although nurses still valued client teaching, they modified their belief that teaching must occur before discharge. Today, referral to a community rehabilitation program or home health agency may be initiated to continue the teaching plan after discharge.

The second perspective is the *symbolic interaction* paradigm, which focuses on the interaction between people in the social system. Specifically, the meaning that is given to acts and symbols forms the basis on which behaviors are selected and roles are constructed. For communication to be effective, symbols must have the same meaning for each person in the interaction (Hardy & Conway, 1988). Mutual understanding of the meaning of symbols controls role-related behavior by either supporting or suppressing it. The responses of others serve to validate behavior. This perspective explains the concept of professional socialization of nurses who learn the role of the professional nurse by observing other nurses' actions, understanding the meaning of their actions, and responding to their reactions. More specifically, a new graduate who is oriented to a position with a preceptor learns the staff nurse role by observing the preceptor's actions and responding to the preceptor's feedback through alteration of the new graduate's own performance.

In nursing, both perspectives are valid. Many nurses function in highly structured settings. A great deal of formalization exists in the form of policies, procedures, job descriptions, evaluation mechanisms, classification systems, and so forth. Thus the structural-functional perspective can be a useful approach for analyzing the formalized aspects of a nurse's role.

As nurses assume caregiver and administrative roles, they interact with a variety of people known as their *role set*. As the symbolic interaction perspective suggests, meaning is assigned to the various interactions between people in the role set as perceived by those individuals. This perspective is useful to analyze the interdependent nature of nursing roles and the process of acquiring behaviors specific to a given nursing role.

TYPES OF ROLES

As discussed earlier, roles evolve from social positions and the context in which they are enacted. Examination of the content of roles reveals that they are derived from personal, social, and occupational domains. Nurses commonly assume positions in all three domains, often simultaneously. For example, a nurse may be a mother or father, a leader in a civic organization, and a nurse educator. Although these roles are not mutually exclusive, they reflect a primary orientation to what we refer to as our personal life, social life, and occupational life.

In most societies the social structure consists of positions that are *reciprocal;* that is, they are dependent on one or more persons for appropriate enactment of the role. Such positions include the roles of mother, father, wife, husband, teacher, nurse, bread-winner, politician, and so forth. Each of these positions brings to mind an image of the person assuming the role, along with an associated set of expected behaviors, and of other people in the social system who are critical to the enactment of the role. Thus the nurse who holds positions in all three domains develops behavior patterns for each role and interacts with a wide range of people with whom interdependent relationships are established. The result is a complex pattern of overlapping social positions and roles, each demanding certain behaviors and relationships that are unique.

THE PROFESSIONAL NURSING ROLE

How do these concepts apply to the role of the professional nurse? The nursing role is a reciprocal one, since it is interdependent with others in the role set, such as clients and families, physicians, and ancillary health care personnel, for its enactment. The nurse's own role expectations and the expectations of individuals in the role set influence the formation of behavior patterns specific to the professional nursing role. Persons in the role set communicate their expectations by sending messages that condemn some behaviors and endorse others. In addition, the role is defined by the context within which it is enacted and by the formalized role prescription designed by the organization. In combination with characteristics and traits of the individual nurse, these factors contribute to the formation of the nursing role as illustrated in Fig. 4-1.

As previously mentioned, the performance of duties and tasks, and the assumption of certain responsibilities form the pattern of behaviors that characterize the professional nurse. The professional role is unique, however, because it is influenced by a *Code of Ethics* that helps to shape professional behavior and frame role expectations. For instance, the nurse is expected to provide high-quality nursing care "with respect for human dignity and the uniqueness of the client, unrestricted by considerations of social or economic status, personal attributes, or the nature of the health problem" (American Nurses' Association, [ANA], 1985, p. 1). The *Code of Ethics* also specifies dimensions and responsibilities of the role, such as accountability, advocacy, competence, delegation, and collaboration. Because nurses are licensed, there are also legal dimensions to the role, as specified in state nurse practice acts. These influences add to the complexity of the professional nursing role by identifying multiple subroles and dimensions of the role that are bounded by organizational, ethical, and legal constraints.

IMPACT OF MULTIPLE ROLES

People in today's society typically assume multiple roles, and nurses are no exception. A woman may be a wife, mother, daughter, daughter-in-law, student, teacher—the list goes on. Similarly, a man may be a husband, father, son, son-in-law, brother, and sportsman and still hold several occupational roles. In addition, each may participate

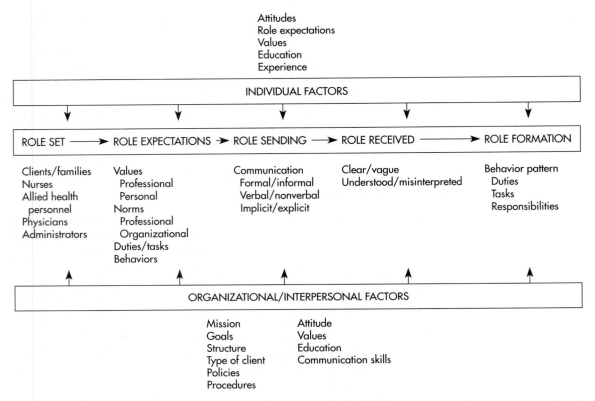

Fig. 4-1   The process of role formation. (Modified from Strader, M.K., & Decker, P.J. [1995]. *Role transition to patient care management.* Norwalk, CT: Appleton & Lange.)

in religious or civic organizations by taking membership or leadership roles that demand a different set of role behaviors.

Often, multiple roles are assumed within different contexts. However, it is possible to assume multiple roles within the same context. Such is the case with the professional nurse, who may be a caregiver, case manager, teacher, advocate, and so forth. When the same person holds several roles with a similar focus, they are referred to as *subroles.* Each subrole may be equally critical to the focal role, or one may be more dominant. For instance, a staff nurse who practices in a setting that employs a number of nonprofessionals to assist with nursing care might see management and supervision of these caregivers as the dominant subroles. As the number and type of roles and subroles held by an individual increases, the risk of role strain also increases.

Role Stress and Strain

Role stress and strain are common phenomena among individuals who hold multiple roles. *Role stress,* generated by the social structure, is said to exist when role obligations are vague, irritating, conflicting, or unrealistic. These conditions are external to the individual, but they may result in role strain, an internal response. *Role strain* is described as an emotional reaction to role stress that may be experienced as feelings of frustration, anxiety, irritability, or distress. When an individual encounters major difficulty in meeting role obligations, role strain is apt to occur (Hardy & Conway, 1988).

What conditions are likely to contribute to role stress and strain in nursing? A number of factors are identified by Hardy and Conway (1988), including changes in the organization and delivery of health care, generation of new nursing roles, economic conditions that result in redefining patient-provider roles, and technological advances. As a result of one or more of these factors, nurses may experience feelings of frustration or anxiety as their role perception and competence are threatened. However, the severity of role stress and strain is individually determined and is dependent on the perceptions of the person assuming the role. This premise was supported in a study of registered nurses (RNs) returning to school (Dick & Anderson, 1993). The investigators found that taking on the additional role of student did not increase the level of stress and strain when the nurses perceived that they had control over their professional career and support from family and colleagues. Personality characteristics were found to partially explain role strain in another sample of RNs returning to school (Lengacher, 1993). Neuroticism, described as feelings of depression, inadequacy, or a poor self-image, was the strongest predictor of role strain among RNs in this study.

The existence of multiple subroles as necessary components of the focal role is another factor that is tied to role stress and strain. In a sample of undergraduate nursing faculty, Lott, Anderson, and Kenner (1993) found that the existence of multiple roles (i.e., nurse, clinician, teacher, advisor, committee member, researcher) was the most prevalent cause of role strain reported by that group. Next were multiple demands on time, followed by multiple role relationships, each with different role obligations. Role stress and strain were manifested by feelings of frustration, anger, inappropriate emotional responses, anxiety, forgetfulness, and fatigue. Although the sample for this study was nursing faculty, staff nurse roles also involve multiple subroles, multiple demands on time, and multiple role relationships that are likely to generate role stress and strain.

Common Role Stressors in Nursing

Role conflict, role ambiguity, role incongruity, and role overload are stressors common to nursing. These stressors may be generated by the changing health care environment in which the nursing role is enacted and a myriad of personal and professional factors. A brief discussion of each of the stressors follows.

Role conflict. When role expectations within or among roles are incompatible with one another, *role conflict* may result. An early study by Corwin (1961) identified alienation in nurses who had both a high professional and a high bureaucratic orientation. This phenomenon has become known as the professional-bureaucratic conflict whereby organizational norms and values dictate behaviors that may be in conflict with professional norms and values. The result is a strain that if not reconciled can result in a response known as *burnout,* an overwhelming inability to adapt to or deal with stressors. Kramer (1974) addressed a similar issue when she discussed *reality shock,* the impact felt by recent nursing graduates who assume positions in highly bureaucratic settings. Selected personality variables, moral behavior, and role concept are some of the factors found to explain professional and bureaucratic role orientations of professional nurses.

The nurse in middle management is a prime candidate for role conflict due to incompatible expectations of staff and administration, such as those identified by Langenfeld (1988). Areas of potential conflict are evident when the manager is expected to "operate from a management perspective, seeing the broad picture in terms of impact for the entire institution" (p. 79) (management expectation) and "understand problems from the employee's point of view, creating 'win-win' situations" (p. 78) (employee expectation). Additional areas of possible role conflict include the base of loyalty (e.g., the organization versus the profession) and the cost-quality dichotomy in terms of what is ideal and what is realistic (Nyberg, 1988).

Role conflict is often thought to be common to the RN who returns to school for advanced education. This individual probably holds a job, has personal and family responsibilities, and, in addition, assumes the role of student (Creasia, 1989). Behavior patterns for each role have already been established, and now a new role is added. Expected behaviors associated with the new role may compete with the established behavior patterns and result in role conflict. Contrary to these notions, a study by Campaniello (1988) found that for a sample of RNs returning to school, the occupancy of multiple roles did not increase their perceived role conflict. For this group, the role of parent more than any other role was a major source of conflict. In another study of RNs returning to school, personality orientation explained the lack of role conflict (Rendon, 1988). The findings suggested that when interpersonal orientation was compliant, rather than detached or aggressive, there was role congruence rather than conflict. Areas of stress and dissatisfaction identified by this group related mostly to economic burdens and disruptions of social and family life.

Role ambiguity. When role expectations are unclear, the stressor is termed *role ambiguity.* Possibly more problematic for nurses than role conflict, "ambiguity for nurses has been related to their diversity of role partners, the lack of clarity in role expectations, and to an uncertainty as to how to initiate subroles of the nursing role" (Hardy & Conway, 1988, p. 202). In addition to these factors, the uncertainty associated with professional practice contributes greatly to role ambiguity. Clinical decision making is one example of uncertainty in which action is taken, possibly based on incomplete information, without certain knowledge of the outcome. While the health care organization may be designed to minimize structurally generated ambiguity, professionals are expected to deal with role ambiguities related to their area of expertise and scope of practice (Hardy & Conway, 1988).

Although role ambiguity has been identified as a construct separate from role conflict, much of the role-related research examining role conflict also measures role ambiguity. In several studies of nurses and organizations, the findings indicated that role ambiguity is more detrimental to role performance, satisfaction, and commitment than is role conflict (Hardy & Conway, 1988). Health care organization and workforce re-design initiatives that are currently underway provide fertile ground for continued role ambiguity in nursing. The extent of role overlap between clinical nurse specialists and nursing unit managers reported by Duffield, Pelletier, and Donoghue (1994) is only one example of role ambiguity in the transitional health care system.

Role incongruity. *Role incongruity* occurs when values are incompatible with role expectations. Refer to the earlier example of the staff nurse who spends much of the time supervising and directing nonprofessional caregivers as a dominant subrole; if the nurse's value system embraces the belief that nursing care should be provided by a nurse rather than by nonprofessionals, then there is a potential for role strain due to role incongruity.

Role transition, the process of assuming and developing a new role, is a form of role incongruity that is familiar to nurses. Kramer and Schmalenberg (1977) describe professional socialization of the graduate nurse who, on assuming a new social position in a health care organization, must assimilate the values and norms of that position as set forth by the organization. A problem arises when these are not in concert with the values and norms the nurse was exposed to as a student. To further complicate the issue, the new graduate must learn the professional nursing role and internalize professional norms and values. Hardy and Conway (1988) note, however, that the strain resulting from role incongruity in this situation may be a prerequisite to learning a new role and may actually facilitate it. When successful transition into the nursing role occurs, it is marked by a sense of role mastery and a feeling of well-being.

It is important to realize that issues related to role incongruity, role transition, and role mastery are not unique to the new graduate. Experienced nurses face the same issues when they are assigned precipitously to an unfamiliar patient care unit or work site. With little opportunity to identify role expectations and clarify values in this new situation, the nurse may experience an increased level of role stress and strain.

"Conditions that may influence the quality of the [role] transition experience and the consequences of transitions are meanings, expectations, level of knowledge and skill, environment, level of planning, and emotional and physical well-being."
Schumacher & Meleis, 1994, p. 119.

Role overload. Finally, when too much work is expected in the allotted time or the role becomes too complex, *role overload* is experienced. This is a common problem for nurses that may be attributed to structural, contextual, or role-related factors. Consider, for example, the nurse who practices in an acute care hospital. Since the beginning of the cost-containment effort in 1983, hospitalized patients as a group are much more acutely ill. Coupled with changes in staffing patterns, the rapid advances in technology, and additional consumer expectations, hospital-based nurses have more responsibilities today than ever before. They often carry a caseload of patients who are more acutely ill and who have very complex care requirements. In addition, they may have to oversee the work of nonprofessionals or professionals who are unfamiliar with the setting and may also be required to perform a variety of nonnursing tasks. By the time the shift is over, nurses are often exhausted, frustrated, and distressed that the quality of care they were able to deliver was less than optimal. The problem is not exclusively that of staff nurses; nurse executives in hospitals also reported a high level of role overload (Burke & Scalzi, 1988).

Role overload is a serious problem in other health care settings as well. As hospitalized patients are discharged earlier, the use of home health services is escalating. Like hospital-based nurses, home health nurses also oversee unlicensed personnel and coordinate the acquisition and delivery of health care services to the client. Their caseload is increasing in both size and complexity as home care becomes more intense and technologically oriented. With the advent of managed care and increased government involvement in health care financing, the amount of paper work also increases, expanding the nurse's role responsibilities and demanding greater amounts of time.

Strategies for Resolving Role Stress and Strain

The appropriate strategies for resolving stress and strain are situation specific and are influenced by the availability of resources, the flexibility of the setting, and/or the position of the nurse in the organization. Consider, for example, a middle manager who seeks to resolve role overload by delegating some managerial functions to an assistant. This strategy can also be used at the staff nurse level to delegate nonnursing functions to available personnel. However, it may be that resources are not sufficient to delegate part of the workload to others. In that case, it becomes necessary to set priorities to make the workload more manageable, with the recognition that less important tasks will not get done.

Modifying contextual or structural conditions is another strategy for relieving role stress and strain. Contextual and structural conditions that may be modified include the setting in which care is delivered, the organization of nursing care delivery, and the control and allocation of resources in the form of money, space, time, materials, or personnel. As these conditions are favorably modified, there is an indirect effect on the type and intensity of role strain experienced.

Role redefinition is a more direct strategy for relieving role strain due to role conflict, ambiguity, or overload. This may be accomplished on either a formal or an informal basis. That is, the role may be redefined in writing, or it may be negotiated with others. While a change in the formal job description is more permanent, negotiating changes in the role is usually a more immediate solution. This latter strategy, derived from the symbolic interactionist perspective, involves mutual understanding between role partners, which results in reprioritizing role expectations, reallocating the workload, and redefining adequate role performance.

Rewriting the job description so that expectations are clearly presented is perhaps the best strategy for reducing role ambiguity. Defining the range of a person's tasks, duties, and responsibilities will diminish the extent to which blurred or overlapping position boundaries can exist. This strategy is especially important when new position titles are bestowed or old roles are blended or combined. Other solutions for reducing role ambiguity include setting one's own performance expectations in writing and sharing them with the supervisor for approval or developing written goals and objectives as part of the performance appraisal mechanism.

Integrating the demands of multiple roles into a larger and meaningful whole and eliminating some of the demands of these roles are both effective strategies for reducing role conflict. For instance, a nurse who works full time and maintains home and family responsibilities is at risk for role conflict when additional roles are added, such as the role of student. Role integration for this nurse may consist of making adjustments in ongoing roles to make the role constellation more manageable. If this same nurse also has been active in community volunteer work, suspending involvement in those activities can reduce role conflict further. These adjustments involve changing the behavior pattern associated with specific roles to a set of behaviors that is more realistic, given the situation. A frequent roadblock to using this strategy is that it usually involves changing the expectations of oneself, a notion that presents major difficulties for some people.

Avoiding situations that conflict with one's value system is the best strategy for reducing the stressful effects of role incongruity. For instance, if a nurse's value system opposes the use of extraordinary means to prolong the life of terminally ill clients, it might be extremely stressful for that nurse to work in the intensive care unit of a large medical center. In that situation, requesting a transfer to another unit is highly recommended. If that cannot be accomplished, negotiating or redefining the role might be an alternative strategy for reducing the level of stress. However, if no middle ground can be reached, assuming a position where role expectations are more compatible with the values of the nurse may be the only recourse.

A theory describing successful *role integration,* a process by which multiple roles are meaningfully organized into a larger whole, was formulated by Hall, Stevens, and Meleis (1992) through a study of women with multiple roles. Role integration reflects the interaction of the individual and the environment on a day-to-day basis, incorporating several distinct roles in a variety of contexts. Nurses who experience a manageable level of role stress and strain may be more successful at integrating multiple roles, thereby feeling less fragmented and frustrated.

ANALYZING PROFESSIONAL NURSING ROLES

Professional nurses assume a number of roles and subroles concurrently as they seek to provide comprehensive care to clients in a variety of health care settings. McClure (1989) describes the role of the nurse as consisting of two subroles: caregiver and integrator. *Caregivers* attend to clients' needs, and *integrators* coordinate services of other specialized departments as clients' needs warrant it. The nurse, drawing from the functional, cognitive, and affective domains, uses a combination of skills, abilities, knowledge, judgment, attitudes, and values to develop and implement a plan for nursing care. As role theory suggests, nursing care is modified by the setting where care is delivered and by the subrole(s) assumed by the nurse. For example, a nurse practicing as a case manager in a community setting may use a different set of competencies than a nursing case manager in an acute care hospital. Similarly, a nurse manager of a community-based clinic uses different competencies than a dialysis nurse practicing in the same clinic. Fig. 4-2 illustrates these relationships.

The theoretical perspectives of roles discussed earlier in this chapter are useful in analyzing the caregiver and integrator facets of the nursing role. Keeping in mind that the setting where care is delivered tends to shape the content of the role, the following section describes selected roles that nurses may assume and identifies some specific responsibilities associated with each.

Caregiver

A fundamental nursing role is that of caregiver (i.e., helping the client and modifying situations that support illness and impede health) (ANA, 1994b). Nurses provide care within three types of nursing systems: wholly compensatory, partly compensatory, and supportive/educative (Orem, 1995). Appropriate nursing actions are selected to provide complete care for the client who is totally dependent, either physically or psychologically, to provide partial care when the client cannot fully assume self-care, and to provide supportive/educative care to assist clients in attaining or maintaining the highest possible level of health. The goal of nursing is to move clients toward responsible self-care at the highest point on the health-illness continuum of which they are capable.

With the client viewed as a biopsychosocial system (Roy, 1989), caregiving is directed toward addressing identified physiological, psychological, social, and spiritual needs. The nurse draws from a repertoire of skills derived from the functional, cognitive, and affective domains to develop nursing interventions appropriate to the caregiver role. Subsumed within the caregiver role are a number of subroles (e.g., teacher, counselor, and advocate), some of which are subsequently discussed in greater depth.

Role responsibilities. McClure (1989) describes the caregiver role as meeting the following client needs: dependency, comfort, monitoring, therapeutic, and educa-

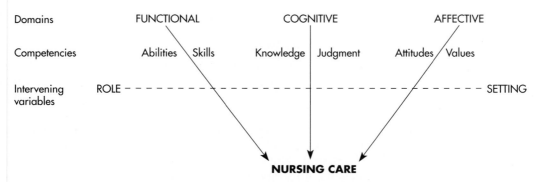

Fig. 4-2   Model for nursing care.

tional. Dimensions of nurse caring include respectful deference to others, assurance of human presence, positive connectedness, professional knowledge and skill, and attentiveness to the other's experience (Wolf et al., 1994). Whether the client is defined as the individual, family, or community, nursing care proceeds along similar lines. Selecting competencies derived from the cognitive, functional, and affective domains and using the nursing process, the nurse:

- Assesses the client
- Analyzes the data
- Identifies the nursing diagnoses
- Develops the nursing care plan
- Implements the plan
- Evaluates the outcomes

Nursing responsibilities can include the provision of direct nursing care or the delegation and supervision of care to other caregivers. Subsumed in the caregiver role are various components of the integrator role, including coordinating the efforts of the multidisciplinary health team, teaching, counseling, discharge planning, and referral. The nurse also makes use of self by exhibiting caring behaviors such as empathy, comfort, and compassion.

Teacher

As clients attempt to execute complex treatment regimens in an effort to cope with chronic disease over extended periods of time, the nurse in both inpatient and outpatient settings frequently assumes the role of teacher. A component of the caregiver role, teaching is also a primary focus of specialized positions, such as that of diabetic educator, cardiac rehabilitation nurse, or wound care specialist. In addition to teaching patients how to live with an existing condition, nurses are also involved in teaching for health promotion and disease prevention (Whitman et al., 1992). Health teaching is the process whereby information is imparted to clients for the purpose of altering cognitive, affective, or psychomotor behavior. A goal of health teaching is to assist individuals in attaining and maintaining healthful lifestyles and practices by preventing, promoting, or modifying a number of health-related behaviors (Redman, 1993). Thus teaching activities are aimed at promoting self-care behaviors, such as adherence to a prescribed treatment regimen, maintenance of a healthful lifestyle, and appropriate use of health care services. It is important for the nurse to have a thorough understanding of the teaching-learning process to facilitate successful client teaching (see Chapter 17).

Role responsibilities. The nurse may either assume an active teaching role or coordinate the teaching efforts of others. When the nurse assumes the active role of teacher/evaluator, responsibilities include:

- Identifying teaching-learning needs
- Assessing the client's motivation and readiness to learn

- Developing educational goals and objectives
- Planning the teaching-learning experience
- Providing information, using appropriate teaching strategies
- Evaluating outcomes of teaching-learning interaction

When several disciplines are involved in educating the client, the nurse may also serve as coordinator of the multidisciplinary team. Responsibilities include:

- Referring teaching-learning needs to appropriate disciplines
- Scheduling teaching sessions to enhance learning
- Reinforcing information provided by others
- Evaluating outcomes

Client Advocate

The role of client advocate is one that lies at the heart of nursing's value system (see Chapter 12). When the nurse assumes the advocacy role, the primary emphasis is on supporting the client emotionally, physically, spiritually, and socially. Curtain (1979) describes advocacy as the philosophical foundation of nursing and not the concept implied in the patient's rights movement or in the legal system. Rather, it is based on mutual understanding between nurses and clients as human beings, taking into account our common needs and our common rights. Advocacy safeguards and advances the interests of the client.

The role of client advocate has three major themes: (1) protector of the client's self-determination, (2) mediator between the client and persons in the client's environment, and (3) actor on the client's behalf (Nelson, 1988). Nursing actions are performed solely to benefit the client. The nurse may provide materials necessary for informed decision making, encourage clients to make health care decisions that they believe are in their best interest, or act directly on behalf of the client. Thus the client advocate runs the risk of conflict with others in the client's personal and/or health care environment (Rushton, 1994).

Role responsibilities. Within each component of the advocacy role, specific responsibilities have been identified. As protector of the client's self-determination, the nurse assists the client in making autonomous and informed decisions by:

- Ensuring that relevant information is available to the client
- Helping the client examine and prioritize values and goals
- Supporting the client in whatever decision is made

As mediator between the client and the environment, the nurse is responsible for:

- Coordinating health care services
- Clarifying communication between the client and community, family, other disciplines, and/or medical services
- Explaining the roles and relationships between various health care providers

As one who acts on the client's behalf, the nurse may intervene directly by:

- Altering the environment to safeguard the client's welfare
- Protecting the client against receiving inadequate care
- Championing the client's rights in the health care, social, and political arenas

Quality Improvement Coordinator

Providing care that is comprehensive and of high quality has long been a basic value of nursing. Attempts to assess health care quality in nursing and other disciplines, however, have been minimally successful, in part, because quality of care is an evolutionary concept that is multidimensional, value laden, dynamic, and changing in response to consumer expectations and technological advances. In addition, many studies lack scientific rigor, and there has been little attempt to relate the process of care to client outcomes. Despite these and other shortcomings, efforts to evaluate the quality of care have gained momentum in recent years because of the increased involvement of the government in health care financing, the concern for accountability rising out of the consumer movement, the proliferation of health care organizations and providers, and the swift pace of advances in health care technologies.

As a result, some health care organizations have created the position of quality improvement coordinator to design and implement studies, review findings, make recommendations for improvement, and coordinate the reevaluation effort. More often, however, nurses in various positions across the organization assume responsibilities of quality improvement as a nursing subrole. Emphasis is placed on improving the system rather than focusing on isolated events. A factual, ongoing, problem-solving approach is used, and statistical trends and variations from the norm are examined (ANA, 1994a). Quality-of-care studies must focus on client outcomes as the ultimate validators of effective care and include nursing-specific indicators to illustrate the nurse's contribution to those outcomes.

Role responsibilities. The quality assurance model proposed by the ANA (1977) guides the quality-of-care evaluation process and thus determines the responsibilities of the nurse evaluator. Individuals across the organization are incorporated into the process of evaluating care while it is ongoing, and the nurse is often the coordinator of these activities. The first step is to identify values that define high-quality care. Standards of nursing practice serve as one source of these values, and to make them explicit, structure, process, and outcome indicators must be identified, along with measurable criteria for each (ANA, 1994a). A task force may assist with selecting criteria for evaluation, setting standards of care against which actual performance will be judged, and identifying measures to use for data collection (Schroeder, 1988). How the study proceeds from this point depends on how the evaluation program is designed. Frequently it is the responsibility of the quality improvement coordinator to develop a method of sampling, identify a time frame for the study, and determine the frequency of monitoring. At the end of the study, the evaluator tabulates the data and compares actual performance against the performance standard. If remedial action needs to be taken, the quality improvement coordinator may be responsible for identifying possible courses of action, developing the plan, and setting a time for reevaluation.

Manager

All nurses function as managers to some extent, and nurses occupy management positions in health care organizations that command roles that vary in breadth, scope, and homogeneity. Positions whose roles are primarily management include clinical manager (head nurse), nursing supervisor, clinical director, and vice president for nursing. Other positions, such as staff nurse and assistant clinical manager, are usually mixed. That is, the position includes aspects of the caregiver role, as well as of the management role.

Nursing management positions demand a diversity of behaviors and strategies for effective role enactment. The set of expected behaviors depends on the perspectives of the people in the role constellation, the placement of the position on the organizational chart, and the relevant issues with which it is concerned. Nurses at higher levels of management are involved with issues such as resource allocation and labor relations, and they make liberal use of problem-solving and decision-making skills. These nurse executives must be flexible, creative, action oriented, and knowledgeable in both business and clinical affairs (Smith et al., 1994). On the other hand, staff nurses who manage and supervise nonprofessional caregivers as a primary nursing subrole use strategies related to personnel management but do not necessarily deal with issues related to the broader organization, such as finances.

The nurse in first-level and middle management is experiencing an expansion of the scope of responsibility and accountability (Mark, 1994). It is predicted that by the year 2000, hospital-based nurse managers will have responsibility for more than one unit, participate in hospital-wide strategic planning, set goals, and plan for effective and efficient use of human, material, and financial resources (Barrett, 1990).

Role responsibilities. Because of the variety of management positions in nursing, it is difficult to come up with a single set of responsibilities that would apply equally. Not only are manager roles highly differentiated within a single organization, but also manager roles at the same administrative level can vary across organizations (Miller & Heine, 1988). Thus the responsibilities outlined here generally relate to positions in middle management, such as clinical manager or supervisor, and are listed in no particular order. Responsibilities of the manager include:

- Establishing operating goals and objectives
- Managing a budget
- Determining staffing standards
- Measuring productivity
- Hiring personnel
- Evaluating performance

- Delegating effectively
- Serving as a clinical resource
- Resolving conflicts
- Promoting team building
- Facilitating communication, both formally and informally
- Serving as a role model and mentor for future managers
- Monitoring interpersonal relations within and between departments
- Enforcing organizational policy
- Promoting high-quality patient care
- Serving on committees to develop policies, procedures, and standards of care
- Using problem-solving and decision-making skills
- Initiating and managing change
- Engaging in coaching and counseling of staff

When asked to identify essential management skills, more than 200 nurse managers identified effective communication and decision-making skills as the most significant for effective role enactment. Other skills receiving high rankings were in problem solving, counseling, staffing, conflict resolution, performance evaluation, team building, and delegating (Chase, 1994).

Researcher

The *Code of Ethics* specifies that the nurse participate "in activities that contribute to the ongoing development of the profession's body of knowledge" (ANA, 1985, p. 1), and the *Standards of Clinical Nursing Practice* (ANA, 1991) identify research utilization as one of the professional performance core competencies. In concert with these mandates, nurses are assuming an increasingly active role in research. In recent years some hospitals and other health care delivery organizations have created the position of nurse researcher. Typically, a doctorally prepared nurse assumes this role for the purpose of coordinating institutional approval of research studies, writing grants, and directing research programs. In addition, the researcher spearheads the involvement of clinical nurses in the research process. The expanding body of research builds the theoretical basis for nursing practice and assists in the understanding of specific client issues related to health and illness, nursing issues related to the professional nursing role, and a broad range of health care delivery issues.

Role responsibilities. Responsibilities of the nurse researcher vary according to the level of research expertise and, frequently, level of education. Although every nurse may not participate fully in the research process, all nurses should be consumers of research. As consumers, nurses must critically evaluate research studies for their quality and relevance to nursing and apply the findings to clinical practice. For those who wish to take a more active role in research, responsibilities include identifying nursing problems for study, participating in nursing research under the guidance of a senior investigator, and directing the scientific investigation of nursing problems (American Nurses Association, 1993).

The research process serves as a framework for identifying specific responsibilities related to the researcher role:

- Identifying the problem
- Reviewing related literature
- Formulating hypotheses
- Determining a suitable research design
- Delimiting the setting and sample
- Selecting and testing measures for data collection
- Collecting data
- Analyzing data and interpreting the results
- Reporting findings

A senior nurse researcher can be fully involved in the entire research process, whereas less-experienced nurses can participate in selected activities under the direction of the senior investigator.

Consultant

As nurses develop specialized areas of expertise, they are often called on to serve as consultants. A consultant is one who draws from personal expertise to advise others, validate current practices, or provide specialized knowledge. Of 270 nurse consultants surveyed, 63% were in independent practice, 30% were employed by business organizations, and 7% were employed by consulting firms (Flaherty & DeMoya, 1989). Consultants can be contracted for such varied services as assisting with research design and data analysis, evaluating new health care products, advising health care professionals and other caregivers on complex client care procedures, designing and evaluating new programs, developing curricula for nursing education, or reviewing records for legal cases. In addition, nurse consultants also serve as expert witnesses in legal cases involving malpractice, environmental hazards, pharmaceuticals, equipment design, and so forth.

Role responsibilities. To ensure its success, marketing must be a major component of the consultant role. This is especially critical for nurses who are in independent practice. Marketing involves identifying the groups who can use the consulting service and then developing a market mix: defining the service, promoting the service, identifying the place where the service will be delivered, and setting a price (Camunas, 1985).

Contracting is a second major responsibility of this role. Contracting should be a formal process that involves outlining the services to be performed, determining a time frame, and setting a fee. If expenses such as transportation, lodging, food, and supplies are to be paid by the contractor, it should be so indicated in the contract. A well-written contract serves as a legal document and protects the nurse consultant against possible negative developments (Scott & Beare, 1993). It is recommended that legal counsel be obtained to review the contract to guard against unforeseeable problems.

Informatics Nurse

A relatively new role in nursing is that of the informatics nurse. Activities involved in identifying, naming, organizing, grouping, collecting, processing, analyzing, storing, retrieving, or managing data and information for nursing and health care are termed *nursing informatics.*

"The practice of nursing informatics includes the development and evaluation of applications, tools, processes, and structures which assist nurses with the management of data in taking care of patients or in supporting the practice of nursing. It includes adapting or customizing existing informatics technology to the requirements of nurses. It involves collaboration with other health care and informatics professionals in the development of informatics products and standards for nursing and health care informatics."
ANA, 1994c, p. 1

Nursing informatics supports the practice of all nursing specialties through the handling of information and spans both clinical and nonclinical domains. The informatics nurse may be at the patient's bedside, teaching in academia, employed by vendors, managing hospital information systems, conducting research, and developing software (Carty, 1994). The nurse may function as a member of a health informatics team to develop integrated systems that serve the information needs of multidisciplinary health care providers. It is important to have a nurse on this team to ensure that the integrated system meets the information needs of practicing nurses.

Role responsibilities. The role of the informatics nurse involves activities related to nursing/health care information systems. These include but are not limited to:

- Designing or implementing nursing informatics applications in nursing practice
- Analyzing and evaluating information requirements for nursing practice
- Evaluating computer and information technologies for their applicability to nursing practice problems
- Developing and teaching theory and practice of nursing informatics
- Consulting and conducting research in the field of nursing informatics
- Collaborating with specialists from nursing and other disciplines in the creation of applications for informatics theory and practice
- Developing strategies, policies, and procedures for introducing, evaluating, and modifying information technology applied to nursing practice (ANA, 1994c)

Case Manager

The role of the professional nurse case manager emerged as an outgrowth of the need for cost-effective and high-quality care in an increasingly complex health care system. The case manager role, according to Barnum (1994), is the most powerful role in health care today. The focus of the case manager role is to mediate client goals or outcomes resulting from activities of interdisciplinary professional care providers. The base of power lies in the fact that these outcomes in turn direct the dollars.

Case management is not easily defined; depending on the circumstances, it may refer to a system, a process, a role, a technology, or a service. Molloy (1994) describes three models of case management: reimbursement based (e.g., third-party payers), social welfare based (e.g., government-funded programs), and hospital/agency based (e.g., hospital or home health programs). Whatever the model of case management, the aim is the same—to ensure access to services that are cost-effective and of high quality. Case management is a way to balance the needs of clients and their families with those of the health care industry and society (Conti, 1989). Using client satisfaction as one indicator of high-quality effective care, the level of satisfaction increased significantly after the implementation of a unit-based model of nursing case management (Brubakken, Janssen, & Ruppel, 1994; Sherman & Johnson, 1994).

As case manager, the nurse uses professional expertise to ensure coordinated and cost-effective care alternatives throughout the course of treatment. A key factor in the case management approach is the identification of outcomes that are specific and time based. This approach facilitates continuous tracking of the client and ongoing evaluation of progress toward expected outcomes, including postdischarge outcomes (Bair, Griswold, & Head, 1989). The case manager is accountable for achieving outcomes within an appropriate length of stay, using resources efficiently, and establishing standards of care (Zander, 1988). Embedded in the role of case manager are the subroles of manager, consultant, clinician, researcher, and educator.

Role responsibilities. The case manager is responsible for assessment, coordination, integration, and evaluation of effectiveness and efficiency of health services. Increasingly, hospitals and home health care agencies are using clinical pathways as tools to designate what care should be provided for a given health problem within a specified time frame. These tools are useful to the case manager for coordinating and integrating client care and determining effectiveness and efficiency of care through analysis of variance reports (see Chapter 5). Among the daily activities of the hospital-based case manager are the following (Meisler & Midyette, 1994):

- Making rounds on each patient
- Assisting nurses with:
  Updating clinical pathways
  Identifying variances
  Evaluating goal achievement
- Developing plans for addressing potential or actual variances
- Meeting with other providers to identify ways to resolve variances
- Reviewing the plan of care with the client
- Updating the family about the client's progress
- Coordinating family conferences and consultations
- Evaluating the chart for duplication of services
- Documenting variations for tracking and summary reporting
- Identifying cost data needed for evaluation of client outcomes

Third-party payers are fully aware of the value of using the case management system to ensure high-quality and cost-effective care. In this situation the case manager monitors the care provided, serves as a gatekeeper by either approving or denying care as professional expertise warrants, or suggests alternatives that might be more cost-effective. Case managers employed by health maintenance organizations (HMOs), case management companies, and cost-containment companies indicated that they were most involved in monitoring service delivery and reviewing needed changes in policies, procedures, and resources (Goodwin, 1994).

Advanced Practice Roles

As it is currently being used, *advanced practice nursing* is an umbrella term that includes nurse practitioners, clinical nurse specialists, certified nurse midwives, and certified nurse anesthetists (ANA, 1994b). Advanced practice nurses (APNs) have a specialized body of knowledge and expanded practice skills acquired through study at the graduate level. They work with individuals, families, and communities to assess health needs, provide and manage care, and evaluate the outcomes of that care. APNs are certified by one of the recognized specialty organizations or the American Nurses Credentialing Center, and their practice is regulated by the state nurse practice act.

"Advanced practice nurses have a greater range, breadth, and depth of competencies that result in a broader repertoire of effective solutions for the needs of individuals, populations, and systems. This knowledge base and skill level render advanced practitioners optimally suited for managing complex, uncertain, and resource-limited situations."
Caterinicchio, 1995, p. 9

Certified nurse midwives (CNMs), approximately 3500 in number, provide prenatal and women's health care; deliver babies in hospitals, homes, and birthing centers; and provide follow-up postpartum care. CNM deliveries accounted for nearly 5% of all births in 1991, and the number is rapidly increasing. Certified RN anesthetists (CRNAs) administer anesthesia for all types of surgery in a variety of settings such as operating rooms, dental offices, and outpatient surgical centers. There are more than 20,000 CRNAs in the United States, and it is estimated that they administer more than 65% of all anesthetics. Clinical nurse specialists (CNSs), about 40,000 in number, provide care in a variety of clinical specialties in both inpatient and outpatient settings. The CNS role is multidimensional and includes direct care, consultation, education, research, administration, and quality-of-care monitoring. Nurse practitioners (NPs) provide primary care related to health promotion and disease prevention in both urban and rural settings. Numbering approximately 25,000, they conduct physical examinations, diagnose and treat common acute illness, provide immunizations, manage chronic conditions, and teach lifestyle modifications for healthy living (American Association of Colleges of Nursing, 1994).

While the roles of nurse midwives and nurse anesthetists are separate and distinct, clinical nurse specialists and nurse practitioners often have blurred or overlapping roles. In a study of CNS and NP role components, Williams and Valdivieso (1994) found that both groups of nurses were involved in education, consultation, administration, and research, but CNSs spent a greater amount of time in those activities than did NPs. On the other hand, NPs spent 63% of their time in direct practice, compared with CNSs, who spent 33% of their time in direct practice. The overlap of roles may be partially due to the fact that more similarities than differences are evident in the graduate educational programs of these two groups. Since 1990, when the NP and CNS advanced clinical practice councils of the ANA merged, consolidation of NP and CNS graduate educational programs into a combined NP/CS program has become increasingly common. There is ongoing debate as to whether this trend should continue (Page & Arena, 1994).

Traditionally, CNSs practiced in acute care settings and NPs practiced in outpatient settings. CNSs were valued for their clinical expertise, and NPs were valued for their role as primary care providers. As these roles are blended, it is expected that the practice settings will become less distinct and the competencies of both groups will be similar. It is anticipated that in the future, nurses in advanced practice will practice concurrently in primary, secondary, and tertiary care settings (Mirr, 1993).

Role responsibilities. Whatever the clinical focus of their work, APNs are expected to (ANA, 1994b):

- Identify individuals, families, or communities at risk.
- Plan and advocate for cost-effective, high-quality care.
- Provide care or manage systems of care.
- Manage acute and chronic health states.
- Assist clients in regaining and maintaining optimal health.
- Prescribe and manage pharmacological interventions.
- Serve as mentor and consultant for other nurses.
- Consult and collaborate with other health professionals.
- Evaluate health programs for populations at risk.
- Participate in professional, organizational, and legislative activities.
- Participate in research to improve client outcomes.
- Develop new cost-effective interventions.
- Advance nursing practice through publication and presentation of scholarly work.

• • •

Nursing's contribution to health care is illustrated by the nature and diversity of nursing roles. While the roles described in this chapter do not constitute an exhaustive list, they are representative of the roles nurses commonly assume. As health care reform becomes a reality, it is anticipated that additional nursing roles will emerge.

Key Points

- The practice of nursing involves assuming a number of diverse roles, some of them simultaneously, in a variety of settings.

- Role theory is useful in understanding the professional nursing role and the problems generated by the social system in which the nurse practices.

- The impact of assuming multiple roles in nursing can result in role stress and strain.

- Strategies to modify role stress and strain are situation specific.

- An examination of nursing roles reveals their diversity and complexity.

- In the caregiver role, the nurse assists clients in modifying situations that support illness and impede health.

- The teaching role focuses on assisting individuals in attaining and maintaining healthy lifestyles.

- In the role of client advocate, the nurse protects the client, mediates between the client and the environment, and acts on the client's behalf.

- As quality improvement coordinator, the nurse coordinates activities to improve the system of care delivery.

- Managerial roles in nursing may be enacted at different levels of the organization and thus vary in content, scope, and responsibility.

- Among the responsibilities associated with the research role are identification of nursing problems for study and application of published research findings to practice.

- The nurse consultant contracts with interested parties to provide services derived from a specialized area of expertise.

- The informatics nurse is involved in the acquisition and management of health care information.

- As case manager, the nurse uses professional expertise to ensure coordinated and cost-effective care alternatives throughout the course of treatment.

- Advanced practice nurses (nurse practitioners, nurse midwives, nurse anesthetists, and clinical nurse specialists) have a specialized body of knowledge and expanded practice skills acquired through study at the graduate level.

Critical Thinking Exercises

1. Select a nursing role of your choice and:
   a. Analyze it according to the symbolic-interactionist perspective and the structure-functionalist perspective.
   b. Describe the role stressors that may be an integral part of the role.
   c. Identify strategies that can be employed to reduce role strain.

2. Identify the sources of role conflict that you are currently experiencing. How can *you* reduce the impact of this conflict? What can *others* do?

3. Describe a situation where you experienced role overload. What were the consequences? How did you resolve the situation? Formulate additional strategies that might have been useful.

4. Describe a situation related to the professional nursing role where role incongruity might be an issue for you. What alternatives can you identify that could result in a satisfactory resolution?

5. Speculate how advanced practice nurses might best be used in your clinical setting. What would be the benefits for the patients? How would the organization benefit from their practice?

References

American Association of Colleges of Nursing. (1994, September). Advanced practice nursing: Extending primary care's reach. *Media Backgrounder,* pp. 1-6.

American Nurses' Association. (1977). *Quality model: A plan for the implementation of the standards of nursing practice.* Kansas City, MO: The Association.

American Nurses' Association. (1985). *Code of ethics with interpretative statements.* Kansas City, MO: The Association.

American Nurses' Association. (1991). *Standards of clinical nursing practice.* Washington, DC: The Association.

American Nurses' Association. (1993). *Education for participation in nursing research.* Washington, DC: The Association.

American Nurses' Association. (1994a). *Implementation of nursing practice standards and guidelines.* Washington, DC: The Association.

American Nurses' Association. (1994b). *Nursing: A social policy statement* [Draft]. Washington, DC: The Association.

American Nurses' Association. (1994c). *The scope of practice for nursing informatics.* Washington, DC: The Association.

Bair, N.L., Griswold, J.T., & Head, J.L. (1989). Clinical RN involvement in bedside-centered case management. *Nursing Economics, 7*(3), 150-154.

Barnum, B.S. (1994). Realities in nursing practice: A strategic view. *Nursing and Health Care, 15*(8), 400-405.

Barrett, S. (1990). *AONE national nurse manager study.* Chicago: American Hospital Association.

Berger, P., & Luckman, T. (1966). *The social construction of reality.* New York: Free Press.

Biddle, B.J. (1979). *Role theory: Expectations, identities and behaviors.* New York: Academic Press.

Brubakken, K., Janssen, W., & Ruppel, D. (1994). CNS roles in implementation of a differentiated case management model. *Clinical Nurse Specialist, 8*(2), 69-73.

Burke, G.D., & Scalzi, C.C. (1988). Role stress in hospital executives and nursing executives. *Health Care Management Review, 13*(3), 67-72.

Campaniello, J.A. (1988). When professional nurses return to school: A study of role conflict and well-being in multiple-role women. *Journal of Professional Nursing, 4*(2), 136-140.

Camunas, C. (1985). Marketing as a nursing skill. In D.J. Mason & S.W. Talbot, *Political action handbook for nurses* (pp. 205-212). Menlo Park, CA: Addison-Wesley.

Carty, B. (1994). The protean nature of the nurse informaticist. *Nursing and Health Care, 15*(4), 174-177.

Caterinicchio, M.J. (1995). Redefining nursing in the midst of health care reform, *Nursing Policy Forum, 1*(1), 8-9.

Chase, L. (1994). Nurse manager competencies. *Journal of Nursing Administration, 24*(48), 56-64.

Christman, L. (1991). Perspectives on role socialization of nurses. *Nursing Outlook, 395,* 209-212.

Conti, R. (1989). The nurse as case manager. *Nursing Connections, 2*(1), 55-58.

Corwin, R. (1961). The professional employee: A study of conflict in nursing roles. *American Journal of Sociology, 66*(6), 604-615.

Creasia, J. (1989). Reducing the barriers to RN educational mobility. *Nurse Educator, 14*(4), 29-33.

Curtain, L. (1979). The nurse as advocate: A philosophical foundation for nursing. *Advances in Nursing Science, 1*(3), 1-10.

Dick, M., & Anderson, S.E. (1993). Job burnout in RN-to-BSN students: Relationships to life, stress, time commitments, and support for returning to school. *Journal of Continuing Education in Nursing, 24*(3), 105-109.

Duffield, C., Pelletier, D., & Donoghue, J. (1994). Role overlap between clinical nurse specialists and nursing unit managers. *Journal of Nursing Administration, 24*(10), 54-63.

Flaherty, Sr. M.J., & DeMoya, D. (1989). An entrepreneurial role for the nurse consultant. *Nursing and Health Care, 10*(5), 259-263.

Goodwin, D.R. (1994). Nursing case management activities: How they differ between employment settings. *Journal of Nursing Administration, 24*(2), 29-34.

Hall, J.M., Stevens, P.E., & Meleis, A.I. (1992). Developing the construct of role integration: A narrative analysis of women clerical workers' daily lives. *Research in Nursing and Health, 15,* 447-457.

Hardy, M.E., & Conway, M.E. (1988). *Role theory: Perspectives for health professionals* (2nd ed.). Norwalk, CT: Appleton & Lange.

Kramer, M. (1974). *Reality shock.* St. Louis: Mosby.

Kramer, M., & Schmalenberg, C. (1977). *The path to biculturalism.* Wakefield, MA: Contemporary Publishing.

Langenfeld, M.L. (1988). Role expectations of nursing managers. *Nursing Management, 19*(6), 78, 80.

Lengacher, C.A. (1993). Development of a predictive model for role strain in registered nurses returning to school. *Journal of Nursing Education, 32*(7), 301-308.

Lott, J.W., Anderson, E.R., & Kenner, C. (1993). Role stress and strain among nondoctorally prepared undergraduate faculty in a school of nursing with a doctoral program. *Journal of Professional Nursing, 9*(1), 14-22.

Mark, B.A. (1994). Emerging role of the nurse manager: Implications for educational preparation. *Journal of Nursing Administration, 24*(1), 48-55.

McClure, M.L. (1989). The nurse executive role: A leadership opportunity. *Nursing Administration Quarterly, 13*(3), 1-8.

Meisler, N., & Midyette, P. (1994). CNS to case manager: Broadening the scope. *Nursing Management, 25*(11), 44-46.

Miller, M., & Heine, C. (1988). The complex role of the head nurse. *Nursing Management, 19*(6), 58-59, 62-64.

Mirr, M.P. (1993). Advanced clinical practice: A reconceptualized role. *Advanced Clinical Practice 4*(4), 599-602.

Molloy, S.P. (1994). Defining case management. *Home Healthcare Nurse, 12*(3), 51-54.

Nelson, M. (1988). Advocacy in nursing: A concept in evolution. *Nursing Outlook, 36*(3), 136-141.

Nyberg, J. (1988). Roles and rewards in nursing administration. *Nursing Administration Quarterly, 13*(3), 36-39.

Page, N.E., & Arena, D.M. (1994). Rethinking the merger of the clinical nurse specialist and the nurse practitioner roles. *Image: Journal of Nursing Scholarship, 26*(4), 315-318.

Orem, D.E. (1995). *Nursing: Concepts of practice* (5th ed.). St. Louis: Mosby.

Redman, B.K. (1993). *The process of patient education* (7th ed.). St. Louis: Mosby.

Rendon, D. (1988). The registered nurse student: A role congruence perspective. *Journal of Nursing Education, 27*(4), 172-177.

Roy, C., Sr. (1989). The Roy adaptation model. In Riehl-Sisca, J.P., *Conceptual models for nursing practice* (3rd ed., pp. 105-114). New York: Appleton-Century-Crofts.

Rushton, C.H. (1994). The critical care nurse as patient advocate. *Critical Care Nurse, 14*(3), 102-106.

Schroeder, P. (1988). UBQA: The system revisited. In S. Pinkerton & P. Schroeder (Eds.), *Commitment to excellence: Developing a professional nursing staff* (pp. 33-41). Rockville, MD: Aspen.

Schumacher, K.L., & Meleis, A.I. (1994). Transitions: A central concept in nursing. *Image: Journal of Nursing Scholarship 26*(2), 119-127.

Scott, L.D., & Beare, P.G. (1993). Nurse consultant and professional liability. *Clinical Nurse Specialist, 7*(6), 331-334.

Sherman, J.J., & Johnson, P.K. (1994). CNS as unit-based case manager. *Clinical Nurse Specialist, 8*(2), 76-80.

Smith, P.M., Parson, R.J., Murray, B.P., Dwore, R.B., Vorderer, L.H., & Okerlund, V.W. (1994). The new nurse executive: An emerging role. *Journal of Nursing Administration, 24*(11), 56-62.

Strader, M.K., & Decker, P.J. (1995). *Role transition to patient care management.* Norwalk, CT: Appleton & Lange.

Whitman, N.I., Graham, B.A., Gleit, C.J., & Boyd, M.D. (1992). *Teaching in nursing practice* (2nd ed.). Norwalk, CT: Appleton & Lange.

Williams, C.A., & Valdivieso, G.C. (1994). Advanced practice models: A comparison of clinical nurse specialist and nurse practitioner activities. *Clinical Nurse Specialist, 8*(6), 311-318.

Wolf, Z.R., Giardino, E.R., Osborne, P.A., & Ambrose, M.S. (1994). Dimensions of nurse caring. *Image: Journal of Nursing Scholarship 26*(2), 107-111.

Zander, K. (1988). Nursing case management: Strategic management of cost and quality outcomes. *Journal of Nursing Administration, 18*(5), 23-30.

The Nursing Process

5

Joan L. Creasia

 ## Objectives

At the completion of this chapter, the reader will be able to:

- Describe the components of the nursing process.
- Analyze the relationship among the components of the nursing process.
- Discuss nursing activities associated with each step of the nursing process.
- Differentiate between evaluating the plan of care and evaluating client outcomes.
- Evaluate the utility of the nursing process as a systematic framework for the delivery of nursing care.

Profile in Practice
Donna Ignatavicius, MS, RN
Author and Consultant,
LaPlata, Maryland

As a practicing nurse and a nurse educator for many years, I used the nursing process as a basis for my clinical teaching and practice. A few years ago when I was teaching a group of nursing students in a local hospital, I had my first encounter with clinical pathways. A consultant was beginning to set up clinical pathways for use in the hospital and, as a nurse educator, I felt the need to incorporate this tool into my teaching. Since I knew little about clinical pathways, I attended seminars and visited hospitals where they were in use. I discovered clinical pathways to be a valuable clinical management tool for nursing because it forces nurses to be outcome oriented rather than task oriented and encourages collaborative practice.

I still believe that the nursing process is useful for beginning nursing students because it provides a structured way of thinking. Once students learn clinical reasoning, however, they should be encouraged to use available tools to spark their thinking and provide cues. The clinical pathway is one such tool. Some clinical pathways have an assessment component that blends nicely with the nursing process. One advantage of using clinical pathways for both students and practicing nurses is that they provide a way to see what has happened with a client and what is expected to happen. This is particularly useful if a nurse or a student is caring for a client in the hospital only once during a 5-day stay. Clinical pathways also facilitate interdisciplinary care by a team of professionals and promote consistency in care. The greatest challenge in the use of clinical pathways is convincing nurses that it is more than a fad. While it is used mainly in hospitals at the present time, it would be a useful tool to coordinate care across the continuum of health care services, thereby improving quality of care and reducing costs.

Perhaps the most widely used practice framework in nursing is the nursing process, a knowledgeable, purposeful series of thoughts and actions that address the nursing needs of specific clients (Duldt, 1995). Described as the core and essence of nursing (Yura & Walsh, 1988), the nursing process offers a specific, organized, and systematic method for the delivery of nursing care. It is central to all nursing actions, relevant in any setting, and applicable within any conceptual reference. It is flexible and adaptable yet sufficiently structured to provide a base from which all systematic nursing actions can proceed. Through the nursing process, the nurse combines the interpersonal, cognitive, and technical skills needed to deliver safe and effective client care.

OVERVIEW OF THE NURSING PROCESS

A systematic process for the delivery of nursing care was first described in the literature by Lydia Hall (1955). Her approach was built around three interrelated spheres of nursing activity: care, core, and cure (Fig. 5-1). The sphere of caring focused on the body—specifically, attention to basic functions and activities of daily living. Therapeutic use of self in providing nursing care was the essence of the core component. Nursing activities related to the cure component included administering specific therapies and supporting the patient and family during the treatment process.

Subsequently, others described a "nursing process," but the model that has withstood the test of time is that developed by Yura and Walsh (1967). They proposed a four-step nursing process model that consisted of assessing, planning, implementing, and evaluating. The current model closely resembles the Yura and Walsh model, but with the addition of a diagnostic component. The five-step nursing process consists of the following elements:

Assessment—identifying client strengths, health status, risk, and concerns
Analysis/diagnosis—processing client data and identifying appropriate nursing diagnoses
Planning—designing strategies to solve identified problems and build on client strengths
Implementation—delivering and documenting the planned care
Evaluation—determining the effectiveness of the care delivered.

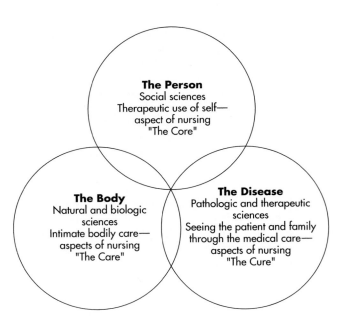

Fig. 5-1   Hall's core, care, and cure diagram. (From Hall L. [1964]. Nursing—What is it? *Canadian Nurse, 60*[2], 151, 1964.)

The American Nurses' Association (ANA) *Standards of Clinical Nursing Practice* (1991) parallel the steps of the nursing process and support its use as illustrated in Table 5-1.

The nursing process is sometimes depicted as a linear model proceeding from assessment through diagnosis, planning, implementation, and evaluation. It is more appropriately conceptualized as a continuous and interactive model (Fig. 5-2), thereby providing a flexible and dynamic approach to client care. This model can accommodate changes in the client's health status and/or failure to achieve expected outcomes through a feedback mechanism. The interactive nature of the model with its feedback mechanism permits the nurse to reenter the nursing process at the appropriate stage to collect additional data, restructure nursing diagnoses, design a new plan, or change implementation strategies. Further examination of the elements of the nursing process reveals the multiple activities embedded in each step.

ASSESSMENT

Assessment "is the deliberate and systematic collection of data to determine a client's current and past health status and functional status and to evaluate the client's present and past coping patterns" (Carpenito, 1993, p. 46). To be useful, data collection must focus on the intended purpose of nursing and the client's health status (Bandman & Bandman, 1995). Data collection centers on the use of multiple sources and types of data, a variety of data collection techniques, and the use of reliable and valid mea-

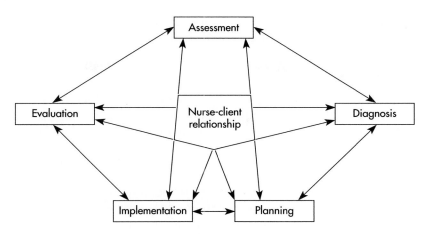

Fig. 5-2 The nursing process feedback system. (Redrawn from Christensen, P.J., and Kenney, J.W. [1995]. *Nursing process: Application of conceptual models* [4th ed.]. St. Louis: Mosby.)

Table 5-1 **Standards of Care**

Standard	Nursing Actions
I. Assessment	The nurse collects client health data.
II. Diagnosis	The nurse analyzes the assessment data in determining diagnoses.
III. Outcome identification	The nurse identifies expected outcomes individualized to the client.
IV. Planning	The nurse develops a plan of care that prescribes interventions to attain expected outcomes.
V. Implementation	The nurse implements the interventions identified in the plan.
VI. Evaluation	The nurse evaluates the client's progress toward attainment of outcomes.

From American Nurses' Association. (1991). *Standards of clinical nursing practice*. Kansas City, MO: The Association.

surement instruments. All of these elements are critical to building a comprehensive database.

Sources of Data

The primary source of data is the client, whether the client is defined as the individual, the family, or the community. Secondary sources of data include written records, other health care providers, and significant others, to name just a few. Using both primary and secondary data sources when assessing the client permits validation of data, helps to reduce bias, and strengthens the overall assessment.

Data Collection Techniques

Assessment techniques include measurement, observation, and interview. *Measurement* is used to determine the dimensions of a given indicator (e.g., blood pressure) or to ascertain such characteristics as quantity, size, or frequency. Measurement may require the use of physical diagnosis instruments, such as a stethoscope or a cardiac monitor, or other kinds of measures to assess functional, behavioral, social, or cognitive domains. Data collection by *observation* requires the use of the senses. In addition to visual observation, tactile and auditory techniques, such as palpation and auscultation, are commonly used. Observation provides a variety and depth of data that may be difficult to obtain by other methods. *Interview,* in either a structured or unstructured format, is used to obtain information such as a health history and demographic data. A *structured interview* is controlled by the nurse and is most effective when specific information is needed, such as in emergency situations. An *unstructured interview* is a more open-ended interview format whereby the nurse engages in active listening, elicits information from the client's perspective, and gains insight into the client's understanding of the problem. This type of interview serves not only to obtain information, but also to build rapport with the client.

Types of Data

Using the above techniques, two types of data are obtained: (1) *objective* or factual data, most often gained through observation and measurement (e.g., reddened tympanic membrane observed through use of an otoscope) and (2) *subjective* or perceptual data, most often gained through interview and active listening (e.g., the client states, "My eardrum hurts"). For a comprehensive assessment, both objective and subjective data must be collected and given equally serious consideration. Care should be taken to avoid personal or biased interpretations of the data, particularly that which is subjective, by recording the data in a very factual way.

Data Collection Instruments

The use of selected data collection measures and instruments can assist the nurse in compiling a comprehensive database and organizing the data into meaningful patterns. Assessment usually begins by taking a nursing history and conducting a physical examination. Many clinical areas have developed nursing history and physical forms specific to the type of agency and the clients served. Regardless of the format, the nursing database should include the following categories of information (Edelman & Mandle, 1994):

- Demographic data
- Current and past medical problems

- Family medical history
- Surgical and (if appropriate) obstetrical history
- Childhood illnesses
- Allergies
- Current medications
- Psychological status
- Social history
- Environmental background
- Physical assessment

The amount of detail may vary; for example, a history obtained in an emergency department may be different from one taken in an extended care facility. The focus of the assessment and history may also vary based on the type of client served. For example, on an oncology unit emphasis may be placed on assessment of pain, social support networks, and coping skills, whereas in a prenatal clinic the focus would be on assessment of fetal growth, knowledge of nutrition, and the need for community resources such as childbirth education classes. Beyond the areas of particular concern, however, it is important to assess all dimensions of the client, including physiological, psychological, sociocultural, developmental, and spiritual aspects (Carpenito, 1993).

It is sometimes desirable to measure specific client characteristics or situations using reliable and valid instruments. For example, the abuse assessment screen presented in Fig. 5-3 is an instrument designed to assess risk of abuse in pregnant women. The FACES pain scale (Fig. 5-4) is used to assess pain in children (Wong, 1995). There are also physiological and behavioral instruments to measure stress, coping, depression, health, and a variety of other variables. Many of these instruments have undergone extensive psychometric testing to estimate their reliability and validity and have been published in compilations (e.g., Waltz and Strickland's [1988] *Measurement of Nursing Outcomes*) and journal articles.

Comprehensive data gathering in the assessment stage is time well spent, since incomplete or inaccurate data may lead to an inappropriate diagnosis and a plan that will only waste valuable time and frustrate both the nurse and the client. The assessment stage is also a time to establish the nurse-client relationship, since the nurse becomes recognized as a caring but organized and purposeful resource for the client. In some situations the assessment stage may also be the time for the nurse to establish a relationship with the client's family and other supportive individuals who may be critical to ensuring effective discharge planning and continuity of care.

ANALYSIS/NURSING DIAGNOSES

Diagnosis involves cognitive activities to cluster cues, evaluate data, and generate hypotheses. According to Gordon (1995), the diagnostic process is a cycle of clinical reasoning, inference, and judgment. Although analysis and nursing diagnosis are conceptualized as one step in the nursing process, two distinct sets of activities actually occur: processing the data and drawing conclusions. Processing the data includes inter-

---

Abuse Assessment Screen

1. Have you ever been emotionally or physically abused by   YES   NO
   your partner or someone important to you?
2. Within the last year, have you been hit, slapped, kicked,   YES   NO
   or otherwise physically hurt by someone?
   If YES, by whom _____
   Number of times _____
3. Since you have been pregnant, have you been hit, slapped,   YES   NO
   kicked, or otherwise physically hurt by someone?
   If YES, by whom _____
   Number of times _____
   Mark the area of injury on the body map.

4. Within the last year, has anyone forced you to have sexual   YES   NO
   activities?
   If YES, by whom _____
   Number of times _____
5. Are you afraid of your partner or anyone you listed above?   YES   NO

Fig. 5-3 Abuse assessment screen. (Developed by Barbara Parker.)

Fig. 5-4 FACES pain scale. (From Wong, D.L. [1995]. *Whaley and Wong's nursing care of infants and children* [5th ed]. St. Louis: Mosby.)

preting information and clustering it. Drawing conclusions culminates in naming the cluster of data, as in identifying a nursing diagnosis.

Analysis

Analysis involves processing the data by organizing, categorizing, and synthesizing the information. The nurse uses critical thinking skills to make inferences in the data from which conclusions can be drawn. (See Chapter 18 for a full discussion of critical thinking.) In the analysis stage, both objective and subjective data are categorized and clustered into patterns. Functional health patterns and human response patterns, presented in Table 5-2, are two typologies that nurses may use to organize and categorize assessment data.

Analysis gives meaning to the data as client strengths, problems, and risks are identified. Client data may be compared against known norms, such as the stages of growth and development or disease-specific behaviors or expectations. Gaps or incongruities in the data are identified, and patterns of behavior are ascertained. Analysis takes place both with the client as the nurse is actively listening and questioning, and later as the nurse processes the information to formulate a plan of care. Analysis is an ongoing process that is called forth when new information is obtained or changes in the client's health status occur. The nursing diagnosis is the end product of data analysis.

Nursing Diagnosis

A *nursing diagnosis* is a definitive statement that describes individual, family, or community health status, risks, or concerns that can be affected by nursing intervention.

Table 5-2   **Typologies to Organize Assessment Data**

Functional Health Patterns (Gordon, 1995)	Human Response Patterns (NANDA, 1986)
Health perception–health management pattern	Exchanging—mutual giving and receiving
Nutritional-metabolic pattern	Communicating—sending messages
Elimination pattern	Relating—establishing bonds
Activity-exercise pattern	Valuing—assigning relative worth
Sleep-rest pattern	Choosing—selecting alternatives
Cognitive-perceptual pattern	Moving—activity
Self-perception–self-concept pattern	Perceiving—reception of information
Role-relationship pattern	Knowing—meaning associated with information
Sexuality-reproductive pattern	Feeling—subjective awareness of information
Coping–stress-tolerance pattern	
Value-belief pattern	

Diagnosis involves drawing conclusions through the use of critical thinking skills from identified patterns in the data (Wilkinson, 1992) and includes the elements of deliberation, inference, interpretation, and choice. Both inductive and deductive reasoning are used to arrive at a nursing diagnosis. *Inductive reasoning* proceeds from the specific to the general (i.e., from a fact or set of facts to a conclusion that is based on high probability) (Bandman & Bandman, 1995). For example, a nurse in the postanesthesia recovery unit observes that patients experience intense pain after a bowel resection. From this observation, the nurse concludes that all postoperative bowel resections probably will have the nursing diagnosis of "pain." *Deductive reasoning,* on the other hand, proceeds from the general to the specific (i.e., from a principle, theory, or idea to an identified fact, set of facts, or predictions). For example, if the premise is accepted as true that pain in the left arm and jaw is a cardinal sign of a myocardial infarction (MI) and Mr. S. comes to the emergency department complaining of left arm and jaw pain, it can be concluded that he is having an MI until it has been proved otherwise. Diagnosis entails back-and-forth movement between these two modes of reasoning.

Nursing diagnoses reflect client problems or risks that can be treated within the scope of nursing practice in any clinical setting. A nursing diagnostic statement differs from a medical diagnosis in both content and context. The *medical diagnosis* describes a pathological condition or symptom that requires treatment aimed at curing the disease or alleviating the symptom. The *nursing diagnosis,* on the other hand, describes the impact of the disease, symptom, or health concern on the activities and lifestyle of the client. A diagnostic statement contains two parts: a description of the problem and the etiology and/or relational factors. Sometimes a third part of the statement is added to reflect signs and symptoms or evidence to clarify the diagnostic statement. For example, a two-part nursing diagnosis for a postsurgical client might be "ineffective breathing pattern related to pain secondary to abdominal surgery." A three-part statement would add the phrase "evidenced by a respiratory rate of 26 and shallow breathing" (Atkinson & Murray, 1995). Nursing diagnoses are intended to promote comprehensive health care and facilitate communication among nurses by providing a common language. An alphabetical listing of nursing diagnoses approved by the North American Nursing Diagnosis Association (NANDA) (1994) is presented in the box on pp. 102-103.

The identification of nursing diagnoses uses the nurse's knowledge, skills, and experience and sets the stage for the remaining steps of planning, implementation, and evaluation. However, judgments and conclusions about the data should be validated with the client before a plan of care is developed or implemented. Inference and interpretation of data are subject to individual bias and are influenced by personal experience, attitudes, and values. Thus the client's interpretation of data may be vastly different from that of the nurse. When the nurse and client do not agree on the diagnosis, then the plan is likely to be ineffective. When they do agree, however, both the nurse and the client can work toward achieving the same outcomes.

PLANNING

Planning involves the development of a plan of action aimed at resolving nursing diagnoses and assisting the client toward the goal of optimal wellness (Yura & Walsh,

1988). In the past, planning for client care was done *by* the nurse *for* the client. More recently, however, plans are often formulated and developed *with* the client. Nevertheless, the client's readiness and willingness to mutually plan with the nurse must be carefully evaluated, since individuals differ in their desire for involvement in the planning process. In addition, some clients want control over some aspects of care but not others. Periodic reassessment of the client's wish for mutual planning is important because the desire for mutual planning may change as the disease condition or circumstances change. Family members and significant others should also be involved in the planning process, since they may be crucial to the implementation of the plan and may serve as support systems to clients who receive care in a community setting. The planning stage includes prioritizing the nursing diagnoses, developing long- and short-term outcomes, defining objectives to serve as measures of progress toward attainment of desired outcomes, and identifying nursing actions to assist the client toward optimal achievement of outcomes.

Setting Priorities

Prioritizing diagnoses consists of ranking them according to importance and labeling them as high, medium, or low priorities. The highest priorities, of course, are basic survival needs, life-threatening client problems, and safety of the client and the nurse. Labeling medium and low priorities may be an area for negotiation between the nurse and the client if the client's perception of importance differs from that of the nurse. A rule of thumb is to focus on the problems the client believes are most important if these priorities do not impede medical treatment (Murray & Atkinson, 1994). Additional considerations in setting priorities are the need for early resolution of health problems that have the potential to impair functioning or normal growth and development; the client's individual needs, values, and overall health status; and constraints of time and resources.

With some clients, the need to reinforce the nurse-client relationship through immediate attainment of a desired outcome may influence the rank of priorities. In other situations, where the client may be feeling helpless or hopeless, a consideration in setting priorities may be the need to select a problem with an easily achievable outcome. These strategies facilitate a sense of accomplishment for both the nurse and the client, demonstrate the value of the nurse to the client, and strengthen the relationship. Such an approach may be especially useful with a client or family who is resistant to interventions or who may have had negative experiences with the health care system in the past.

Identifying Outcomes

Once priorities are established, desired outcomes must be identified. Common categories of outcomes are those that reflect the attainment of an optimal level of health, alleviation of a problem, or modifications of lifestyle. Since outcomes occur along a time line, some may be achieved quickly, whereas others may take longer to become apparent.

NANDA Diagnoses, 1995-1996

Activity intolerance
Activity intolerance, risk for
*Adaptive capacity, decreased: in-
  tracranial
Adjustment, impaired
Airway clearance, ineffective
Anxiety
Aspiration, risk for
Body image disturbance
Body temperature, altered, risk for
Bowel incontinence
Breastfeeding, effective
Breastfeeding, ineffective
Breastfeeding, interrupted
Breathing pattern, ineffective
Cardiac output, decreased
Caregiver role strain
Caregiver role strain, risk for
Communication, impaired verbal
*Community coping, potential for
  enhanced
*Community coping, ineffective
*Confusion, acute
*Confusion, chronic
Constipation
Constipation, colonic
Constipation, perceived
Coping, defensive
Coping, family: potential for growth
Coping, ineffective family: compro-
  mised
Coping, ineffective family: disabling
Coping, ineffective individual
Decisional conflict (specify)
Denial, ineffective
Diarrhea
Disuse syndrome, risk for
Diversional activity deficit
Dysreflexia
*Energy field disturbance

*Environmental interpretation syn-
  drome: impaired
*Family processes, altered: alcoholism
Family processes, altered
Fatigue
Fear
Fluid volume deficit
Fluid volume deficit, risk for
Fluid volume excess
Gas exchange, impaired
Grieving, anticipatory
Grieving, dysfunctional
Growth and development, altered
Health maintenance, altered
Health-seeking behaviors (specify)
Home maintenance management,
  impaired
Hopelessness
Hyperthermia
Hypothermia
Incontinence, functional
Incontinence, reflex
Incontinence, stress
Incontinence, total
Incontinence, urge
*Infant behavior, disorganized
*Infant behavior, disorganized: risk for
*Infant behavior, organized: potential
  for enhanced
Infant feeding pattern, ineffective
Infection, risk for
*Injury, perioperative positioning: risk
  for
Injury, risk for
Knowledge deficit (specify)
*Loneliness, risk for
*Management of therapeutic regimen,
  community: ineffective
*Management of therapeutic regimen,
  families: ineffective

*Indicates a diagnosis new to the 1995-1996 taxonomy.

NANDA Diagnoses, 1995-1996—cont'd

*Management of therapeutic regimen, individuals: effective

Management of therapeutic regimen, individuals: ineffective

*Memory, impaired

Mobility, impaired physical

Noncompliance (specify)

Nutrition, altered: less than body requirements

Nutrition, altered: more than body requirements

Nutrition, altered: risk for more than body requirements

Oral mucous membrane, altered

Pain

Pain, chronic

*Parent/infant/child attachment, altered risk for

Parental role conflict

Parenting, altered

Parenting, altered, risk for

Peripheral neurovascular dysfunction, risk for

Personal identity disturbance

Poisoning, risk for

Post-trauma response

Powerlessness

Protection, altered

Rape-trauma syndrome

Rape-trauma syndrome: compound reaction

Rape-trauma syndrome: silent reaction

Relocation stress syndrome

Role performance, altered

Self-care deficit, bathing/hygiene

Self-care deficit, dressing/grooming

Self-care deficit, feeding

Self-care deficit, toileting

Self-esteem disturbance

Self-esteem, chronic low

Self-esteem, situational low

Self-mutilation, risk for

Sensory/perceptual alterations (specify) (visual, auditory, kinesthetic, gustatory, tactile, olfactory)

Sexual dysfunction

Sexuality patterns, altered

Skin integrity, impaired

Skin integrity, impaired, risk for

Sleep pattern disturbance

Social interaction, impaired

Social isolation

Spiritual distress (distress of the human spirit)

*Spiritual well-being, potential for enhanced

Suffocation, risk for

Swallowing, impaired

Thermoregulation, ineffective

Thought processes, altered

Tissue integrity, impaired

Tissue perfusion, altered (specify type) (renal, cerebral, cardiopulmonary, gastrointestinal, peripheral)

Trauma, risk for

Unilateral neglect

Urinary elimination, altered

Urinary retention

Ventilation, inability to sustain spontaneous

Ventilatory weaning process, dysfunctional

Violence, risk for: self-directed or directed at others

*Indicates a diagnosis new to the 1995-1996 taxonomy.

Long-term outcomes. A *long-term outcome* reflects expected client behavior that indicates that a concern or condition specified by the nursing diagnosis has been alleviated. Long-term outcomes flow from the descriptive portion of the nursing diagnosis and may focus on health promotion, health maintenance, or health restoration (Christensen & Kenney, 1995). Expected outcomes are "desirable and measurable health states, including biological or physiological, psychological, sociocultural, and spiritual aspects, and the knowledge or skills related to these health states" (McFarland & McFarlane, 1993, p. 17). Outcomes must be realistic and achievable, taking into account a number of factors, such as the client's strengths, limitations, lifestyle, and resources. As with setting priorities, outcomes may be mutually determined by the nurse and the client. The nurse, with a greater knowledge base than the client, may need to assist the client in selecting appropriate and achievable outcomes.

As sometimes happens, the client makes decisions about health care that are likely to result in less than optimal outcomes. For example, a hypertensive client may agree to take antihypertensive drugs but refuse to alter his diet despite being advised by the nurse of the potentially adverse consequences of that decision. The nurse must accept the fact that the client has chosen to be the ultimate decision maker in this aspect of his care and must identify other treatment modalities and outcomes that might be mutually acceptable (e.g., increasing the level of exercise).

Intermediate outcomes. *Intermediate outcomes* are a series of objectives that are sequential and progressive, and that lead to attainment of the long-term outcome. An *objective* describes the intended result of a particular nursing action or set of actions and must be stated in specific and measurable terms. In general, three to six objectives are needed for each long-term outcome to reflect a logical, incremental progression toward attainment. To be truly measurable, an objective must be stated in behavioral terms and have three characteristics: performance, conditions, and a criterion. *Performance* is the activity expected by the client, such as listing sources of food high in calcium or demonstrating administration of insulin. *Conditions* describe the circumstances under which the client performs the activity, such as in the home setting, without assistance, or within a particular time frame. A *criterion* is the standard by which the performance is evaluated and may include measures such as speed, the degree of accuracy, the quality of the behavior, a time frame, or a criterion-reference, such as a standard of the American Heart Association. An example of a measurable behavioral objective is presented in Table 5-3.

A common error is to state objectives using the nurse as the frame of reference instead of the client. If the objective begins with the phrase "the client will," then the objective reflects expected client behavior. Sometimes this phrase is not explicitly stated, so it is a good idea to test the appropriateness of the objectives by inserting the phrase "the client will." If the objective cannot accommodate this phrase, then it is probably a nursing action and not a client outcome. As an example, the objective in Table 5-3 correctly reflects an expected client behavior. However, exchanging the words "the client will" for "encourage to" changes this client objective into a nursing action (i.e.,

Table 5-3   **Example of a Measurable Behavioral Objective**

Objective	Characteristic
The client will walk	Performance
One half the length of the hall	Criterion
Unassisted	Condition
On the second postoperative day	Condition

"encourage to walk one half the length of the hall unassisted by the second postoperative day").

Nursing Actions

Each objective must be accompanied by one or more nursing actions aimed at helping the client achieve the objective. These actions are defined by the professional role of the nurse in a particular setting and the legal scope of nursing practice as specified in the state's nurse practice act. *Independent* nursing actions are those that the nurse has the knowledge, skill, and legal right to perform. *Dependent* nursing actions are those that require supervision or direction by another health care professional, often a physician. Some nursing actions are *interdependent* (i.e., they require collaboration with other health professionals).

The full range of nursing actions (independent, dependent, interdependent) is represented in the categories of nursing activities identified by Maibusch (1987):

- Surveillance/observation
- Supportive measures
- Assistive measures
- Treatment/procedures
- Emotional support
- Teaching
- Coordination of care

The recently developed Nursing Interventions Classification (NIC) system provides the nurse with more than 300 intervention labels, definitions, and related activities to assist in planning and implementing care (McCloskey & Bulechek, 1996). A sample set of interventions from the NIC system is presented in the box on p. 106.

When selecting a specific nursing action, the nurse must consider the characteristics of the nursing diagnosis, the scientific basis for the intervention, the feasibility of implementing the action, its acceptability to the client, and the level of nursing expertise required (Bulechek & McCloskey, 1987). Nursing actions may be performed by the nurse or delegated to assistive personnel as appropriate. However, the ultimate accountability for nursing actions rests with the nurse.

Nursing Interventions for Medication Management

Definition: Facilitation of safe and effective use of prescription and over-the-counter drugs.

Activities

Determine what drugs are needed and administer according to prescriptive authority and/or protocol.

Determine patient's ability to self-medicate, as appropriate.

Monitor effectiveness of the medication administration modality.

Monitor patient for the therapeutic effect of the medication.

Monitor for signs and symptoms of drug toxicity.

Monitor for adverse effects of the drug.

Monitor for nontherapeutic drug interactions.

Review periodically with the patient and/or family types and amounts of medications taken.

Facilitate changes in medication with physician, as appropriate.

Determine factors which may preclude the patient from taking drugs as prescribed.

Develop strategies with the patient to enhance compliance with prescribed medication regimen.

Consult with other health care professionals to minimize the number and frequency of drugs needed for a therapeutic effect.

Teach patient and/or family members the expected action and side effects of the medication.

Provide patient and family members with written and visual information to enhance self-administration of medications as appropriate.

Obtain physician order for patient self-medication, as appropriate.

Establish a protocol for the storage, restocking, and monitoring of medications left at the bedside for self-medication purposes.

Investigate possible financial resources for acquisition of prescribed drugs as appropriate.

Determine impact of medication use on patient's lifestyle.

Provide alternatives for timing and modality of self-administered medications to minimize lifestyle effects.

Assist the patient and family members in making necessary lifestyle adjustments associated with certain medications as appropriate.

Instruct patient when to seek medical attention.

Identify types and amounts of over-the-counter drugs used.

Provide information about the use of over-the-counter drugs and how they may influence the existing condition.

Determine if the patient is using culturally based home health remedies and the possible effects on use of over-the-counter and prescribed medications.

Provide patient with a list of resources to contact for further information about the medication regimen.

Contact patient and family post-discharge as appropriate to answer questions and discuss concerns associated with the medication regimen.

From McCloskey, J.C., & Bulechek, G.M. (1996). *Nursing interventions classification (NIC)* (2nd ed., p. 383). St. Louis: Mosby.

Plan of Care

At this point, a plan of care is formulated. Nursing diagnoses, long- and short-term outcomes, and nursing actions are incorporated into a written or printed format that guides nursing care. The formal care plan also serves as a communication tool between nurses and other health professionals to ensure that the care is individualized, consistent, and goal directed, and that it meets standards.

Individually constructed handwritten care plans are becoming somewhat of a rarity as nurses rely more on standardized and computer-generated plans of care. Standardized care plans, once scorned as lacking individuality and promoting assembly-line care, are now viewed more favorably. The content is usually developed by clinical experts, and the plan can be individualized to reflect unique considerations, innovative approaches, or specific treatment routines.

As health care agencies move toward full implementation of information systems, computerized care plans are becoming commonplace. Computerized care plans can be generated according to the nursing diagnosis or the medical diagnosis, or they can be individually constructed. Some computerized care plans use a menu of appropriate outcomes and interventions from which the nurse (and sometimes the client) can select (Brider, 1991). The fact that computerized care plans can be quickly generated and easily updated are distinct advantages of these systems.

Two newer alternatives to the traditional care plan are the clinical pathway tools and the CareMap. The clinical pathways include both medical and nursing interventions for clients in a particular diagnosis-related group (DRG) classification along a specified time line. The clinical pathway is individualized if the client's condition warrants it, but it is anticipated that an established clinical pathway will be appropriate for 75% of the clients in that DRG (Murray & Atkinson, 1994). The CareMap includes nursing diagnoses, as well as clinical path interventions that lead to desired outcomes along a specified time line. This tool has an accompanying variance sheet that nurses use to document changes in the standard intervention or in the time line. A sample CareMap and variance sheet are illustrated in Figs. 5-5 and 5-6.

Perhaps some of the new, innovative types of care plans will be more appealing and useful to nurses than those used in the past. A recent study of 1096 nurses found that less than 30% liked the way care planning was done in their hospitals (Martin et al., 1994). A smaller study conducted earlier contained similar findings (Hildman, 1992).

IMPLEMENTATION

Implementation "is the initiation and completion of actions necessary to accomplish the defined goal of optimal wellness for the client" (Yura & Walsh, 1988, p. 154). During implementation the nurse uses intellectual, interpersonal, and technical skills to provide care that is client focused and goal oriented, and that meets the physical and psychosocial needs of the client. Implementation includes actions taken by the nurse, other members of the health team, and the client and/or family members. It involves executing the plan of care by undertaking the previously identified nursing actions, supervising others in providing care, and documenting the care.

CareMap: Congestive Heart Failure

	Day 1 ER 1-4 hours	Day 1 Floor Telemetry or CCU 6-24 hours	Day 2 Floor	Day 3 Floor	Day 4 Floor	Day 5 Floor	Day 6 Floor
Location				Benchmark Quality Criteria			
Problem							
1) Alteration in gas exchange/profusion and fluid balance due to decreased cardiac output, excess fluid volume	Reduced pain from admission or pain free; Uses pain scale; O$_2$ sat. improved over admission baseline on O$_2$ therapy	Respirations equal to or less than on admission	O$_2$ sat = 90; Resp 20-22; Vital signs stable; Crackles at lung bases; Mild shortness of breath with activity	Does not require O$_2$; Vital signs stable; Crackles at base; Respirations 20-22; Mild shortness of breath with activity	Does not require O$_2$ (O$_2$ sat on room air 90%); Vital signs stable; Crackles at base; Respirations 20-22; Completes activity with no increase in respirations; No edema	Can lie in bed at baseline position; Chest X-ray clear or at baseline	No dyspnea
2) Potential for shock	No signs/symptoms of shock	No signs/symptoms of shock	No signs/symptoms of shock	No signs/symptoms of shock; Normal lab values	No signs/symptoms of shock	No signs/symptoms of shock	No signs/symptoms of shock
3) Potential for consequences of immobility and decreased activity: skin breakdown, DVT	No redness at pressure points; No falls	No redness at pressure points; No falls	Tolerates chair, washing, eating, and toileting	Has bowel movement; Up in room and bathroom with assist	Up ad lib for short periods	Activity increased to level used at home without shortness of breath	Activity increased to level used at home without shortness of breath
4) Alteration in nutritional intake due to nausea and vomiting, labored		No c/o nausea; No vomiting; Taking liquids as offered	Eating solids; Takes in 50% each meal	Taking 50% each meal	Taking 50% each meal; Weight 2 lbs from patient's normal baseline	Taking 75% each meal	Taking 75% each meal
5) Potential for arrhythmias due to decreased cardiac output: decreased irritable foci, valve problems, decreased gas exchange	No evidence of life-threatening dysrhythmias	Normal sinus rhythm with benign ectopy	K(WNL); Benign or no arrhythmias	Digoxin level DNL; Benign or no arrhythmias	Digoxin level WNL; Benign or no arrhythmias	Digoxin level WNL; Benign or no arrhythmias	Digoxin level WNL; Benign or no arrhythmias
6) Patient/family response to future treatment & hospitalization	Patient/family expressing concerns; Following directions of staff	Patient/family expressing concerns; Following directions of staff	Patient/family expressing concerns; Following directions of staff	States reasons for and cooperates with rest periods; Patient begins to assess own knowledge and ability to care for CHF at home	Patient decides whether he/she wants discussion with physician about advanced directives	States plan for 1-2 days postdischarge as to meds., diet, activity, follow-up appointments; Expresses reaction to having CHF	Repeats plans; States signs and symptoms to notify physician/ER; Signs discharge consent
7) Individual problem:							

Assessments/Consults	Vital signs q 15 min Nursing assessments focus on lung sounds, edema, color, skin integrity, jugular vein distention Cardiac monitor Arterial line if needed Swan Ganz Intake & output	Vital signs q 15 min-1 hr Repeat nursing assessments Cardiac monitor Arterial line Swan Ganz Daily weight Intake & output	Vital signs q 4 hrs Repeat nursing assessments D/C cardiac monitor Arterial line D/C arterial and Swan Ganz 24 hr Daily weight Intake & output	Vital signs q 6 hrs Repeat nursing assessments Daily weight Intake & output	Vital signs q 6 hrs Repeat nursing assessments Daily weight Intake & output Nutrition consult	Vital signs q 6 hrs Repeat nursing assessments Daily weight Intake & output	Vital signs q 6 hrs Repeat nursing assessments Daily weight Intake & output
Specimens/Tests	Consider TSH studies Chest X-ray EKG CPK q 8 hr × 3 ABG if pulse Ox: (range) Lytes, Na, K, Cl, CO_2, Glucose, BUN, Creatinine Digoxin: (range)	B/G	Evaluate for ECHO Lytes, BUN, Creatinine			Chest X-ray Lytes, BUN, Creatinine	
Treatments	O_2 or intubate IV or Heparin lock	O_2 IV or Heparin lock	IV or Heparin lock	DC pulse Ox if stable D/C IV or Heparin lock			
Medications	Evaluate for Digoxin Nitrodrip or paste Diuretics IV Evaluate for antiemetics Evaluate for antiarrhythmics	Evaluate for Digoxin Nitrodrip or paste Diuretics IV Evaluate for pre-load/afterload reducers K supplements Stool softeners	D/C Nitrodrip or paste Diuretics IV or PO K supplements Stool softeners Evaluate for nicotine patch	Change to PO Digoxin PO diuretics K supplements Stool softeners Nicotine patch if consent	PO diuretics K supplement Stool softeners Nicotine patch if consent	PO diuretics K supplement Stool softeners Nicotine patch if consent	PO diuretics K supplement Stool softeners Nicotine patch if consent
Nutrition	None	Clear liquids	Cardiac, low-salt diet	Cardiac, low-salt diet	Cardiac, low-salt diet	Cardiac, low-salt diet	
Safety/Activity	Commode Bedrest with head elevated Reposition patient q 2 hrs Bedrails up Call light available	Commode Bedrest with head elevated Dangle Reposition patient q 2 hrs Enforce rest periods Bedrails up Call light available	Commode Enforce rest periods Chair with assist ½ hr with feet elevated Bedrails up Call light available	Bathroom privileges Chair × 3 Bedrails up Call light available	Ambulate in hall × 2 Up ad lib between rest periods Bedrails up Call light available	Encourage ADLs that approximate activities at home Bedrails up Call light available	Encourage ADLs that approximate activities at home Bedrails up Call light available
Teaching	Explain procedures Teach chest pain scale and importance of reporting	Explain course, need for energy conservation Orient to unit and routine	Clarify CHF Dx and future teaching needs Orient to unit and routine Schedule rest periods Begin medication teaching	Importance of weighing self every day Provide smoking cessation information Review energy conservation schedule	Cardiac rehab level as indicated by consult Provide smoking cessation support Dietary teaching	Review CHF education material with patient	Reinforce CHF teaching
Transfer/Discharge Coordination	Assess home situation: notify significant other If no arrhythmias or chest pain, transfer to floor Otherwise transfer to ICU	Screen for discharge needs Transfer to floor	Consider Home Health Care referral		Evaluate needs for diet and anti-smoking classes Physician offers discussion opportunities for advanced directives	Appointment and arrangement for follow-up care with Home Health Care nurses Contact VNA	Reinforce follow-up appointments

Fig. 5-5 Sample CareMap for congestive heart failure. (Courtesy The Center for Case Management, South Natick, MA. CareMap is a registered trademark of the Center for Case Management.)

Date	Description	Prob	Path	Source	Action	Initials
1-Feb	Son unavailable: out of town on business		8	A3	Ask ICU to call 2/2	AB
1-Feb	Afib O$_2$ sat + 85% Glucose 250 No Swan Ganz	5 1	• • • 1	A1 A1 A1 B6	Transfer ICU Lasix, O$_2$ 6L Diabetic regime	CD
2-Feb	Unable to transfer to floor Afib	• 5		C9 • A1	Order to drop pt. to general care rate Benign	CD
2-Feb	Echo not done Hct 34, Hgb 13		2	C9	Schedule for Monday Begin FeSO$_4$	CD
3-Feb	Unable to get home med delivery	6		D14	Provide pharmacy list to pt.	EF
3-Feb	Nutrition consult early		1	B7	Begin teaching	EF
4-Feb	Wt 135 Ankle edema	4 4		A1 A1	Continue lasix Elevate feet Inc. ambulation Encourage rhythmic exercises in bed	EF
5-Feb	Complaining about CHF diet and doesn't want to make plans	6		A1	Arrange for VNA follow-up for 3 visits	GH
6-Feb	Requests nicotine patch			A2	Notify physician to order before she leaves. Call pharmacy to begin instruction	JK

Variance Source Codes

A	**Patient/Family**	
	1	Condition
	2	Decision
	3	Availability
	4	Other
B	**Clinician**	
	5	Order
	6	Decision
	7	Response Time
	8	Other
C	**Hospital**	
	9	Bed/Appt. Availability
	10	Info/Data Availability
	11	Other
D	**Community**	
	12	Placement/Home Care
	13	Transportation
	14	Other

Fig. 5-6 Variance sheet to accompany the CareMap for congestive heart failure. (Copyright 1992, The Center for Case Management, South Natick, MA.)

Nursing Roles in Implementation

As the plan of care is implemented, the nurse may assume a variety of roles, such as practitioner, educator, collaborator, coordinator, advocate, and evaluator. When the client is actively involved in the implementation process, the role of the nurse shifts to that of facilitator. Regardless of the role(s) assumed, the nurse must focus on the client, being constantly aware of the client's response to the intervention. Cues from the client should direct the implementation. For example, if the nurse is teaching a client how to change a surgical dressing and the client is experiencing pain, it would be better to discontinue the teaching plan for the moment and focus on controlling the pain.

Documentation

The final stage of implementation is careful documentation. The system of documentation may be agency specific, but the content should reflect the client's concerns and the nursing process. Whatever the form of documentation, certain information should be included in the record:

- A description of the nursing action that was performed
- The client's observed response to the intervention
- Any new data that may have emerged
- Progress (or lack of it) toward achievement of outcomes and objectives

Documentation should also include a description of planned interventions that did *not* occur and the reasons why.

EVALUATION

Evaluation is an ongoing activity that occurs at each stage of the nursing process. By definition, *evaluation* involves "placing value or worth," so both the client and the care provider should have input into the process. Together, the nurse and client make a judgment about the extent to which the nursing diagnoses were appropriate, the plan was effective, and the outcomes were achieved.

Purposes of Evaluation

The overall purpose of the evaluation phase of the nursing process is to determine the client's progress toward the attainment of preselected outcomes. Evaluation of outcomes is accomplished by comparing actual outcomes with predicted outcomes. However, it is important to recognize that evaluation is a multistage process that occurs throughout the episode of care. During the assessment phase, evaluation focuses on the appropriateness of data sources and methods used for data collection, as well as on the comprehensiveness of the database. During analysis and diagnosis, evaluation centers on whether the data are appropriately clustered, whether the nursing diagnoses reflect the data and the client's health concerns, and whether the nursing diagnoses are clear, concise, and relevant. During the planning process, evaluation activities are directed toward determining the appropriateness of the intermediate and long-term outcomes, nursing diagnosis priorities, and selected nursing actions. During the implementation stage, evaluation focuses on the relevance and effectiveness of specific nursing activities. The nurse and client continue to evaluate these components until the client's health concerns are resolved, the outcomes are achieved, and/or the episode of care ends.

Another way to focus evaluation activities is to judge the appropriateness, adequacy, effectiveness, and efficiency of the plan of care and its implementation. An *appropriate* plan of care is relevant to the client's health concerns and focuses on mutually desirable outcomes. An *adequate* plan is one that is suitable and sufficient in terms of the amount and quality of care. An *effective* plan of care is one that achieves desired outcomes within the specified time frame, and an *efficient* plan is one that maximizes the use of client, provider, and agency resources.

Types of Evaluation

Evaluation of nursing care is both formative and summative. *Formative evaluation* is an ongoing process, appraising the client's movement toward achievement of desired outcomes. It occurs throughout the nursing process and serves as a feedback mechanism. Formative evaluation involves a judgment about the appropriateness and adequacy of the plan of care and the degree of success in facilitating achievement of intermediate outcomes. *Summative evaluation* occurs at a specified point in time or at the conclusion of the episode of care and involves a judgment about the extent to which desired outcomes are achieved. Summative evaluation also appraises the effectiveness and efficiency of the plan of care in terms of the resources used to achieve the desired outcomes.

Guidelines for Evaluation

As previously mentioned, evaluation includes comparing actual outcomes against predicted outcomes and evaluating the nursing care plan. If the outcomes are not as expected, the nurse and client must determine the reason. Questions that might be asked are:

- Were the assessment data appropriate and complete?
- Were the data interpreted correctly?
- Were nursing diagnoses appropriate?
- Were outcomes and objectives realistic, attainable, and measurable?
- Was the nursing care plan directed toward resolution of nursing diagnoses?
- Was the implementation of the plan individualized in accordance with the client's strengths and limitations?
- Were both the nurse and the client working toward the same outcomes?

Based on the answers to these questions, it may be necessary to reenter the nursing process at the appropriate point and try again.

CRITICAL THINKING AND THE NURSING PROCESS

To effectively use the nursing process, the nurse must engage in critical thinking that is disciplined, logical, and reflective. The critical thinker consciously thinks about his or her own thinking while it is occurring so that it is more clear, precise, accurate, relevant, consistent, and fair (Paul, 1988). Throughout the nursing process, the nurse uses a combination of abilities to sort and categorize data, identify patterns in the data, draw inferences, develop hypotheses that are stated in the form of outcomes, test these hypotheses as care is delivered, and make criterion-based judgments of effectiveness. Such critical thinking can distinguish between fact and fiction, thereby providing a rational basis for the delivery of nursing care. While one may argue that the nursing process constrains critical thinking because of its structured format, there is general agreement that critical thinking skills and subskills are evident throughout the nursing process, as illustrated in Table 5-4. Although the components of the nursing process are described as separate and distinct steps, they become an integrated way of thinking as nurses gain more clinical experience.

THE UTILITY OF THE NURSING PROCESS

The nursing process provides a deliberate and systematic approach to planning, implementing, and evaluating client care. A recent study of nurses' knowledge of and at-

---

Table 5-4   **Overview of Critical Thinking Throughout the Nursing Process**

Nursing Process	Critical Thinking Skills
Assessment	Observing Distinguishing relevant from irrelevant data Distinguishing important from unimportant data Validating data Organizing data Categorizing data
Analysis/diagnosis	Finding patterns and relationships Making inferences Stating the problem Suspending judgment
Planning	Generalizing Transferring knowledge from one situation to another Developing evaluative criteria Hypothesizing
Implementation	Applying knowledge Testing hypotheses
Evaluation	Deciding whether hypotheses are correct Making criterion-based evaluations and judgments

From Wilkinson, J.M. (1992). *Nursing process in action.* Redwood City, CA: Addison-Wesley.

titude toward the nursing process revealed that nurses were knowledgeable and attitudes were generally positive (Martin et al., 1994). This study underscores the utility of the nursing process as a framework for nursing practice. The fact that most nurses are knowledgeable about the nursing process facilitates communication between them and provides a consistent approach to care for the client. The widespread acceptance of the nursing process as a framework for nursing practice is reflected in the finding that nurses hold a positive view of the nursing process. Its utility can be further underscored by its demonstrated relevance across multiple clinical settings and with a variety of client groups.

 ## Key Points

- The nursing process is an interactive model consisting of five interrelated components.

- Assessment focuses on data collection using a variety of methods and techniques for the purpose of building a comprehensive client database.

- Analysis and diagnosis center on processing and synthesizing the data, drawing conclusions, and validating them with the client.

- Planning involves mutual decision making between the nurse and the client to identify desired outcomes and select strategies to achieve them.

- Implementation is the initiation and completion of actions taken by the nurse, the client, or others to execute the plan of care and to document the actions.

- Evaluation focuses on the extent to which expected client outcomes are achieved and on the effectiveness and efficiency of the plan of care.

- The nursing process offers a systematic framework for the delivery of nursing care.

- Critical thinking skills are used throughout the nursing process.

 ## Critical Thinking Exercises

1. "The nursing process is described as a systematic framework for the delivery of nursing care that is widely accepted and useful in any clinical setting." Formulate arguments to defend *and* refute this statement.

2. Differentiate the sources of data that are appropriate and necessary to plan care for a client in a hospital setting and to plan care for a client in a community setting.

3. Evaluate the nursing assessment instrument used in your current area of practice in terms of its adequacy for your clinical setting, usefulness in other clinical settings, and comprehensiveness. What additional data would be useful, and how might you collect this information?

4. Select a client and conduct a thorough assessment:
   a. Use the typologies presented in Table 5-2 to organize data collected during the assessment. Which of these typologies did you find most useful? Explain why.
   b. Based on the data, identify the nursing diagnosis with the *highest* priority and develop a long-term outcome. Construct three *measurable* objectives that reflect a logical progression toward that outcome.

5. Evaluation has been described as the most neglected stage of the nursing process. Present your arguments to support or refute that statement and provide clinical examples to illustrate your points.

References

American Nurses' Association. (1991). *Standards of clinical nursing practice.* Kansas City, MO: The Association.

Atkinson, L.D., & Murray, M.E. (1995). *Clinical guide to care planning.* New York: McGraw-Hill.

Bandman, E.L., & Bandman, B. (1995). *Critical thinking in nursing* (2nd ed.). Norwalk, CT: Appleton & Lange.

Brider, P. (1991) Who killed the nursing care plan? *American Journal of Nursing, 91*(5), 35-38.

Bulechek, G.M., & McCloskey, J.C. (1987). Nursing interventions: What they are and how to choose them. *Holistic Nursing Practice, 3*(3), 38.

Carpenito, L. (1993). *Nursing diagnosis: Application to clinical practice* (5th ed.). Philadelphia: J.B. Lippincott.

Christensen, P.J., & Kenney, J.W. (1995) *Nursing process: Application of conceptual models* (4th ed.). St. Louis: Mosby.

Duldt, B.W. (1995). The nursing process: The science of nursing in the curriculum. *Nurse Educator, 20*(1), 24-26.

Edelman, C.L., & Mandle, C.L. (1994). *Health promotion throughout the lifespan* (3rd ed.). St. Louis: Mosby.

Gordon, M. (1995). *Manual of nursing diagnoses: 1995-1996.* St. Louis: Mosby.

Hall, L. (1955, June). Quality of nursing care. *Public Health News,* New Jersey State Department of Health.

Hildman, R. (1992). Registered nurses' attitudes toward the nursing process and written/printed nursing care plans. *Journal of Nursing Administration, 22*(5), 5.

Maibusch, R.M. (1987). *The nursing minimum data set: Benefits and implications for clinical nurses* (NLN Publication No. 41-2199). New York: National League for Nursing.

Martin, P.A., Dugan, J., Freundl, M., Miller, S.E., Phillips, R., & Sharritts, L. (1994). Nurses' attitudes toward the nursing process as measured by the Dayton Attitude Scale. *Journal of Continuing Education in Nursing, 25*(1), 35-40.

McCloskey, J.C., & Bulechek, G.M. (1996). *Nursing interventions classification (NIC)* (2nd ed.). St. Louis: Mosby.

McFarland, G.K., & McFarlane, E.A. (1993). *Nursing diagnosis and intervention.* St. Louis: Mosby.

Murray, M.E., & Atkinson, L.D. (1994). *Understanding the nursing process: The next generation.* New York: McGraw-Hill.

North American Nursing Diagnosis Association. (1986). 21 new diagnoses and a taxonomy. *American Journal of Nursing, 86,* 1414-1415.

North American Nursing Diagnosis Association (1994). *NANDA nursing diagnoses: Definitions and classification 1995-1996.* Philadelphia: The Association.

Paul, R. (1988). *What, then, is critical thinking?* Paper presented at the eighth annual and sixth international conference on critical thinking and educational reform. The Center for Critical Thinking and Moral Critique, Sonoma State University, Rohnert Park, CA.

Waltz, C.F., & Strickland, O.L. (1988). *Measurement of nursing outcomes: Vol I. Measuring client outcomes.* New York: Springer.

Wilkinson, J.M. (1992). *Nursing process in action.* Redwood City, CA: Addison-Wesley.

Wong, D.L. (1995). *Whaley and Wong's nursing care of infants and children* (5th ed.). St. Louis: Mosby.

Yura, H., & Walsh, M.B. (1967). *The nursing process: Assessing, planning, implementing, evaluating,* (1st ed.). New York: Appleton-Century-Crofts.

Yura, H., & Walsh, M.B. (1988) *The nursing process: Assessing, planning, implementing, evaluating* (5th ed.). Norwalk, CT: Appleton & Lange.

Client Systems

6

Gail O. Mazzocco

 ## Objectives

At the completion of this chapter, the reader will be able to:

- Identify and describe the elements of general systems theory.

- Apply general systems theory to the assessment of the individual, family, community, or population.

- Analyze data, plan, implement and evaluate nursing care based on general systems theory.

Profile in Practice

Barrie Gleason Carveth, MSN, RN
Family Nurse Practitioner,
Westhaven Nursing Clinic,
University of Virginia,
Charlottesville, Virginia

Knowledge and understanding of client systems was critical in establishing our nursing clinics in Virginia. Before we applied for funding, we did a thorough community assessment that included identification of needs perceived by the community's residents. The assessment was done by University of Virginia nursing students, who conducted a door-to-door survey asking residents what their health needs were and what services they thought were needed in their community. We also identified community leaders and asked them to serve on an advisory board. Our first two clinics are located in public housing communities. One is in a high rise for disabled and elderly residents, and the other is a mixture of young families and independent seniors. In each site we have monthly meetings of our community advisory board. We also now have a third nursing clinic located in a rural school district.

In these clinics, which serve low-income families, we provide physical examinations, immunizations, prescriptions, health screening, and referrals. In addition, we have a toy-lending library where parents can borrow age-appropriate toys for their children. A key feature in our success is the community advisory board, which keeps us in touch with what is happening in the community.

Nursing is currently faced with changes that are as significant as any in its history. For the first time, compassion and clinical competence are not the most significant measures of an expert nurse. High-quality nursing care must also contribute to reduced health care costs. If these often contradictory ends are to be achieved, health care providers must work together to coordinate and consolidate care. General systems theory successfully combines humanistic and scientific perspectives in a single model—one that can be used by all health professionals. This chapter focuses on three types of client systems: individuals, families, and communities or populations at risk. All three are typical of living systems, since they are goal directed and display complex behaviors.

GENERAL SYSTEMS THEORY

General systems theory was developed in response to the tendency of modern science to explain complex phenomena by dividing them into their component parts. While that approach worked reasonably well in the physical sciences, it was less successful when it was used to explore behavior. With the assistance of a number of other scientists, von Bertalanffy (1956) developed general systems theory as a new analytical approach—one that is based on integration and holism.

"General systems theory is a set of related definitions, assumptions, and propositions which deal with reality as an integrated hierarchy" (Miller, 1978, p. 9). Systems theory focuses on each system as a whole but pays particular attention to the way in which its parts or subsystems work together. This perspective makes systems theory especially helpful in recognizing patterns and dealing with complexity (Tonges & Madden, 1993). Because it is so widely applicable, the theory also has the potential to improve communication between the members of the health team. These general attributes make systems theory particularly helpful to nurses.

Most nurses are employed in institutions that use a body systems or "medical model" approach to health care. A client's health problems are identified and treated based on a health history, physical examination, and diagnostic tests. The specific body system or systems that are malfunctioning are then treated in an attempt to improve the client's health status. While education and social support are often included in the treatment plan, they are generally secondary services.

Consider the effect of this approach on the most common of clients, a 74-year-old woman who enters the hospital with congestive heart failure. While her immediate problems may be well served by treating her cardiovascular and respiratory symptoms, long-term success is rarely the result of intervention with either of those systems. In fact, this approach frequently results in repeated admissions to the hospital. Most nurses are all too familiar with this expensive and dysfunctional pattern.

A general systems model examines individual functioning as reflected by physiological, psychosocial, and educational needs. Because it attempts to meet all of those needs, the model can help this client improve her condition and remain out of the hospital. The nurse who uses systems theory evaluates the individual, family, community, or population group as a whole and simultaneously considers the relationship between parts. For that reason, the theory can serve as the foundation for a comprehensive assessment and analysis of human systems (LaMonica, 1985). Because the theory is general, information is easy to share with nurses in a variety of settings, as well as with other health professionals.

Systems Terminology

A *system* may be defined as a unit whose parts work together toward a specific goal (Gillies, 1994). *Input,* in the form of matter, energy, and information, enters the system and is used by the system's parts or *subsystems* in a process known as *throughput.* The system then releases matter, energy, and information into the environment as *output.* While most of the output remains in the environment, part of it returns to the system as *feedback.* This operation allows a system to monitor itself in an attempt to move closer to a steady state known as *equilibrium* or *homeostasis.* Every system is surrounded by a *boundary* that separates it from the environment and determines what enters the

---

Systems Terminology

Boundary The separation between the system and what lies outside. The boundary also determines what enters and leaves the system.

Entropy The tendency toward disorder or chaos.

Environment All larger systems that either influence or are influenced by the system under study.

Equilibrium A steady state.

Feedback Output that is returned to the system and that allows it to monitor itself over time in an attempt to move closer to a steady state known as equilibrium or homeostasis.

Homeostasis A condition of balance within the range of normal.

Input Matter, energy, and information that enter a system.

Negentropy The tendency toward order.

Output Matter, energy, and information that leave a system.

Subsystems The subparts of the system.

Suprasystems The next larger organized entity of which a system is a part.

System A group of elements that interact with one another in order to achieve a goal (von Bertalanffy, 1956).

Throughput The process by which the system processes input and releases it as output.

system. The environment can also be subdivided into a *suprasystem,* the next larger grouping of which the system is a part. And beyond that are a series of larger and more complex systems (Fig. 6-1).

An individual is a system because he or she takes in matter, energy, and information in the form of food, fluids, oxygen, data, and sensations as input and then uses biological, psychological, and sociocultural subsystems to process that input. The individual then returns matter, energy, and information to the environment in the form of both physical and psychosocial behaviors. Some of that output returns to the human system as feedback, which allows the individual to determine how well he or she is functioning. The amount of feedback that is accepted is partially controlled by the individual (Yura & Walsh, 1978). In the human, a boundary extends beyond the skin to an area of personal space and separates the individual system from that of the family, which is usually the individual's suprasystem.

Common Characteristics of All Systems

Each system has common characteristics that influence its ability to operate. The first of these is related to the system's structure and function. *Structure* refers to a system's visible physical parts, whereas *function* represents those activities that a system carries out to achieve its goals (Helvi, 1991). *Structure and function are not separate entities. Rather, they are so closely related that a change in one causes a change in the other* (Helvi, 1991). For example, a person has physical structures that process all input. Those structures include relatively complex nervous and endocrine systems that work together to coordinate both physical and psychosocial behaviors. A structural change in the nervous system alters the way in which the individual functions.

A second characteristic is related to boundary permeability. *Each system is surrounded by a boundary that may range from being completely open to the environment to being completely closed to it.* However, few systems are found at the extremes, since most require

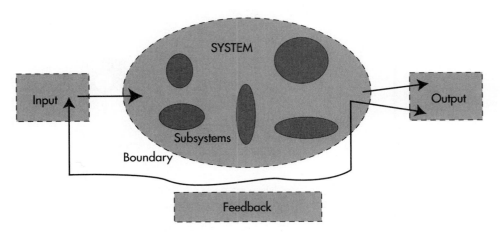

Fig. 6-1   The environment as a system.

a moderate amount of environmental input in order to function. Without that input, a system becomes increasingly disordered, or *entropic*. For example, a family with a school-aged child receives input from the school indicating that their 9-year-old has difficulty reading. A family whose boundary is open reviews the information and takes steps to correct the situation. A family with a less permeable boundary may discount or ignore the information and allow the situation to deteriorate.

Finally, *systems are hierarchically arranged within an environment* (Christensen & Kenney, 1995). In other words, there is an organizational scheme in which simple systems precede those that are more complex. As a result, most systems are a part of larger, more complex systems (suprasystems) and contain smaller, simpler systems (subsystems). For example, a family is part of a community, and that community is part of a state or region. However, the family also has individual members who function as individual systems themselves (Fig. 6-2). Surrounding the system is the environment, which is composed of all those elements that impact on the system being studied. While it may be more accurate to think of the environment as a series of increasingly complex systems, it generally is simpler to view it as a single unit.

Special Characteristics of Behavioral Systems

The generalizations that have been made thus far apply to all systems, closed or open, living or nonliving. However, the nurse is primarily concerned with living or behavioral systems. These systems have some additional characteristics that reflect their vital nature.

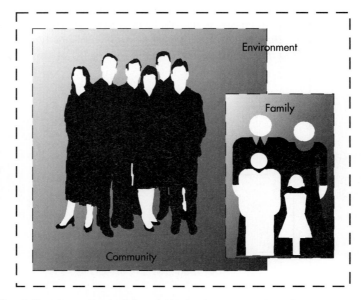

Fig. 6-2   The individual family as a subsystem within the community.

Perhaps because it has the physical and chemical characteristics of life, a behavioral system operates as more than just a collection of specialized subsystems. As they work together to achieve system goals, the subsystems become an efficient and functional unit. Therefore *a living system performs as a unified whole rather than as merely the sum of its parts* (Byrne & Thompson, 1978). Common purpose is the fuel for this cooperative effort.

Because common purpose is so important, *a living system must be goal directed.* The specific goal varies with the system, but goals direct the function and structure of every system. An individual, as a complex behavioral system, may select and later alter some goals. Those alterations require the individual to overcome the forces that operate to maintain the system's status quo.

A living system continually takes in matter, energy, and information from the environment and so never reaches true equilibrium. Instead, a human works toward *homeostasis,* a condition of balance within the range of normal (von Bertalanffy, 1956). To maintain that balance, a living system must adapt to environmental changes. Homeostatic regulators must sometimes be overcome in order to stimulate alterations in the system's internal processes and to change its level of functioning (Kast & Rosenzweig, 1981). This process is not easy, particularly when the system's goals and those of the environment are at odds. For example, an individual may be totally committed to life in a small town, where employment is unavailable. If he or she is to survive economically, it may be necessary to move to a less desirable location. In spite of the environmental pressure, that move may be impossible if the individual cannot change his or her level of functioning.

Fortunately, *a living system is always open to the environment* (LaMonica, 1985). The continual intake of new matter, information, and energy, when combined with feedback, provides ample opportunity for a system to become aware of the need to change its goals. Equally important, *input allows the system to become increasingly complex and organized.* This increasing organization is called *negentropy* (Helvi, 1991). The ability to absorb input is essential both for system growth and for goal achievement. In fact, living systems will become disordered, or entropic, if they are unable to obtain sufficient input.

A final characteristic that is also related to goal achievement is *equifinality.* This refers to living systems' ability to reach the same goal from different initial conditions and by different routes (von Bertalanffy, 1956). It was difficult for systems theorists to explain how open systems, which began with differing resources and in different environments, could achieve similar goals. von Bertalanffy suggests that this ability results from the dynamic interaction of the subsystems involved, which allows for creative approaches to goal achievement.

SYSTEMS THEORY AND THE INDIVIDUAL

Systems theory can help the practicing nurse deliver humane, clinically proficient health care. However, that goal will be reached more easily if the nurse keeps several suggestions in mind. These hints will help both new and experienced users of systems theory avoid some of the pitfalls that can result when any theory is applied in a practical setting.

First, it is best to work with the system that seems to be the source of the problem. The divisions between subsystem, system, and suprasystem are sometimes arbitrary. For example, in a tightly knit or fused family, the family group may carry on some functions that commonly belong to the individual. Infants and small children are very dependent on their families for basic needs. In these and similar cases, it may be difficult to decide where the individual ends and the family begins. In such situations, it is usually best to focus on the system in which the problem resides.

Second, systems theory is a general theory that can be used across disciplines. As a result, the approach is most helpful in dealing with problems broadly and in focusing on the relationship between subsystems. It works best as a general guide rather than as a blueprint for nursing action.

An Approach to Assessment

The following case study is used to illustrate the application of systems theory throughout the nursing process.

Hilda Muller is a 71-year-old woman who lives in a small city located about 100 miles from a major metropolitan area. Mrs. Muller lives in the house where she was born and where she and her 72-year-old husband, Thomas, have lived since their marriage almost 50 years ago. They have three children, all of whom are married and live within 2 hours of their parents. In addition, they have a number of close friends in their neighborhood and are very active in a local church. Mr. and Mrs. Muller enjoy traveling and own a small camper that they use to travel around the United States. Until early this year, things were going well for the family. In February Mr. Muller went to a local auto service center, but was unable to find his way home. The incident forced Hilda to admit that her husband had been increasingly forgetful over the last several months. When he became lost again last week, Hilda and Tom made an appointment with their family physician.

The visit to the doctor seemed uneventful. Except for the recent episodes, neither member of the couple could recall any change in Tom's health. Tom described the two incidents as "strange. I knew where I was, but had no idea how to get home. I must have waited for 20 minutes before someone came to help me." Mr. Muller also indicated that he was sometimes unable to recall his best friend's name but did know that he was a friend. Tom could recall no syncope, seizures, speech problems, tremors, weakness, clumsiness, or paralysis. He has had no mood changes, depression, or problems with sleeping, and he takes only ibuprofen for arthritis. He uses no alcohol or other drugs. He has had no major illnesses but does have arthritis and an enlarged prostate. He eats well, is 5 feet 8 inches tall, and weighs 167 pounds.

Tom is a high school graduate who was employed by the railroad for 41 years and never missed a day of work, something of which he is quite proud. His mother is still alive at age 91, is in a nursing home, and has had Alzheimer's disease for 4 years. Tom continues to drive near home, but he and his wife have decided to postpone a trip to Florida until after Tom's problem is identified.

Assess the individual's input. Input includes the quantity and quality of matter, energy, and information that cross the individual's boundary.

Tom eats a normal diet, uses ibuprofen, does not use alcohol or illegal drugs, has many friends, and receives active support from his family and community. Friends call daily, and his children call weekly and visit often. Tom reads the local newspaper daily but rarely watches television. He knows the location of a local senior citizen's center, but has never been inside the building.

Assess the individual's output. The individual's observable behaviors, both physical and psychosocial, are output. These include what we commonly call signs and symptoms.

Tom has few symptoms of health problems, except for his transient confusion, and follows a regular daily routine that includes getting together with friends and helping to maintain the church building. He has been retired from the railroad for 6 years and really enjoys this period of life. He is friendly, outgoing, sexually active, and very involved in the community. Tom likes to travel and generally enjoys life.

Consider the individual's throughput mechanisms. The way in which the subsystems process matter, energy, and information is suggested by system output and the relationship between input and output. For example, an individual may have signs or symptoms of illness, such as shortness of breath or edema (output), or may be losing weight in spite of eating adequately (imbalance between input and output).

In spite of the fact that Tom is taking in and putting out sufficient matter, energy, and information, he is forgetful. This suggests a processing, or throughput, problem with his physiological and/or behavioral subsystems.

Assess the individual's feedback mechanisms. An individual's output that returns to the system in order to monitor it is known as feedback. Problems with the sensory subsystem, such as poor hearing, may make it impossible for some feedback to reenter the system. A client may have difficulty monitoring his or her own behavior when an accurate perception of feedback is frightening or would require a change in a valued behavior. For example, a 39-year-old man who has a strong family history of heart disease may ignore episodes of chest pain (feedback) because he is afraid of having a myocardial infarction.

Tom appears to have no difficulty with hearing but does wear bifocals. He immediately recognized his problem and sought help for it. His mother has Alzheimer's disease, and Tom is familiar with the progression of her disease.

Assess the individual's boundary. Its boundary must be selectively permeable if a system is to function adequately. Selective permeability refers to the boundary's ability to determine specifically what matter, energy, and information can enter or leave the system. In some instances, system boundaries completely break down. Physiologically, boundary failure is often the result of the failure of a subsystem. For example, when one's kidneys fail, the entire system loses the ability to control some output. Psychosocial boundary failures are more difficult to describe. Certainly, the schizophrenic client who cannot tell where he or she ends and the outside world begins has a problem with boundary integrity.

Tom has no obvious problems with moving input or output through his boundary. In fact, interacting with the larger world is an important part of his life. He has no major health problems that would affect permeability. He is 72 years old, appears to view his life as productive and happy, and has achieved a sense of balance in life (Ebersole & Hess, 1994). He shows no signs of disengaging or of letting go.

Assess the individual's environment. The environment includes both the immediate suprasystem (usually the family) and the larger world. In some instances, problems that seem to belong to the client are actually problems with resources in the larger environment. Since the difficulty did not begin within the client, its solution is apt to be found in the environment from which the problem arose.

Tom is rich in certain resources. He has family and friends, and he is active in a church that is also supportive. His mother's illness may also have provided him with information regarding health care assistance in the community and the state. However, it is unclear from the history whether the resources Tom may need are readily accessible.

Assessment and analysis are reciprocal activities. As data are gathered, they are interpreted and analyzed. The specific questions one asks in the assessment stage are, to some degree, determined by an analysis of previous answers. Therefore, while assessment and analysis are generally described separately, they actually occur almost simultaneously.

Analysis

Analysis is the process of drawing inferences that are based on the raw data that have been gathered. It is not simple, since it requires the nurse to apply knowledge and experience to a particular client. In fact, the ability to combine knowledge and experience, as well as client and sensory cues, into a unified sense of the client's condition is the mark of a skilled nurse (Benner, Tanner & Chesla, 1992). It is clear that in spite of the challenges involved, a holistic analysis is essential to the provision of competent nursing care.

Healthy functioning requires the client to meet both biological and psychosocial goals. The individual's subsystems should operate together in a way that contributes to goal achievement. As a first step in the process of analyzing data, the nurse should describe and evaluate the interaction between the subsystems.

Homeostasis requires the individual to balance the matter, energy, and information that enters the system with that which leaves. A disparity between input and output may suggest a problem with maintaining a steady state. A number of physiological and psychological difficulties, such as fluid volume excess or deficit, ineffective breathing patterns, and some appetite disorders fall into this category. In some instances, internal processes are working so inefficiently that they prevent effective use of environmental input. As a second step in analysis, the nurse should indicate how well the client is able to maintain homeostasis.

Finally, any individual must adapt to internal and external changes. That process requires energy, which must be imported or diverted from other system activities. The final step in analysis requires the nurse to describe how well the individual is adjusting to internal and environmental changes.

Tom's biological and psychosocial subsystems are functioning well. In particular, his respiratory and cardiovascular systems are in excellent condition, as are his hearing and speech. He has no problems with major organs or with his immune response. He does have some degenerative arthritis in his hands, knees, and back, but this has not affected his mobility. He has had no sensory, motor, or coordination problems but has had transient problems with orientation. He is cheerful, friendly, and alert. He wears bifocals for presbyopia, but his vision has not worsened over the last 4 years. Based on this analysis, problems with other body systems do not account for his orientation problem. Rather, he seems to have a throughput, or processing, problem. He appears to be maintaining homeostasis, even in the face of a threat. Because the source of the problem has not been identified, Tom's need to change has been slight. However, he has been reasonably adaptable in the past.

Planning, Implementation, and Evaluation

Planning, implementation, and evaluation are considered together in this section. Because systems theory is general, the following suggestions apply to all three of these phases. The focus of this section is on the nurse as a member of the health care team. Since the use of an interdisciplinary team should improve care while it decreases cost, it is likely to be used increasingly in the future. For this reason, every nurse needs to work cooperatively with other health professionals. General systems theory is an effective vehicle by which to reach that end because of its holistic nature.

In general, a systems design is similar to other theoretical approaches to planning, implementation, and evaluation. In addition, the method can be used effectively by a team of health care professionals who have differing educational and clinical backgrounds. The client and the team cooperatively determine which problems are amenable to intervention and develop goals and objectives that focus on those problems. The group identifies the roles of each member, executes the plans that have been developed, evaluates success or failure, and alters the plan as needed.

There are four characteristics of open systems that are particularly helpful to those who are planning, implementing, and evaluating care. These are holism, equifinality, homeostasis, and adaptation.

Holism. A focus on the whole individual, *holism* emphasizes the uniqueness of that individual. While nursing has almost universally emphasized the need for individualized client care, personalized care occurs relatively rarely in practice settings. Systems theory reminds us to develop plans that address the client as a whole, rather than as a collection of illnesses. In fact, if the health care team does not consider the client as a whole, it is likely that planning and intervention will be less than effective.

Equifinality. A second characteristic allows providers to be flexible in responding to a client's unique needs during the development and implementation of plans of care. *Equifinality* suggests that a client's health care goals may be reached by a number of different routes. Therefore planning and implementing care can be an accommodative process—one that meets the needs of the client, effectively uses the skills of team members, and recognizes a range of approaches to meet those needs.

Homeostasis. Planning and implementation should attempt to maintain or improve homeostatic mechanisms. A client who has unmet health needs often has difficulty maintaining a stable energy supply. This may occur either because the demands that are made on his or her system require increased energy or because normal energy sources (food, oxygen, etc.) are insufficient. Therefore the team and client should develop, implement, and evaluate plans that attempt to reduce energy needs or to increase available energy, both biological and physiological.

Adaptation. Maintaining homeostasis does not preclude adapting to new circumstances. Many common health problems require increased energy merely to maintain a steady state. Positive changes, such as gathering new information or altering habit patterns require even more energy. Adapting to internal or environmental change means that energy must either be imported by the system or transferred from some other activity. Plans that center on adaptation or change should always include some consideration of whether the energy required for that change is available. If this is not done, goals that focus on these areas are likely to fail.

Tom needs further assessment in order to identify his problem and its source. It is likely that the process will involve his family physician, a nurse, a psychologist, and perhaps a gerontologist. Once his problem is identified, other health team members may have to work in concert with Tom and his wife.

It is clear that the nursing process will be more successful if it is used in conjunction with systems concepts. These concepts strengthen assessment, analysis, planning, implementation, and evaluation for the nurse. They are particularly helpful in today's health care climate, where shared responsibility is increasingly important. The inexperienced student can use systems theory as he or she learns about the nursing process.

Meanwhile, the experienced practitioner can apply the concepts in the workplace in a flexible, realistic way. Whether this means working independently or with a health care team, it increases the likelihood that the client will be a part of a health care system that is both humane and scientifically sound.

Applied Research

Research that applies general systems theory concepts and principles to the care of the individual is limited. Systems theory serves as a foundation for many nursing theories. For example, Johnson, King, Orem, Rogers, and Neuman all base their theoretical models, at least in part, on general systems theory. While elements of these theories have been tested, only a few studies have been conducted where all of the criteria for theory testing were met. Between the years of 1952 to 1985, Silva (1986) found that only 9 of 62 studies that purported to test nursing theories actually met the criteria. This may be due to several factors. Any theory is difficult to test in the workplace, but it is particularly difficult to translate systems theory's abstract concepts into concrete and measurable terms (Reed, 1993). In addition, theory testing must be the explicit goal of the research, the theory must be the underlying guide for the study, the relationships between the theory and research must be clear, and the research findings must draw explicit conclusions regarding the adequacy of the theory (Fawcett, 1993).

Another problem is related to the fact that clinical nurse researchers do most of their applied research in areas other than theory testing (Knafl, Bevis, & Kirchhoff, 1987). In spite of these difficulties, a number of authors have been successful in applying nursing theory directly to the care of clients. For example, a reliable and valid instrument that evaluates behavioral change in cancer patients is based on the Johnson behavioral system model (Derdiarian, 1983).

FAMILY SYSTEMS

Most of us are born into, live out our lives, and die within families, and may limit our analysis to the quirks of our own families. General systems theory provides a framework that helps the nurse assess other families, identify their relevant patterns, and plan, implement, and evaluate family interventions (Feldstein & Rait, 1992). General systems theory is sufficiently broad to accommodate the perspectives of a number of family theorists. These viewpoints are particularly helpful in family assessment, since they focus on family characteristics and behaviors that influence family functioning.

The family is defined as "an open system of interacting personalities composed of interrelated positions and roles" (Fawcett, 1975). It is a living system in which there are "a series of interlocking . . . subsystems [where] a change in one part will produce a change in another" (Bowen, 1974). The family system takes in matter, energy, and information as input, processes it, and either retains it or releases it into the environment as output. The family uses feedback to determine whether it is meeting its goals and evaluates activities as simple as monitoring a savings account balance or as complex as monitoring a child. Every family has a boundary, but because it is emotional rather than physical, it may be difficult to identify. Finally, the family exists within an environment, usually the community.

An Approach to Assessment

Review the Muller family case study that was presented in the section on individual assessment. The same case study is the basis for family assessment and provides an example of how one can alter the definition of a system.

Assess the family's input. A family obtains most of its matter, energy, and information from the community. Resources include a range of assets that strengthen a family's ability to cope, whereas stressors reflect insufficient assets, as well as environmental demands that diminish family resources.

The Muller family has sufficient income, including Social Security, railroad retirement, and savings. They own their own home, car, and travel trailer. They have three children and a large group of friends. They belong to a church association, and they travel for pleasure. Their children are all doing well; each is married, and two of the three have young children. Mr. Muller's mother is not well, and they visit her at least twice a week. Her nursing home bills are paid for from her savings and retirement income, which are sufficient to cover current costs.

Assess the family's output. Every family demonstrates a range of observable behaviors to the community and to each other. The activities in which the members participate and the home where they live reflect family resources and values. Families develop both functional and dysfunctional patterns of behavior as they attempt to resolve problems and reduce tensions.

The Mullers attend church regularly and describe themselves as "true believers." They used to bowl, but they stopped when Tom's knees began bothering him. Hilda said that she really misses bowling but would never go without Tom. However, Tom rarely mentions bowling. Both Tom and Hilda are covered by Medicare and supplementary insurance coverage. They see their family physician regularly, get flu shots every fall, and see the dentist every 6 months. They indicate that they haven't told their children about the episode in the service center, but once there is a diagnosis, they'll "get the family together and discuss things."

Assess the family's throughput mechanisms. The way a system processes information is suggested by the relationship between the system's input and output. However, there are specific issues that directly influence system functioning. Each of these should be considered individually.

The first of these are family set factors. *Set factors* are those enduring family characteristics that predispose a family to behave in a particular way. They include religion, educational level, socioeconomic class, ethnocultural background, and values. The nurse should pay particular attention to the relationships between these characteristics, since many of them are interconnected. For example, education, socioeconomic class, and values tend to reflect and may predict one another.

The second consideration is family structure. Over the last 25 years, the idea of what constitutes a family has changed dramatically. Family arrangements include a broad range of married, single-parent, and multiadult households, with or without children (Stanhope & Lancaster, 1992). Structural elements include the family composition, value systems, communication network, role system, and power structure (Friedman, 1992).

A third issue is family developmental stage. Developmental theorists suggest that families change in predictable ways over time (Friedman, 1992). These normal changes result from internal and environmental experiences that typically occur as a family matures. Until quite recently, developmental stage was based on childbearing and child-rearing responsibilities such as those described by Duvall (1977) and presented in Table 6-1.

Similarly, Stanhope and Lancaster (1992) identified six stages of growth in traditional families. These include the following:

1. Between families: the unattached young adult
2. The newly married couple
3. Families with young children
4. Families with adolescents
5. Launching children and moving on
6. Families in later life

Because some families do not include children, theorists have also described less-child-oriented stages that can apply to all families. Generally, these stages focus on the following: (1) the initiation of family, (2) the formation of a family identity, (3) increasing family integration with or without childbearing, and (4) an actualizing period when the focus is on the mature, adult family (Stanhope & Lancaster, 1988). Regardless of the approach used, the nurse must attempt to determine whether the family is carrying out the functions that are appropriate to its developmental stage.

A final issue, strongly influenced by structure, is family functioning, or the way the family operates as a unit. Family functioning includes an analysis of its ability to carry out those activities that are traditionally its responsibility, including family communication patterns, decision-making skills, and family roles. *Roles* refer to the behavior expected of an occupant of a particular position in the family and include both rights and responsibilities (Rosenkoetter, 1993). Since roles within a family significantly influence how the family functions, much information about how a family operates can be obtained by assessing those roles.

Family structure, developmental stage, roles, communication, and decision-making patterns collectively influence the way a family works together. While a weakness in one area may be compensated for by strengths in another, a family with multiple weaknesses often suffers from severely compromised functioning. A systems approach is a practical way to consider how these factors together influence family functioning. At least one assessment tool, the Feetham Family Functioning Survey, measures the ability of the family to function as an open system. This tool has demonstrated both reliability and validity (Roberts & Feetham, 1982).

Table 6-1   **Duvall's Eight-Stage Family Life Cycle and Family Developmental Tasks**

Stage	Family Life Cycle Stage	Family Developmental Tasks
I	Beginning families (married couples without children)	Establishing a mutually satisfying marriage Adjusting to pregnancy and the promise of parenthood Fitting into the kin network
II	Childbearing families (oldest child birth through 30 months)	Having, adjusting to, and encouraging the development of infants Establishing a satisfying home for both parents and infant(s)
III	Families with preschool children (oldest child 2½ to 6 years of age)	Adapting to the critical needs and interests of preschool children in stimulating, growth-promoting ways Coping with energy depletion and lack of privacy as parents
IV	Families with school-age children (oldest child 6 to 13 years of age)	Fitting into the community of school-age families in constructive ways Encouraging children's educational achievement
V	Families with teenagers (oldest child 13 to 20 years of age)	Balancing freedom with responsibility as teenagers mature and emancipate themselves Establishing postparental interest and careers as growing parents
VI	Families launching young adults (first child leaving home through last child leaving home)	Releasing young adults into work, college, marriage with appropriate rituals and assistance Maintaining a supportive home base
VII	Middle-aged parents (empty nest to retirement)	Rebuilding the marriage relationship Maintaining kin ties with older and younger generations
VIII	Family during retirement and aging (retirement to death of both spouses)	Adjusting to retirement Closing the family home or adapting it to aging Coping with bereavement and living alone

From Duvall, E.M. (1977). *Marriage and family development* (5th ed.). New York: HarperCollins.

The Mullers are a middle class, Protestant family of German ancestry, and they are a nuclear family without children at home. Both members are high school graduates. Developmentally, they are a family in later life. The family is close knit and supportive, but values independence. The family has successfully met the developmental tasks of aging until this point. They have loving relationships with their adult children, enjoy retirement, and seem to find meaning in life; however, some of life's more challenging tasks are ahead of them: adjusting to changes in health, to altered living arrangements, or to the loss of a spouse, for example (Friedman, 1992).

The family discusses everything, although Hilda says that she is the "chatterbox in the family." Tom and Hilda have discussed the possibility that Tom may have "the same prob-

lem as his mother does." It was that concern that caused them to seek medical advice, a decision that both agreed was an easy one. While Tom sometimes appears to be the family manager, he states that it is actually Hilda who manages their daily lives, including their money. However, Tom is a skilled carpenter and does household repairs for his family and for several elderly neighbors.

Assess the family's feedback mechanisms. While individuals commonly use both physical and psychosocial data as they evaluate themselves, families primarily use psychosocial measures. In some families, goal accomplishment is determined mainly by external measures of success, such as income or status, whereas other families measure success internally, based on personal values. Families differ in their responses to evidence that they are not meeting their goals, and they may change their behavior or their goals, or both.

The Mullers believe that success isn't measured by money. Instead, they value their good name, good friends, and family, and believe that living according to God's will is true success. The last is the most important; therefore they do not necessarily accept feedback that is based on secular societal values.

Assess the family's boundary. While an individual's boundary may be easy to identify, a family's boundary is often more difficult to detect (Helvi, 1991). It may surround only the family members who live in the home, or it may include other, not so obvious, members. Boundaries vary in both permeability and integrity. One of the functions of a boundary is to exclude matter, energy, and information that the system does not need. In some families, that function is severely compromised. If substances that could be harmful to members are allowed to enter freely, then the boundary is not functioning effectively.

The Muller family includes two members: Hilda and Tom. Once their children married, they formed their own families and are now considered to be part of the extended family. All three children have keys to their parents' home. Friends are frequent visitors. In spite of their welcoming attitude, Hilda and Tom are careful about locking the doors and are cautious with strangers.

Assess the family's environment. Normally, the community in which the family lives is considered to be the suprasystem. Many of the family's resources must be obtained from the suprasystem. Often, a family's developmental stage helps to determine what resources are most significant to its members. An elderly family may be particularly concerned about health care services but care little about schools, whereas a family with growing children may have different priorities. A mixed-age community requires a balance of services that can meet the needs of all residents.

The Mullers live in a mixed-age community that has a range of health care and social service options for the elderly. Public transportation is limited, although some door-to-door transportation is available for the elderly. Generally, residents drive private cars. The family's church has a nurse who is employed to make home visits and a part-time volunteer driver who provides transportation to those in need.

Analysis

Analysis is the process of making sense of the information about the family that the nurse has gathered. The nurse must make inferences that are based on adequate data and arise from a combination of experience and a strong knowledge base. While many nurses have developed unique approaches to analysis, the abilities to achieve family goals, maintain homeostasis, adapt to change, and manage environmental stressors are reasonable expected outcomes on which to base nursing inferences.

A functioning family should be able to meet its goals successfully. These goals include both the responsibilities that the society asks of any family and those more personal decisions about how time, money, and energy should be spent. Set factors, developmental stage, communication, decision-making patterns, and roles influence a family's ability to function. It is essential to use the gathered data as a basis for describing how well the family is functioning and to draw conclusions about why a family is or is not successful in achieving its goals.

A second measure of a functional family is its ability to maintain homeostasis. To do so, it must take in sufficient matter, energy, and information to balance that which it uses with that which it returns to the community. Since it is the boundary that regulates what enters and leaves the system, a family that is relatively closed to its environment may have difficulty obtaining what it needs to maintain homeostasis. On the other hand, a family may give so much to the community that it has insufficient energy to meet its own needs. A large disparity between input and output suggests that a family is having difficulty maintaining its balance. When a family requires significant community support and still has difficulty functioning, something may be wrong with its internal processes. Stressors such as illness or a developmental or role change may demand increased resources or may impair a family's ability to effectively use the resources it has. Any family must be able to adapt to a variety of changes. The nurse should begin by focusing on the family's specific developmental stage. Each stage brings with it predictable family challenges that require the use of adaptive energy. In addition, there are environmental stressors with which the family must cope. Because of the environment's unpredictability, these stressors may require a surplus of adaptive energy. A combination of developmental and environmental stressors may tax the resources of even the most functional family.

The Mullers seem to be meeting their family goals, as defined by both society and themselves. Their success may be attributable to a variety of factors. The couple communicates openly with one another, even in stressful, potentially frightening situations. They see one another as supportive friends and have long-established roles that have helped them to manage the early stresses of aging. Decisions are generally shared, and the family rarely avoids diffi-

cult or frightening decisions. The future may bring with it greater challenges than the present. In particular, greater role flexibility may be needed if one member becomes ill. While the family has handled Tom's immediate problem effectively, they may have to consider the long-range implications of his condition. The Mullers do have considerable resources to help them, including extended family, friends, and community.

The family is able to maintain homeostasis. Tom's condition may represent a stressor that is a real challenge to the family. However, the Mullers seem to have the adaptive energy that change requires. If they continue to use that energy and internal and environmental resources effectively, they should maintain their balance.

Planning, Implementation, and Evaluation

Planning, implementation, and evaluation are based on family needs and represent the action segments of the nursing process. They give the nurse who is working with a family the opportunity to cooperatively and thoughtfully develop, carry out, and evaluate the process. Because the three steps are so closely connected that they are often reciprocal, they are discussed together here. As is true for the individual, this process requires cooperation between family, health team members, and community resources.

A systems approach to planning, implementation, and evaluation has some unique features. Because the family is goal directed, its participation is essential to achieve health-related goals (Foust, 1994). The family should clearly identify the goals its members are willing to pursue and, with the health team, determine how to meet them. While the nurse may be aware of particular strategies that may be helpful, a range of possible approaches, any of which may achieve the goal, should be considered (equifinality). This requires the active participation of the family, the health team, and other resource people.

Nursing actions should focus on supporting or improving the family's homeostatic mechanisms. When a family is overwhelmed by demands, it is often helpful to identify and reduce the number of stressors with which the members are dealing. The family may have to alter its behavior in order to return to or maintain a steady state. It is during periods of stress that the family has the opportunity to experiment with new approaches to solving problems in order to make permanent adaptations. The nurse should encourage healthy changes that increase family stability.

In addition, the nurse may help the family adapt to change or increase the permeability of its boundary. Increasing boundary permeability has a dual purpose: to help the family identify external resources and then help them to actually use them (Miller & Janosik, 1980). A wide range of coping strategies may be used in the process (see box on p. 134).

Finally, because systems theory is especially useful to examine the relationship between subsystems, research that explores the relationship between family members may suggest effective strategies for specific families. For example, studies that explore feedback between mother and child (Anderson, 1981) or mothers' perceptions during childbirth (Mercer, Hackley, & Bostrom, 1983) support the use of general systems theory in family-centered maternity settings.

Increasing Family Coping	
Within the Family	**Outside the Family**
Family support	Seeking information
Family humor	Maintaining community relations
Sharing of experiences	Seeking support, both social and
Redefining the problem	spiritual
Shared problem solving	
Role flexibility	

Modified from Friedman, M. (1992). *Family nursing: Theory and practice.* Norwalk, CT: Appleton & Lange.

COMMUNITY/POPULATION–FOCUSED SYSTEMS

Many people think of a community as an environment with physical or political boundaries. Community health nursing, however, defines the term more broadly to reflect concern with the health of groups or populations of individuals (Clark, 1992). Communities are composed of population groups—collections of individuals with shared characteristics (Clemen-Stone, Eigsti, & McGuire, 1994). These population groups may be defined by the areas where they live (inner city, suburb) but are more commonly composed of subgroups of the general population (the elderly, school-age children). While community health nursing is concerned about improving the health of the entire population, it is especially concerned about groups that are at special risk for illness. Fig. 6-3 illustrates both a traditional community and a population group.

Assessment

The primary reason to assess a community is to identify and change those negative factors that influence its health status. This process requires the nurse, often in concert with others, to gather data from a variety of sources in order to develop an accurate and comprehensive picture of the group involved. This may seem overwhelming to even an experienced community health nurse. A systematic approach can help to make the process more manageable.

Assess the community's input. The matter, energy, and information to which the community has access influences its health status. This includes health care and non–health care resources from both public and private sources. For example, while the elderly have more chronic illnesses than other age groups, they also have access to health care provided by the federal government and access to a potent political action group, the American Association of Retired Persons (AARP). Newspapers, radio, and television reflect and shape community opinion, whereas state and national policy help to determine community resources.

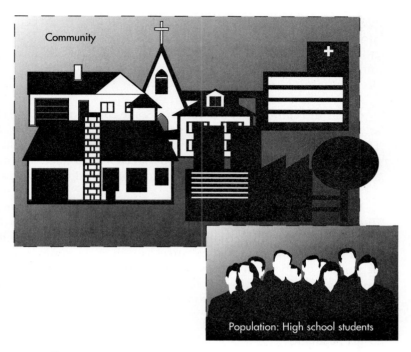

Fig. 6-3   A traditional community and population group.

Assess the community's output. A community's goals and the degree to which they are achieved represent its output. Regardless of the unique features of the population, two goals are almost always present. All groups work to ensure their own survival and to achieve self-fulfillment for themselves and for their members. Demographic, morbidity, and mortality statistics describe a community's characteristics, as well as its health outcomes. These data help to identify illness patterns or public health problems that are unique to the group. In some communities, osteoporosis is a serious problem, whereas other communities are more concerned about teenage pregnancy.

Assess the community's throughput mechanisms. Throughput refers to the way in which a community processes its input. This includes the ways that information is communicated between members. For example, are there formal communication networks, or do informal systems predominate? Are there newspapers or newsletters? What recreational and other interactional opportunities are there? Does the population take advantage of them?

Health and health-related programs may be provided by the community itself, the state, or the nation. These programs may treat existing disease or may attempt to ensure that a group remains healthy, both physically and emotionally. In either case, social services, programs, and activities are targeted at specific geographical regions and population groups.

Assess the community's feedback mechanism. Every community has the opportunity to evaluate its own goal achievement, especially in the area of health. Healthy groups should attempt to realistically evaluate feedback that relates to its health goals and then make an effort to respond to the data appropriately. This may require an entire community to change its behavior.

Assess the community's boundary. Some communities have clearly defined boundaries that are determined by age, gender, socioeconomic status, or place of residence. These boundaries may be defended rigidly or loosely, depending on the purposes of the community. It is essential that boundaries allow necessary matter, energy, and information to enter and that they exclude that which is unnecessary.

Assess the community's environment. Because communities are not self-sufficient, they depend on their environment to function effectively. This dependence on others requires negotiation and cooperation, in both the private and public sectors. However, some groups have abundant resources within their community and are therefore less dependent on the external environment. Most community nursing texts contain survey tools that include the preceding information. These tools may be helpful to those who undertake a community assessment.

Data Analysis

The purpose of analyzing population data is to identify group health needs. To do this, the nurse must draw conclusions about the data that have been gathered. There are a number of approaches to data interpretation that can facilitate the inferential process. In any case, the community involved must be an active participant in the process. A systems approach is particularly helpful in identifying the relationships between subsystems:

1. Review the data in each category and summarize the information, describing both strengths and weaknesses. Support your conclusions with statistical evidence.
2. Identify gaps, omissions, or inconsistencies in your data. Gather additional information as needed.
3. Make inferences about community health problems based on the data (Anderson & McFarlane, 1988). This is generally done by comparing the data with the data of the larger population or by using measures that reflect a desired group outcome or goal (U.S. Department of Health and Human Services, 1991).
4. Develop a priority list to indicate the order in which problems should be addressed.

Planning, Implementation, and Evaluation

The same skill and knowledge that help the nurse plan, implement, and evaluate care with the individual and the family are used with larger populations. However, there are some special abilities that are essential to the community health nurse. Resolving a group health problem is rarely accomplished by one person. Instead, it requires the concerted action of all those who are concerned about health. As a result, the nurse must work cooperatively with other professional groups, as well as with governmental and voluntary agencies and organizations. This cooperative planning requires patience, negotiation, compromise, and more patience. The outcome is a plan that reflects group input and is therefore more likely to be successively implemented. It may, however, be quite different from the one the nurse originally envisioned.

Evaluation is the weak link in many population-focused health plans. Because planning and implementation require so much energy, there is often little inclination to rework those steps when they are ineffective. Therefore evaluation should begin early in the process, when alterations are simpler and less costly. However, because many population-focused plans address complex problems, it remains necessary to measure long-term outcomes despite the difficulty involved.

In spite of the challenges inherent in addressing population-based health problems, it can be an extremely rewarding process for the nurse. It encourages the development of new skills that can be used to help clients in a wide variety of settings. More important, the process can have a tremendous impact on the health of population groups, the state, and the nation.

Key Points

- Systems theory is especially useful to nursing because it focuses on the whole but pays particular attention to the way the parts work together.

- Systems theory is a broadly applicable interdisciplinary approach that can be used by nurses in most settings, with all types of clients, and by all members of the health care team.

- The theory is applicable in all phases of the nursing process and is particularly useful in the analysis of data.

- The case study illustrates how general systems theory can serve as a useful framework for assessing and providing care for individuals and families.

- Care for communities and populations at risk can be accommodated within the general systems theory framework.

Critical Thinking Exercises

1. Discuss the major advantages of using general systems theory as a basis for client care. What, if any, are the disadvantages?

2. Apply the following concepts to the family in which you were raised: input, throughput, output, boundary, environment, homeostasis, and suprasystem.

3. Select an individual client and:
   a. Use general systems theory as a framework for assessment and data analysis.
   b. Describe your findings according to the principles and concepts of general systems theory.

4. One of the most challenging parts of family assessment is assessing the family's throughput. Describe a family (your own or other) in terms of its set factors, structure, developmental stage, and functioning. How might that family process information?

5. Compare and contrast the use of systems theory to assess, plan, implement, and evaluate care with a population group and a geographical community.

References

Anderson, C. (1981). Enhancing reciprocity between mother and neonate. *Nursing Research, 30*(2), 89-93.

Anderson, E.T., & McFarlane, J.M. (1988). *Community as client.* Philadelphia: J.B. Lippincott.

Benner, P., Tanner, C., & Chesla, C. (1992). From beginner to expert: Gaining a differentiated clinical world in critical care nursing. *Advances in Nursing Science, 14*(3), 13-28.

Bowen, M. (1974). Bowen on triangles. *Workshop Monograph,* Center for Family Learning.

Byrne, M., & Thompson, L. (1978). *Key concepts for the study and practice of nursing* (2nd ed.). St. Louis: Mosby.

Christensen, P.J., & Kenney, J. (1995). *Nursing process: Application of conceptual models* (4th ed.). St. Louis: Mosby.

Clark, M.J. (1992). *Nursing in the community.* Norwalk, CT: Appleton & Lange.

Clemen-Stone, S., Eigsti, D.G., & McGuire, S.L. (1994) *Comprehensive family and community health nursing: Family, aggregate, and community practice.* (4th ed.). St. Louis: Mosby.

Derdiarian, A. (1983). An instrument for theory and research development using the behavioral systems model for nursing: The cancer patient. *Nursing Research, 32*(4), 196-200.

Duvall, E.M. (1977). *Marriage and family development* (5th ed.). New York: J.B. Lippincott.

Ebersole, P., & Hess, P. (1994). *Toward healthy aging: Human needs and nursing response* (4th ed.). St. Louis: Mosby.

Fawcett, J. (1975). The family as an open, living system: An emerging conceptual framework for nursing. *International Nursing Review, 22,* 113-116.

Fawcett, J. (1993) *Analysis and evaluation of nursing theories.* Philadelphia: F.A. Davis.

Feldstein, M.A., & Rait, D. (1992). Family assessment in an oncology setting. *Cancer Nursing, 15*(3), 161-168.

Foust, J.B. (1994). Creating a future for nursing through interactive planning at the bedside. *Image: Journal of Nursing Scholarship 26*(2), 129-131.

Friedman, M. (1992). *Family nursing: Theory and practice.* Norwalk, CT: Appleton & Lange.

Gillies, D.A. (1994). *Nursing management: A systems approach* (3rd ed.). Philadelphia: W.B. Saunders.

Helvi, C. (1991). *Community health nursing.* New York: Springer.

Kast, F., & Rosenzweig, J. (1981). General systems theory: Applications for organizations and management. *Journal of Nursing Administration, 81*(8), 32-40.

Knafl, K., Bevis, M., & Kirchhoff, K. (1987). Research activities of clinical nurse researchers. *Nursing Research, 36*(4), 249-252.

LaMonica, E. (1985). *The humanistic nursing process.* Belmont, CA: Wadsworth Health Science Division.

Mercer, R., Hackley, K., & Bostrom, A. (1983). Relationship of psychosocial and perinatal variables to perception of childbirth. *Nursing Research, 32*(4), 202-207.

Miller, J. (1978). *Living systems.* New York: McGraw-Hill.

Miller, J., & Janosik, E. (1980). *Family focused care.* New York: McGraw-Hill.

Reed, K. (1993). Adapting the Neuman systems model for family nursing. *Nursing Science Quarterly, 6*(2), 93-97.

Roberts, C., & Feetham, S. (1982). Assessing family functioning across three areas of relationships. *Nursing Research, 31,* 231-235.

Rosenkoetter, M. (1993). The influence of pats on life patterns in the home. In G. Wegner & R. Alexander (Eds.), *Readings in family nursing* (pp. 299-308). Philadelphia: J.B. Lippincott.

Silva, M. (1986). Research testing nursing theory: State of the art. *Advances in Nursing Science, 9*(1), 1-11.

Stanhope, M., & Lancaster, J. (1988). *Community health nursing: Process and practice for promoting health* (2nd ed.). St. Louis: Mosby.

Stanhope, M., & Lancaster, J. (1992). *Community health nursing: Process and practice for promoting health* (3rd ed.). St. Louis: Mosby.

Tonges, M., & Madden, M.J. (1993). "Running the vicious cycle backward" and other system solutions to nursing problems. *Journal of Nursing Administration, 23*(1), 39-44.

U.S. Department of Health and Human Services (1991). *Healthy people 2000* (DHHS Publication No. [PHS] 91-50213). Rockville, MD: The Department.

von Bertalanffy, L. (1956). General systems theory. In B.D. Ruben & J. Kim (Eds.), *General systems theory and human communication* (pp. 7-16). Rochelle Park, NJ: Hayden.

Yura, H., & Walsh, M. (1978). *The nursing process.* New York: Appleton-Century-Crofts.

Theories and Frameworks for Professional Nursing Practice

7

Joan L. Creasia

Joan L. Creasia

🍂 Objectives

At the completion of this chapter, the reader will be able to:

- Distinguish between a concept, theory, conceptual framework, and model.
- Identify and define the four central concepts of nursing theories.
- Compare and contrast the main precepts of selected theories of nursing.
- Examine criteria for evaluating the utility of a specific nursing theory for its relevance to practice, education, or research.
- Identify theories from related disciplines that have application to nursing.

Profile in Practice

Martha Raile Alligood, PhD, RN
College of Nursing,
University of Tennessee,
Knoxville, Tennessee

After graduating from a diploma program and practicing nursing for a few years, I became interested in missionary nursing. I completed my BSN degree to prepare for a 3-year term as director of the nursing program at Christian Hospital, Mashoko Mission, Rhodesia (now Zimbabwe), Africa.

During my BSN program at the University of Virginia, I learned about theory-guided nursing practice. The content was theory based, using theories from other disciplines, such as Selye's stress theory, Erikson's human development theory, and Maslow's theory of motivation and personality. I saw an immediate benefit of using theory to guide the reasoning process in practice; it explained many puzzles from my first 10 years in nursing. When I completed the degree and looked back over that experience, my thought was "What we really need is *nursing theory* to guide nursing practice." Although a few nurse theorists had published their works by that time, I was not aware of them. It was when I returned from Africa and was teaching psychiatric nursing in a diploma program that I learned of Orem's *Concepts of Practice* and incorporated her ideas into the course. A particular focus was to let patients maintain responsibility for their care or help them regain that capacity.

Because I also found King's theory useful, I was drawn to a master's degree program at Ohio State University that organized the curriculum according to King's interacting systems framework. King's theory guided the content for core courses in nursing of individuals (personal system), family and small groups (interpersonal system), and communities (social systems). Theory-based practice was required in the clinical courses (in my case, nursing of adults). I had my first experience using a nursing framework to guide my thoughts and actions in practice. Even as feeble as those first efforts were, the contrast between my former practice and that guided by King's framework was obvious at once. King's concepts formed a framework for me to view orthopedic patients as whole persons in family and social contexts. King not only changed my role and that of the patient, but also guided the information I collected, shaped the mutual process of the nurse-patient relationship, and directed my nursing actions.

My fascination with nursing theory soon led me to New York University for my doctorate, where I learned Rogerian nursing science from Martha Rogers herself. I used her worldview of the mutual simultaneous process of people and their environments as the basis for my hypothesis that creative changes in developmental actualization were related to empathy as a "feeling attribute" of the developmental process. This middle-range theory, when tested, explained the importance of creative expression in adult development and the risk to health in the elderly when creative expression is thwarted.

My personal experiences with both King's and Rogers' theories reinforced my belief in the value of theory-based practice and research.

---

*"Theory is the poetry of science. The poet's words are familiar, each
standing alone, but brought together they sing, they astonish, they teach"*
Levine, 1995, p. 14.

Theories and conceptual frameworks consist of the theorist's words brought together to form a meaningful whole. Theories and frameworks provide direction and guidance for structuring professional nursing practice, education, and research. In practice, theories and frameworks help nurses to describe, explain, and predict everyday experiences, and they also serve to guide assessment, intervention, and evaluation of nursing care. In education, a conceptual framework provides the general focus for curriculum design and guides curricular decision making. In research, the framework offers a systematic approach to identifying questions for study, selecting appropriate variables, and interpreting findings. The importance of theory in building a body of nursing knowledge is emphasized by Chinn and Jacobs (1987), who state, "Nursing theory ought to guide research and practice, generate new ideas, and differentiate the focus of nursing from other professions" (p. 145). Fig. 7-1 illustrates these relationships.

Many nurse theorists have made substantial contributions to the development of a body of nursing knowledge. Offering an assortment of perspectives, the theories vary in their level of abstraction and their conceptualization of the client, health, illness, and nursing. From a historical perspective, nursing theories reflect the influence of the larger society and illustrate increased sophistication in the development of nursing ideas. Table 7-1 presents a chronology of events related to the development of nursing theories.

TERMINOLOGY ASSOCIATED WITH THEORETICAL PERSPECTIVES

To understand the structure of nursing knowledge, it is necessary to define the main components of theoretical perspectives. The most fundamental component of a theory is a *concept,* which is defined as an idea or word that describes an object, event, or property and brings forth a mental image of the phenomenon being described (Fawcett & Downs, 1992). Since a concept is an abstract representation of the real world, it is important to realize that concepts embedded in a theory represent the theorist's perspective of reality (Keck, 1994). The fact that a theorist's perspective may be different from that of the reader does not invalidate the theory. Rather, a different perspective offers an alternative way of viewing the world of nursing.

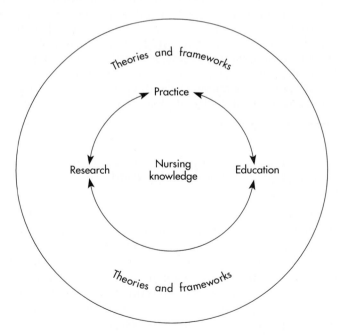

Fig. 7-1   Relationship between theories and frameworks and nursing education, research, and practice.

Concepts must be related to one another in order for a theory to exist. *Theoretical statements,* also called *propositions,* describe the relationship between two or more concepts (Hickman, 1995). One theoretical statement, or several theoretical statements taken together, can constitute a theory. A *theory,* then, is a statement or group of statements that describe, explain, or predict relationships between concepts (i.e., objects, events, or properties). Theories may be broad or limited in scope, thus varying in their ability to describe, explain, or predict. Theories that are the broadest in scope are called *grand theories* and are composed of relatively abstract concepts and relationships that cannot readily be tested in research. *Middle-range theories,* on the other hand, encompass a limited number of concepts that are relatively concrete and more easily tested.

A theory is based on a set of *assumptions,* (i.e., statements that are commonly held to be true). Assumptions may be either implicitly or explicitly stated by the theorist. Assumptions that are *implicit* require the reader to infer their existence, as in Orem's Self-Care Deficit Theory, where it must be presumed that individuals desire self-care. Assumptions that are *explicit,* on the other hand, are in the form of clear statements, as in Johnson's Behavioral System Model, which describes an individual as a set of behavioral subsystems.

A *conceptual framework* serves as a guide to theory development by providing an orienting scheme or world view that helps focus our thinking. A conceptual framework may be visualized as an umbrella under which many theories can exist. The major distinction between a conceptual framework and a theory is the level of abstraction, with a conceptual framework being more abstract than a theory. The term conceptual framework is often used interchangeably with conceptual model, although the term *model* is generally used to refer to a graphic illustration of theoretical relationships. Without attempting to justify the classification of individual theoretical perspectives included in this chapter, the term to which each is most commonly referred (i.e., theory, model, framework) is used.

COMPONENTS OF NURSING THEORIES

A nursing theory is a "relatively specific and concrete set of concepts and propositions that purports to account for or characterize phenomena of interest to the discipline of nursing" (Fawcett, 1989, p. 23). Four central concepts of interest to the discipline of nursing are person, environment, health/illness, and nursing. *Persons* are the recipients of nursing care and include individuals, families, and communities. *Environment* refers to the surroundings of the client, internal factors affecting the client, and the setting where nursing care is delivered. *Health and illness* describe the client's state of well-being. *Nursing* is the discipline from which client care actions are derived. Most nursing theories define or describe these central concepts, either explicitly or implicitly. In addition to these concepts, many theories include assumptions about the nature of the client and the environment, theoretical statements describing the relationships between the major concepts, and definitions of concepts specific to a particular theory.

In keeping with this organizational scheme, descriptions of the theoretical perspectives presented in this chapter include a brief overview, basic assumptions about the individual and the environment, definitions of health and illness, a description of nursing including the goal of nursing, and definition of concepts and subconcepts specific to each theory. Some theories are more amenable to this scheme than others because of their degree of specificity or stage of development. When the needed information is not explicitly detailed by the theorist, inferences are made based on what seems to be implicitly stated. Because most of the theories are quite global, condensing them into discrete and somewhat restrictive categories obscures some of the true essence of the relationships. Thus the reader is encouraged to consult the primary source to gain a full appreciation of the depth, scope, and extent of the relationships put forth.

OVERVIEW OF SELECTED NURSING THEORIES

Theories and frameworks selected for inclusion in this chapter are those that exemplify the evolution of nursing from early times (e.g., Nightingale) to more recent ones (e.g., Parse) as illustrated in Table 7-1.

"Exploring a variety of nursing theories ought to provide nurses with new insights into patient care, opening nursing options otherwise hidden, and stimulating innovative interventions. But it is imperative that there be variety—for there is no global theory of nursing that fits every situation."
Levine, 1995, p. 13.

Nightingale's Environmental Theory

Florence Nightingale conceptualized disease as a reparative process and described the nurse's role as manipulating the environment to facilitate and encourage this process. Her directions regarding ventilation, warmth, light, diet, cleanliness, variety, and noise are discussed in her classic nursing textbook *Notes on Nursing* (1859).

Brief overview. The environment is critical to health, and the nurse's role in caring for the sick is to provide a clean, quiet, peaceful environment to promote healing. Nightingale's intent was to describe nursing and provide guidelines for nursing education.

Assumptions about the individual. Individuals are responsible, creative, in control of their lives and health, and desire good health.

Environment. The environment is external to the person but affects the health of both sick and well persons. One of the chief sources of infection, the environment must include pure air, pure water, efficient drainage, cleanliness, and light.

Health and illness. Health is described as a state of being well and using one's powers to the fullest. Illness or disease is the reaction of nature against the conditions in which we have placed ourself. Disease is a reparative mechanism, an effort of nature to remedy a process of poisoning or of decay.

Table 7-1   **History of Nursing Theory Development**

Events	Year	Nurse Theorists
	1860	Florence Nightingale Described nursing and environment
	1952	Hildegard E. Peplau Nursing as an interpersonal process: patients with felt needs
Scientific era: nurses questioned purpose of nursing	1960	Faye Abdellah (also 1965; 1973) Patient-centered approaches
	1961	Ida Jean Orlando Nurse-patient relationship; deliberative nursing approach
Process of theory development discussed among professional nurses	1964	Ernestine Wiedenbach (also 1970; 1977) Nursing: philosophy, purpose, practice, and art
	1966	Lydia E. Hall Core (patient), care (body), cure (disease)
	1966	Virginia Henderson (also 1972; 1978) Nursing assists patients with 14 essential functions toward independence
Symposium: theory development in nursing	1967	Myra Estrin Levine (also 1973) Four conservation principles of nursing
Symposium: nature of science and nursing	1968	
Dickoff, James, and Weidenbach wrote "Theory in a Practice Discipline" in *Nursing Research*		
Symposium: nature of science in nursing	1969	
First nursing theory conference		
Second nursing theory conference	1970	Martha E. Rogers (also 1980) Science of unitary man: energy fields, openness, pattern, and organization
Consensus on nursing concepts: nurse/nursing, health, client/patient/individual, society/environment	1971	Dorothea E. Orem (also 1980; 1985) Nursing facilitates patients' self-care
Discussion on what theory is: the elements, criteria, types, and levels, and the relation to research	1971	Imogene King (also 1975; 1981) Theory of goal attainment through nurse-client transactions
NLN required conceptual frameworks in nursing education	1973	

Modified from Christensen, P.J., & Kenney, J.W. (1995). *Nursing process: Application of conceptual models* (4th ed.). St. Louis: Mosby.
Continued

Table 7-1   **History of Nursing Theory Development—cont'd**

Events	Year	Nurse Theorists
Borrowed theories from other disciplines Expanded theories from other disciplines	1974	Sister Callista Roy (also 1976; 1980; 1984) Roy's adaptation model: nurse adjusts patient's stimuli (focal, contextual, or residual) Betty Neuman Health-care systems model: a total person approach
Recognized problems in practice and developed theories to test and use in practice	1976	Josephine Paterson and L. Zderad Humanistic nursing
Second nurse educator conference on nursing theory	1978	Madeleine Leininger (also 1980; 1981) Transcultural nursing Caring nursing
Articles on theory development in *ANS, Nursing Research, and Image*	1978 1979	Jean Watson (also 1985) Philosophy and science of caring; humanistic nursing
Books written for nurses on how to critique and develop theory, and describing application of nursing theories Graduate schools of nursing develop courses in how to analyze and apply nursing theories	1980	Dorothy E. Johnson Behavioral system model for nursing
Research studies in nursing identified nursing theories as framework for study	1981	Rosemarie Rizzo Parse (also 1987) Man-living-health: a theory of nursing
Numerous books published on analysis, application evaluation, and/or development of nursing theories	1982-present	

Nursing. Nursing is a service to mankind intended to relieve pain and suffering. Nursing's role is to promote or provide the proper environment for patients, including fresh air, light, pure water, cleanliness, warmth, quiet, and appropriate diet. The goal of nursing is to promote the reparative process by manipulating the environment.

Key Concepts. *Environment* refers to conditions external to the individual that affect life and development (i.e., ventilation, warmth, light, diet, cleanliness, and noise). Three major relationships are identified: the environment to the patient, the nurse to the environment, and the nurse to the patient. Examples of these follow:

The need for light, particularly sunlight, is second only to the need for ventilation. If necessary, the nurse should move the patient "about after the sun according to the aspects of the rooms, if circumstances permit, [rather] than let him linger in a room when the sun is off" (p. 48).

Nursing's role is to manipulate the environment to encourage healing. Nursing "ought to signify the proper use of fresh air, light, warmth, cleanliness, quiet, and the proper selection and administration of diet" (p. 6).

The sine qua non of all good nursing is to never allow a patient to be awakened, intentionally or accidentally. "A good nurse will always make sure that no blind or curtains should flap. If you wait till your patient tells you or reminds you of these things, where is the use of their having a nurse?" (p. 27).

Variety is important for patients to divert them from dwelling on their pain. "Variety of form and brilliancy of color in the objects presented are actual means of recovery" (p. 34).

Peplau's Interpersonal Process

Hildegard Peplau published the book *Interpersonal Relations in Nursing* in 1952 in which she described a partial theory for nursing practice. The book described the phases of the interpersonal process in nursing, roles for nurses, and methods for studying nursing as an interpersonal process. Numerous papers were published over the years, and her book was reprinted in 1988.

Brief overview. The focus of Peplau's model is on the goal-directed interpersonal process. "Psychodynamic nursing is being able to understand one's own behavior to help others identify felt difficulties, and to apply principles of human relations to the problems that arise at all levels of experience" (1952, p. xiii). The interpersonal relationship "has a starting point, proceeds through definable phases and, being time-limited, has an end point" (1992, p. 4).

Assumptions about the individual. The individual is an organism that "strives in its own way to reduce tension generated by needs" (1952, p. 82).

Environment. Although the environment is not explicitly defined, it can be inferred that the environment is the "existing forces outside the organism and in the context of culture" (1952, p. 163).

Health and illness. Health is a "word symbol that implies forward movement of personality and other ongoing human processes in the direction of creative, constructive, productive, personal, and community living" (1952, p. 12). By implication, illness is a condition that is marked by no movement or by backward movement in these areas.

Nursing. Nursing is a therapeutic interpersonal process because it involves the interaction between two or more individuals who have a common goal. For individuals who are sick and in need of health care, it is a healing art. Six nursing roles emerge in the various phases of the nurse-patient relationship: stranger, resource person, teacher, leader, surrogate, and counselor.

Key concepts. The nurse-patient relationship consists of four phases:

Orientation. The patient seeks professional assistance with a problem. The nurse and patient meet as strangers, and recognize, clarify, and define the existing problem.

Identification. The patient learns how to make use of the nurse-patient relationship and responds selectively to people who can meet his or her needs; the patient and nurse clarify each other's expectations.

Exploitation. The patient takes advantage of all available services. The nurse helps the patient to maintain a balance between dependence and independence and to use the services to help solve the current problem and work toward optimal health.

Resolution. The patient is free to move on with his or her life as old goals are put aside and new goals are adopted. The patient becomes independent of the nurse, and the relationship is terminated.

Henderson's Complementary-Supplementary Model

Virginia Henderson views nursing as an art and a discipline separate from medicine. In *The Nature of Nursing* (1966), she indicated that the "unique function of the nurse is to assist the individual, sick or well, in the performance of those activities contributing to the health or its recovery (or a peaceful death) that he would perform unaided if he had the necessary strength, will, or knowledge" (p. 15).

Brief overview. The nurse's role is that of a substitute for the patient, a helper to the patient, and a partner with the patient. Fourteen basic patient needs constitute components of nursing care.

Assumptions about the individual. The mind and body being inseparable, a person must maintain physiological and emotional balance. An individual requires assistance in order to achieve health and independence or a peaceful death. Individuals will achieve or maintain health if they have the necessary strength, will, or knowledge (1966, p. 15). The individual and family should be viewed as a unit.

Environment. The environment is "the aggregate of all the external conditions and influences affecting the life and development of an organism" (1978, p. 829).

Health and illness. Health is a quality of life basic to human functioning. Although not specifically stated, health seems to be equated with independence. Conversely, it can be inferred that illness is a lack of independence.

Nursing. Nursing has a unique function to assist sick or well individuals in a supplementary or complementary role. The goals of nursing are to help the individual gain independence as rapidly as possible and to promote health (1971).

Key concepts. Fourteen basic patient needs constitute the components of nursing care (1966):

1. Breathe normally.
2. Eat and drink adequately.
3. Eliminate body wastes.
4. Move and maintain a desirable position.
5. Sleep and rest.
6. Select suitable clothes.
7. Maintain the body temperature within normal range by adjusting clothing and modifying the environment.
8. Keep the body clean and well-groomed to protect the integument.
9. Avoid dangers in the environment and avoid injuring others.
10. Communicate with others in expressing emotions, needs, fears, or opinions.
11. Worship according to one's faith.
12. Work in such a way that there is a sense of accomplishment.
13. Play or participate in various forms of recreation.
14. Learn, discover, or satisfy the curiosity that leads to normal development and health and use the available health facilities.

Rogers' Science of Unitary Human Beings

First presented as *The Theoretical Basis for Nursing* in 1970, Martha Rogers' conceptualizations, dating back to the 1960s, evolved into the current science of unitary human beings. She posited that humans are dynamic energy fields who are integral with the environment and who are continuously evolving. She viewed nursing as a science and art that focuses on the nature and direction of human development and human betterment. Nursing scholars who subscribe to Rogers' theory are committed to continuing her work (see box on p. 150).

Brief overview. The individual is viewed as an irreducible energy field who is integral with the environment. The nurse seeks to promote symphonic interactions between humans and their environments.

Assumptions about the individual. The individual is a unified irreducible whole, manifesting characteristics that are more than, and different from, the sum of his or her parts, and is continuously evolving irreversibly and unidirectionally along a space-time continuum. Pattern and organization of humans are directed toward increasing complexity rather than maintaining equilibrium. The individual "is characterized by

---

She Is Missed...

Sarah Hall Gueldner, DSN, RN, FAAN
Professor and Director of Doctoral Studies,
College of Nursing, Medical University of South Carolina,
Charleston, South Carolina;
Past President, Society of Rogerian Scholars

   Dr. Martha E. Rogers, one of nursing's first theorists and a world-class scholar, died at her home in Phoenix, Arizona, on March 13, 1994, at the age of 79. Her contributions to nursing science were immense. Her exquisitely written purple book, *An Introduction to the Theoretical Basis of Nursing* (1970), heralded the beginning of nursing's now fevered pursuit of its theoretical base. Noting her death, the *New York Times* (March 18, 1994) wrote, "Rogers drew on many disciplines, including psychology, sociology, biology, history, and literature, to postulate a humanistic nursing science." Her classic written works and the continuing scholarship of the many individuals who studied with her are a lasting memorial to this great nurse scholar. Dr. Rogers leaves a legacy of visionary thinking that will take nurse scientists into the next millennium.

---

the capacity for abstraction and imagery, language and thought, sensation and emotion" (1970, p. 73).

Environment. The environment is an irreducible pandimensional energy field identified by pattern and integral with the human energy field (Rogers, 1994). The individual and the environment are continually exchanging matter and energy with one another, resulting in changing patterns in both the individual and the environment.

Health and illness. Health and illness are value laden, arbitrarily defined, and culturally infused notions. They are not dichotomous but are part of the same continuum. Health seems to occur when patterns of living are in harmony with environmental change, whereas illness occurs when patterns of living are in conflict with environmental change and are deemed unacceptable.

Nursing. A science and an art, nursing is unique in its concern with unitary human beings as synergistic phenomena. The science of nursing should be concerned with studying the nature and direction of unitary human development integral with the environment and with evolving descriptive, explanatory, and predictive principles for use in nursing practice. The new age of nursing science is characterized by a synthesis of fact and ideas that generate principles and theories (Rogers, 1994). The art of nursing is the creative use of the science of nursing for human betterment (Rogers, 1990). The goal of nursing is the attainment of the best possible state of health for the individual who is continually evolving by promoting symphonic interactions between humans and environments, strengthening the coherence and integrity of the human field, and directing and redirecting patterning of both fields for maximum health potential.

Key concepts. The concepts describe the individual and environment as energy fields that are in constant interaction. The nature and direction of human development form the basis for the principles of nursing science:

Energy field—the fundamental unit of the living and nonliving. Energy fields are dynamic, continuously in motion, and infinite. They are of two types:

Human energy field—more than the biological, psychological, and sociological fields taken separately or together; an irreducible, indivisible, pandimensional whole identified by pattern and manifesting characteristics that cannot be predicted from the parts.

Environmental energy field—an irreducible, indivisible, pandimensional energy field identified by pattern and integral with the human field.

Openness—continuous change and mutual process as manifested in human and environmental fields.

Pattern—the distinguishing characteristic of an energy field perceived as a single wave.

Pandimensionality—replaces the earlier term *four-dimensionality* and is a nonlinear domain thought to characterize human and environmental fields without spatial and temporal attributes.

Principles of nursing science—postulate the nature and direction of unitary human development; also called principles of homeodynamics, which are as follows:

Helicy—"the continuous, innovative, probabilistic, increasing diversity of human and environmental field patterns characterized by repeating rhymicities" (1989, p. 186).

Resonancy—"the continuous change from lower to higher frequency wave patterns in human and environmental fields" (1989, p. 186); the process of change is one of increasing diversity.

Integrality—replacing the earlier concept of complementarity, it is "the continuous mutual human and environmental field process" (1989, p. 186).

Orem's Self-Care Deficit Theory

Foundations of Dorothea Orem's theory were introduced in the late 1950s, but it was not until 1971 that the first edition of *Nursing: Concepts of Practice* was published. The second, third, fourth, and fifth editions were published in 1980, 1985, 1991, and 1995, respectively, and show evidence of development and refinement of the theory. Orem focuses on nursing as deliberate human action and notes that all individuals can benefit from nursing when they have health-derived or health-related limitations for engaging in self-care or the care of dependent others.

Brief overview. The individual practices self-care, a set of learned behaviors, to sustain life, maintain or restore functioning, and bring about a condition of well-being. The nurse assists the client with self-care when there is a deficit in his or her ability to perform.

Assumptions about the individual. The individual is viewed as a unity whose functioning is linked with the environment and who, with the environment, forms an integrated, functional whole. The individual functions biologically, symbolically, and socially.

Environment. The environment is linked to the individual, forming an integrated system. It is implied that the environment is external to the individual.

Health and illness. Health, which has physical, psychological, interpersonal, and social aspects, is a state in which human beings are structurally and functionally whole. Illness occurs when an individual is incapable of maintaining self-care as a result of structural or functional limitations.

Nursing. Nursing involves assisting the individual with self-care practices to sustain life and health, recover from disease or injury, and cope with their effects (1985). The nurse chooses deliberate actions from nursing systems (see below) designed to bring about desirable conditions in persons and their environments. The goal of nursing is to move a patient toward responsible self-care or meet existing health care needs of those who have health care deficits.

Key concepts. The concepts focus on self-care in terms of requisites, demands, and deficits, and delineate the nurse's role in client care:

Self-care—activities that individuals initiate and perform on their own behalf to maintain life, health, or well-being.
Self-care requisites—three categories:
   Universal—common to all human beings; concerned with the promotion and maintenance of structural and functional integrity. These include air, water, food, elimination, activity and rest, solitude and social interaction, prevention of hazards, and promotion of human functioning.
   Developmental—associated with conditions that promote known developmental processes at each stage of the life cycle.
   Health-deviation—genetic and constitutional defects and deviations that affect integrated human functioning and impair the individual's ability to perform self-care.
Therapeutic self-care demands—based on the notion that self-care is a human regulatory function; the totality of self-care actions performed by the nurse or self in order to meet known self-care requisites.
Self-care deficits—gaps between known therapeutic self-care demands and the ability to perform self-care.
Nursing systems—systems of concrete actions, which are of three types:
   Wholly compensatory—the nurse compensates for the individual's total inability to perform self-care activities.
   Partly compensatory—the nurse compensates for the individual's inability to perform some (but not all) self-care activities.

Supportive-educative—with the individual able to perform all self-care activities, the nurse assists the client in decision making, behavior control, and the acquisition of knowledge and skill.

Subsystems of each nursing system:

Social—the complementary and contractual relationship between the nurse and the client.

Interpersonal—the nurse-client interaction.

Technological—"diagnosis, prescription, regulation of treatment, and management of nursing care" (1985, p. 160).

King's Theory of Goal Attainment

Although the foundation for her theory was developed in 1964, it was not until her 1971 publication *Toward a Theory for Nursing* that Imogene King presented her entire conceptual framework and identified the concepts of social systems, health, perception, and interpersonal relations. The theory was refined in *A Theory for Nursing: Systems, Concepts, Process* (1981), where King identified the focus of nursing as being on people interacting with their environments, leading to a state of health, which is the ability to function in roles. The theory is derived from a systems framework and is concerned with human transactions in different types of environments (King, 1995a).

Brief overview. The individual is viewed as an open system and as one component of a nurse-client interpersonal system whose interactions lead to the attainment of mutually agreed-on goals.

Assumptions about the individual. Human beings are open systems in transaction with the environment and are conceptualized as social, sentient, rational, perceiving, controlling, purposeful, action-oriented beings.

Environment. As an open system, it is implied that the individual and the environment interact and that both the internal and external environments generate stressors.

Health and illness. Health is described as an individual's ability to function in social roles. This implies optimal use of one's resources to achieve continuous adjustment to internal and external environmental stressors. Illness is a deviation from normal, an imbalance in a person's biologic structure, psychological makeup, or social relationships.

Nursing. A process of action, reaction, and interaction, the nurse and client communicate, set goals, and explore means to achieve those goals. "The domain of nursing includes promoting, maintaining and restoring health, caring for the sick and injured and caring for the dying" (1981, p. 4). The goal of nursing is to help individuals to maintain their health so they can function in their roles. "The goal of the nursing system, as a whole, is health for individuals, health for groups, such as the family, and health for communities within a society" (1995b, p. 24).

Key Concepts. Two sets of concepts are subsumed in the theory, one relating to the parties involved in the nurse-client relationship and the other pertaining to the process of goal attainment:

Concepts related to the nurse-client relationship:
   Personal system—an individual.
   Interpersonal system—two or more interacting individuals.
   Social system—communities and societies.
Concepts related to goal attainment:
   Communication—process of giving information from one person to another.
   Interaction—process of perception between the person and environment or one or more persons, represented by verbal and nonverbal behaviors that are goal directed.
   Perception—an individual's representation of reality.
   Transaction—observable behavior or individuals interacting with their environment.
   Role—a set of behaviors displayed by the individual, who occupies a given position in a social system.
   Stress—a dynamic state of interaction with the environment to maintain balance for growth, development, and performance.
   Growth and development—"continuous changes in individuals occurring at molecular, cellular, and behavioral levels" (1981, p. 148).
   Time—a duration between one event and another.
   Space—defined by "gestures, postures, and visible boundaries erected to mark off personal space" (1981, p. 148).

Roy's Adaptation Model

Sister Callista Roy has continuously expanded her model from its inception in the 1960s to the present time. She focuses on the individual as a biopsychosocial adaptive system and describes nursing as a humanistic discipline that "places emphasis on the person's own coping abilities" (1984, p. 32). The individual and the environment are sources of stimuli that require modification to promote adaptation.

Brief overview. The individual is a biopsychosocial adaptive system, and the nurse promotes adaptation by modifying external stimuli.

Assumptions about the individual. The individual is in constant interaction with a changing environment, and to respond positively to environmental change, a person must adapt. The person's adaptation level is determined by the combined effect of three classes of stimuli—focal, contextual, and residual. The individual uses both innate and acquired biological, psychological, or social adaptive mechanisms and has four modes of adaptation.

Environment. All conditions, circumstances, and influences surrounding and affecting the development and behavior of persons and groups constitute the environment. Having both internal and external components, the environment is constantly changing.

Health and illness. "Health and illness are one inevitable dimension of a person's life" (1989, p. 106). Health is a process of being and becoming an integrated and whole person. Conversely, illness is a lack of integration.

Nursing. An external regulatory force, nursing acts to modify stimuli affecting adaptation by increasing, decreasing, or maintaining stimuli. The goal of nursing is to promote the person's adaptation in the four adaptive modes, thus contributing to health, the quality of life, and dying with dignity.

Key concepts. The concepts describe and define adaptation in terms of the individual's internal control processes, adaptive modes, and adaptive level:

Adaptation—the individual's ability to cope with the constantly changing environment.

Adaptive system—consists of two major internal control processes:

Regulator—receives input from the external environment and from changes in the person's internal state and processes it through neural-chemical-endocrine channels.

Cognator—receives input from external and internal stimuli that involve psychological, social, physical, and physiological factors and processes it through cognitive pathways.

Adaptive modes—ways a person adapts. There are four modes:

Physiological—determined by the need for physiological integrity derived from the basic physiological needs.

Self-concept—determined by the need for interactions with others and psychic integrity regarding the perception of self.

Role function—determined by the need for social integrity; refers to the performance of duties based on given positions within society.

Interdependence—involves ways of seeking help, affection, and attention.

Adaptive level—determined by the combined effects of stimuli:

Focal stimuli—that which immediately confronts the individual.

Contextual stimuli—all other stimuli present.

Residual stimuli—beliefs, attitudes, or traits that have an indeterminate effect on the present situation.

Neuman's Systems Model

Betty Neuman developed her systems model in 1970 in response to student requests to focus on breadth rather than depth in understanding human variables in nursing problems. First published in 1972, it was refined to its present form and published in *The Neuman Systems Model* (1989, 1995). Neuman believes that nursing encompasses a wholistic client systems approach to help individuals, families, communities, and society reach and maintain wellness. Neuman's focus on the whole system explains her use of the term "wholistic."

Brief overview. This theory offers a wholistic view of the client system, including the concepts of open system, environment, stressors, prevention, and reconstitution. Nursing is concerned with the whole person.

Assumptions about the individual. The client is a whole person, a dynamic composite of interrelationships between physiological, psychological, sociocultural, developmental, and spiritual variables. "The client is viewed as an open system in interaction with the environment" (1989, p. 68). The client is in "dynamic constant energy exchange with the environment" (1989, p. 22).

Environment. Both internal and external environments exist, and the person maintains varying degrees of harmony between them. The environment includes all internal and external factors affecting and affected by the system (1995). Emphasis is on all stressors—interpersonal, intrapersonal, extrapersonal—that might disturb the person's normal line of defense.

Health and illness. "Health is equated with optimal system stability" (1989, p. 33). Disharmony among parts of the system is considered illness. "The wellness-illness continuum implies that energy flow is continuous between the client system and the environment" (1989, p. 33).

Nursing. Nursing is a "unique profession in that it is concerned with all of the variables affecting the individual's response to stress" (1982, p. 14). The major concern of nursing is in "keeping the client system stable through accuracy in both the assessment of effects and possible effects of environmental stressors and in assisting client adjustments required for an optimal wellness level" (1989, p. 34). Nursing goals are determined by "negotiation with the client for desired prescriptive changes to correct variances from wellness" (1989, p. 73).

Key concepts. The nurse is concerned with all the variables affecting an individual's response to stressors:

Concepts related to client system stability:
> *Flexible line of defense*—outer boundary that ideally prevents stressors from entering the system.
> *Normal line of defense*—represents a range of responses to environmental stressors when the flexible line of defense is penetrated (1995).
> *Lines of resistance*—protect the basic structure of the client and become activated when the normal line of defense is invaded by environmental stressors.
> *Interventions*—purposeful nursing actions that help clients retain, attain, and/or maintain system stability. There are three levels of intervention:

Primary prevention—reduces the possibility of encounter with stressors and strengthens the flexible lines of defense.

Secondary prevention—relates to appropriate prioritizing of interventions to reduce symptoms resulting from invasion of environmental stressors; protects the basic structure by strengthening the internal lines of resistance.

Tertiary prevention—focuses on readaptation and stability. A primary goal is to strengthen resistance to stressors by reeducation to help prevent recurrence of reaction or regression. "Tertiary prevention tends to lead back, in a circular fashion, toward primary prevention" (1989, p. 73).

Leininger's Cultural Care Theory

Drawing from a background in cultural and social anthropology, Madeleine Leininger's contribution to nursing knowledge is related to transcultural nursing and caring. Her book, *Transcultural Nursing: Concepts, Theories and Practice* (1978), presented her conceptual framework for cultural care and health. She continues to explicate the linkages between nursing and anthropology as she identifies and defines concepts such as care, caring, culture, cultural values, and cultural variations (1984, 1991).

Brief overview. Transcultural nursing focuses on a comparative study and analysis of different cultures and subcultures in the world with respect to their caring behavior, nursing care, health-illness values, and patterns of behavior with the goal of developing a scientific and humanistic body of knowledge in order to derive culture-specific and culture-universal nursing care practices (1978).

Assumptions about the individual. Clients are caring and cultural beings who perceive health, illness, caring, curing, dependence, and independence differently. The social structure, world view, and values of people vary transculturally.

Environment. The environment is defined as a social structure, the "interrelated and interdependent systems of a society which determine how it functions with respect to certain major elements, namely: the political (including legal), economic, social (including kinship), educational, technical, religious, and cultural systems" (1978, p. 61).

Health and illness. Perceptions of health and illness are culturally infused and therefore cannot be universally defined. "Health refers to a state of well-being that is culturally defined, valued, and practiced, and which reflects the ability of individuals (or groups) to perform their daily role activities in culturally expressed, beneficial, and patterned lifeways" (1991, p. 48). World views, social structure, and cultural beliefs influence perceptions of health and illness and cannot be separated from them. For example, some cultures perceive illness to be largely a personal and internal body experience, whereas others view illness as an extrapersonal or cultural experience.

Nursing. Nursing is a learned humanistic and scientific profession that focuses on personalized (individual and group) care behaviors, functions, and processes that have physical, psychocultural, and social significance or meaning. The goal of nursing is to assist, support, facilitate, or enable individuals or groups to regain or maintain their health in a way that is culturally congruent, or to help people face handicaps or death (1991).

Key concepts. Among the core concepts of transcultural nursing theory are:

Care—phenomena related to assistive, supportive, or enabling behavior toward or for another individual with evident or anticipated needs to ease or improve a human condition.

Caring—actions directed toward assisting, supporting, or enabling an individual (or group) to ameliorate or improve the human condition or lifeway.

Culture—values, beliefs, norms, and lifeway practices of a particular group that guides thinking, decisions, and actions in patterned ways.

Cultural care—the cognitively known values, beliefs, and patterned lifeways that assist, support, or enable another individual or group to maintain well-being, improve a human condition or lifeway, or deal with illness, handicaps, or death.

> *Cultural care diversity*—the variability of meaning, patterns, values, lifeways, or symbols of care that are culturally derived for health or to improve a human condition.

> *Cultural care universality*—common, similar or uniform care meanings, patterns, values, lifeways, or symbols that are culturally derived for health or to improve a human condition.

Cultural-congruent care—assistive, supportive, facilitative, or enabling acts or decisions that fit individual, group, or institutional cultural values, beliefs, and lifeways (1991).

> *Cultural care preservation or maintenance*—professional actions and decisions that help people of a particular culture to retain and/or preserve relevant care values.

> *Cultural care accommodation or negotiation*—professional actions and decisions that help people of a designated culture adapt to or negotiate with others for a beneficial or satisfying health outcome.

> *Cultural care repatterning or restructuring*—professional actions and decisions that help a client change or modify their lifeway to improve health while still respecting the client's cultural values and beliefs.

Watson's Philosophy and Science of Caring

Jean Watson's theoretical formulations focus on the philosophy and science of caring, the core of nursing. With an aim toward reducing the dichotomy between nursing theory and practice, the framework was first published in 1979 and further developed in her 1985 and 1988 publications. Watson draws from multiple disciplines to derive carative factors that are central to nursing and describes concepts as they relate to the pivotal theme of caring.

Brief overview. Caring, a moral ideal rather than a task-oriented behavior, is central to nursing practice and includes aspects of the actual caring occasion and the transpersonal caring relationship. An interpersonal process, caring results in the satisfaction of human needs.

Assumptions about the individual. Individuals (i.e., both the nurse and the client) are nonreducible and are interconnected with others and nature (1985, p. 16).

Environment. The client's environment contains both external and internal variables. The nurse promotes a caring environment, one that allows individuals to make choices relative to the best action for him or her at that point in time.

Health and illness. Health is more than the absence of illness, but because it is subjective, it is an illusive concept. "Health refers to unity and harmony within the mind, body, and soul" (1985, p. 48). Conversely, illness is disharmony within the spheres of the person.

Nursing. The practice of nursing is different from curing and consists of ten carative factors as described below. The goal of nursing is to help persons attain a higher degree of harmony by offering a relationship that the client can use for personal growth and development.

Key concepts. The caring relationship and ten carative factors form the core of nursing and delineate the domain of nursing practice:

Transpersonal caring—an intersubjective human-to-human relationship in which the nurse affects and is affected by the other person (client). Caring is the moral ideal of nursing where there is the utmost concern for human dignity and preservation of humanity (1985).
Carative factors (1979):
   1. Formation of a humanistic-altruistic system of values
   2. Instillation of faith-hope to promote wellness
   3. Cultivation of sensitivity to self and to others
   4. Development of a helping-trust relationship
   5. Promotion and acceptance of the expression of positive and negative feelings
   6. Systematic use of the scientific problem-solving method for decision making
   7. Promotion of interpersonal teaching-learning
   8. Provision for a supportive, protective, and/or corrective mental, physical, sociocultural, and spiritual environment
   9. Assistance with the gratification of human needs
  10. Allowance for existential-phenomenological forces

In addition to the carative factors, nurses must facilitate clients' development in the area of health promotion through teaching preventive health actions.

Johnson's Behavioral System Model

Originally presented as a paper at Vanderbilt University in 1968, Dorothy Johnson did not personally publish her theory of nursing until 1980. However, her early paper was widely cited, and published interpretations of it appeared in 1974 (Grubbs, 1974) and 1976 (Auger, 1976). Johnson views the individual as a behavioral system that is continually striving for balance. The nurse fosters "efficient and effective behavioral functioning...to prevent illness and during and following illness" (1980, p. 207).

Brief overview. The individual is viewed as a collection of interrelated behavioral subsystems whose response patterns form an organized and integrated whole. The nurse serves as an external regulatory force to preserve and maintain system balance.

Assumptions about the individual. A behavioral system composed of a set of behavioral subsystems, the individual strives to attain and maintain behavioral system balance, sometimes requiring adaptation and modification to return to a steady state. The individual is characterized by organization, interaction, interdependency, and integration of the parts and elements (subsystems).

Environment. The natural forces impinging on the individual constitute the environment in which the behavioral system exists. There are both internal and external environments, but these are not defined.

Health and illness. It may be inferred that health is a state of balance in which the behavioral system is self-maintaining and self-perpetuating, and interrelationships between the subsystems are harmonious. Conversely, illness is a state of disorganization and dysfunction of the system.

Nursing. Described as an external regulatory force, the practice of nursing imposes external controls to fulfill the functional requirements of the subsystems. The goal of nursing is "to restore, maintain or attain behavioral system balance and stability at the highest possible level for the individual" (1980, p. 214).

Key concepts. The concepts describe the individual as a set of subsystems that, together, form a behavioral system:

Behavioral system—composed of seven behavioral subsystems that are integrated and that characterize each person's life.
Behavioral subsystem—a formed set of behavioral responses that seem to share a common drive but that are modified over time through maturation or learning. The seven subsystems are:
Affiliative—security as a consequence of social inclusion, intimacy, and the formation and maintenance of a strong social bond.
Dependency—succoring behavior that calls for the response of nurturing and has as its consequence approval, attention, or physical assistance.

Ingestive—appetite satisfaction as it is governed by social and psychological considerations.

Eliminative—elimination of body wastes as a learned behavior that strongly influences purely biological eliminative acts.

Sexual—procreation and gratification with responses originating with gender role identity and the broad range of behaviors dependent on one's biological sex.

Achievement—mastery or control over some aspect of the self or environment; includes intelligence, physical, creative, mechanical, care-taking, and social skills.

Aggressive—protection and preservation of self and society within the limits imposed by society.

Parse's Theory of Human Becoming

Rosemarie Rizzo Parse developed a philosophical model that focuses on the inseparable concepts of man-living-health as nursing's concern. Taking an existential approach, she derived three principles that center on the idea of man-living-health always moving toward greater diversity and "becoming" (1981).

Brief overview. Always in the process of becoming, man-living-health are inseparable. Nursing is a human science that focuses on man and health.

Assumptions about the individual. The individual is an open being, coexisting with the environment. Man freely chooses meaning in situations and bears responsibility for decisions. As life progresses, individuals become more complex and diverse, forming new patterns of relating.

Environment. The environment is inseparable from the individual. Both man and the environment interchange energy, unfold together toward greater complexity and diversity, and influence one another's rhythmical patterns of relating.

Health and illness. Health is an open process of becoming and is a rhythmically co-constituting process of the man-environment interrelationship. Illness is not the opposite of health but rather a pattern of man's interrelationship with the world (1981). Both health and illness are lived experiences.

Nursing. A human science, nursing focuses on man as a living unity and his participation in health experiences. The goal of nursing is to illuminate and mobilize family (human) interrelationships.

Key concepts. The concepts are incorporated into three major principles that focus on meaning, rhythmicity, and cotranscendence. Within each principle, succeeding concepts build on preceding ones.

Meaning—arises from man's interrelationship with the world and refers to happenings to which we attach varying degrees of significance.
Imaging—a process that structures the meaning of an experience.
Valuing—a process of confirming cherished beliefs.
Languaging—expressing valued images.
Rhythmicity—the movement of man and environment toward greater diversity.
    Revealing-concealing—disclosing of some aspects of self and hiding of others all at once.
    Enabling-limiting—the result of making choices; in choosing, one is both enabled in some things and limited in others.
    Connecting-separating—a simultaneous process; connecting with some phenomena results in separating from others.
Cotranscendence—the process of reaching out beyond the self.
    Powering—a process of moving toward all future possibilities.
    Originating—creating unique ways of living; distinguishing self from others.
    Transforming—an ongoing process of change; moving toward greater diversity by transcending the present.

APPLICATION TO NURSING PRACTICE

It is evident that the nursing theories and frameworks discussed here offer a variety of perspectives. For example, some are process oriented and dynamic, such as Peplau's interpersonal process, King's theory of goal attainment, Rogers' science of unitary human beings, and Parse's human becoming. Others are more outcome oriented, such as Roy's adaptation model, Johnson's behavioral system model, and Orem's self-care deficit theory. Rogers' and Neuman's models focus on the wholeness of the individual and conceptualize nursing as one component of the individual's life process. King's theory is directed toward the interaction between the nurse and the client, who are inseparable. Leininger, Nightingale, and Henderson developed humanistic perspectives, since they focus on personalized, individualized care for all. Johnson and Roy conceptualize the nurse as an external regulator whose function is to promote system balance or adaptation. Orem views the nurse as one who assists the individual with self-care practices when the individual is unable to effectively care for himself or herself.

Most of the nursing theories presented in this chapter are too extensive to be used in their entirety in a given nursing care situation. For example, Orem describes three types of nursing systems, but for a client who is in the intensive care unit and on life support, only the wholly compensatory nursing system is relevant. Similarly, with Neuman's three levels of prevention, only clients with symptoms resulting from invasion of environmental stressors are appropriate recipients of secondary prevention. However, the theories can guide nursing assessment in terms of what questions to ask and what areas to assess. For instance, a nurse using Roy's adaptation model would assess the biological, psychological, and social aspects of the client. Similarly, the nurse who uses Johnson's behavioral system model would assess the seven subsystems for evidence of system balance or imbalance. The type of client, the setting where care is delivered, and the goal of nursing are what influence the selection of an appropriate theoretical framework for practice. The more specific theories can be readily adapted for use in a practice setting. The more global theories may better serve as frameworks for research, the findings of which can then be applied to practice.

EVALUATING THE UTILITY OF NURSING THEORIES AND FRAMEWORKS

Not all theories and frameworks are equally comprehensive or equally useful in every situation; nor are they meant to be, as discussed in this chapter. The definition of the client and the setting where care is delivered limit the utility of some of the theories and frameworks presented here. To be useful in practice, a theory must work in a specific setting. Its concepts must be operationalized in ways that promote application and facilitate nursing activities in that setting (Barnum, 1994). It is important to examine a theory's utility for the intended use and the consistency of its internal structure. The value and logical structure of a theory can be evaluated by asking questions proposed by Fawcett (1989, 1993), such as:

1. Are the assumptions inherent in the theory clearly stated?
2. Are the relationships between the concepts clearly explained?
3. Is the theory stated clearly and concisely?
4. Are there conflicting views within the structure of the theory?
5. Can relationships between concepts be tested in research (i.e., observed and measured) and applied to practice?
6. Does the theory lead to nursing activities that meet societal expectations (social congruence)?
7. Does the theory lead to nursing activities that are likely to result in favorable client outcomes (social significance)?
8. Does the theory include explicit rules for use in practice, education, or research (social usefulness)?

THEORIES FROM RELATED DISCIPLINES

Several nursing theories derived their conceptual basis from theories developed by related disciplines and adapted to specific situations. Many of these theories are useful and relevant to nursing in their original form. For example, systems theory (von Bertalanffy, 1956) is useful as an approach to assess individuals, families, and communities as described in Chapter 6. General adaptation syndrome (GAS), a theory of adaptation to stress, describes three phases of adjustment to stress: alarm reaction, stage of resistance, and stage of exhaustion (Selye, 1974, 1982). This theory can be applied to clients who are suffering not only psychological or social stress, but physiological stress as well. Theories of coping have been developed by Lazarus and Folkman (1984) and by McCubbin and Patterson (1981), who agree that coping is the process that leads to adaptation. For clients experiencing an intense level of stress, nursing interventions designed to promote and support the coping process can be derived from the relationships specified by this theory. Both coping and adjustment are embedded in Duvall's (1977) stages of family life and developmental tasks, which can serve as the framework for delivering age-specific or situation-specific nursing interventions. Aguilera (1994) provides a theory and framework for successful resolution of a crisis situation.

These theories are only a sample of those developed by related disciplines that can be useful to nursing. One or more of these theories can serve as a framework for designing interventions for clients throughout the life cycle, developing and implementing research studies, and framing educational curricula. In combination with nursing theories, there is a wide array of theoretical perspectives in various stages of development from which to choose.

 ## Key Points

- A theory is a group of statements that describe the relationship between two or more concepts.

- The main components of nursing theories are persons, environment, health/illness, and nursing.

- Nightingale's theory focuses on nursing's role in manipulating the environment.

- Peplau's theory centers on the interpersonal process in nursing.

- Henderson identifies 14 basic patient needs that constitute the components of nursing care.

- According to Rogers, the nurse seeks to promote coherence between individuals and their environments.

- According to Orem, the nurse assists the individual with self-care practices when there is a deficit in the client's own ability for self-care.

- King conceptualizes the nurse and the client as components of an interpersonal system who seek to attain mutually agreed-on goals.

- Roy's theory describes the client as a biopsychosocial adaptive system and the nurse as one who modifies stimuli to promote adaptation.

- Three levels of nursing intervention—primary, secondary, and tertiary prevention—are specified in Neuman's systems model.

- Leininger's theory centers on providing culturally congruent nursing care.

- Watson identifies the caring relationship and 10 carative factors that form the core of nursing.

- Johnson's theory describes the nurse as an external regulatory force whose goal is to restore behavioral system balance.

- Parse describes nursing as a human science that focuses on man and health.

- The more specific theories, in whole or in part, can be readily adapted for use in any practice setting.

- The more global theories may better serve as frameworks for research, the findings of which can then be applied to practice.

- Theories from related disciplines also have relevance to nursing practice, education, and research.

- All theories have the potential to make substantial contributions to the nursing profession by enhancing the development of a unique body of nursing knowledge.

 ## *Critical Thinking Exercises*

1. "An individual is in constant interaction with the environment." Apply this statement to the client in each of the following settings and discuss the implications for nursing practice:
   a. A community mental health clinic
   b. An intensive care unit
   c. An extended care facility
   d. A well-baby clinic

2. How do Florence Nightingale's ideas apply to nursing practice in the current health care system?

3. Defend or refute the following statement: "We should have only one nursing theory, rather than several, to guide education, practice, and research."

4. Compare and contrast the definitions of health and illness in two nursing theories, citing similarities and differences. Which one of these is most closely aligned with your own definitions of health and illness?

References

Aguilera, D.C. (1994). *Crisis intervention: Theory and methodology* (7th ed.). St. Louis: Mosby.

Auger, J.R. (1976). *Behavioral systems and nursing.* Englewood Cliffs, NJ: Prentice Hall.

Barnum, B.J.S. (1994). *Nursing theory: Analysis, application, evaluation* (4th ed.). Philadelphia: J.B. Lippincott.

Chinn, P.L. & Jacobs, M.K. (1987). *Theory and nursing: A systematic approach* (2nd ed.). St. Louis: Mosby.

Christensen, P.J., & Kenney, J.W. (1995) *Nursing process: Application of conceptual models* (4th ed.). St. Louis: Mosby.

Duvall, E.M. (1977). *Marriage and family development* (5th ed.). New York: J.B. Lippincott.

Fawcett, J. (1989). *Conceptual models of nursing* (2nd ed.). Philadelphia: F.A. Davis.

Fawcett, J. (1993). *Analysis and evaluation of nursing theories.* Philadelphia: F.A. Davis.

Fawcett, J., & Downs, F. (1992). *The relationship of theory and research* (2nd ed.). Philadelphia: F.A. Davis.

Grubbs, J. (1974). An interpretation of the Johnson behavioral system model. In J.P. Reihl, & C. Roy, *Conceptual models for nursing practice* (pp. 160-197). New York: Appleton-Century-Crofts.

Henderson, V. (1966). *The nature of nursing: A definition and its implications for practice, research, and education.* New York: Macmillan.

Henderson, V. (1971). Health is everybody's business. *Canadian Nurse, 67,* 31-34.

Henderson, V., & Nite, G. (1978). *The principles and practice of nursing.* New York: Macmillan.

Hickman, J.S. (1995). An introduction to nursing theory. In J.B. George, *Nursing theories: The base for professional practice* (4th ed., pp. 1-14), Norwalk, CT: Appleton & Lange.

Johnson, D.E. (1980). The behavioral system model for nursing. In J.P. Reihl, & C. Roy, *Conceptual models for nursing practice* (2nd ed., pp. 207-215). New York: Appleton-Century-Crofts.

Keck, J. (1994). Terminology of theory development. In A. Marriner-Toomy, *Nursing theorists and their work* (3rd ed., pp. 17-36). St. Louis: Mosby.

King, I. (1971). *Toward a theory for nursing.* New York: John Wiley & Sons.

King, I. (1981). *A theory for nursing: Systems, concepts, process.* New York: John Wiley & Sons.

King, I. (1995a). A systems framework for nursing. In M.A. Frey & C.L. Sieloff (Eds.), *Advancing King's systems framework and theory of nursing* (pp. 14-21). Thousand Oaks, CA: Sage Publications.

King, I. (1995b). The theory of goal attainment. In M. Frey & C.L. Sieloff (Eds.), *Advancing King's systems framework and theory of nursing* (pp. 23-32). Thousand Oaks, CA: Sage Publications.

Lazarus, R.S., & Folkman, S. (1984). *Stress appraisal and coping.* New York: Springer.

Leininger, M. (1978). *Transcultural nursing: Concepts, theories and practices.* New York: John Wiley & Sons.

Leininger, M. (Ed.) (1984). *Care: The essence of nursing and health.* Thorofare, NJ: Charles B. Slack.

Leininger, M. (1991). *Culture, care, diversity and universality: A theory of nursing* (NLN Publication No. 15-2402). New York: National League for Nursing.

Levine, M.E. (1995). The rhetoric of nursing theory. *Image: Journal of Nursing Scholarship 27*(1), 11-14.

McCubbin, H.I., & Patterson, J.M. (1981). *Family stress: Resources and coping.* St. Paul, MN: University of Minnesota.

Neuman, B. (1982). *The Neuman systems model: Application to nursing theory and practice* (1st ed.). Norwalk, CT: Appleton-Century-Crofts.

Neuman, B. (1989). *The Neuman systems model* (2nd ed.). Norwalk, CT: Appleton & Lange.

Neuman, B. (1995). *The Neuman systems model* (3rd ed.). Norwalk, CT: Appleton & Lange.

Neuman, B.M., & Young, R.J. (1972). A model for teaching total person approach to patient problems. *Nursing Research, 21,* 264-269.

Nightingale, F. (1946). *Notes on nursing: What it is and what it is not.* Philadelphia: Edward Stern. (Original work published 1859).

Orem, D.E. (1980). *Nursing: Concepts of practice* (2nd ed.). New York: McGraw-Hill.

Orem, D.E. (1985). *Nursing: Concepts of practice* (3rd ed.). New York: McGraw-Hill.

Orem, D.E. (1991). *Nursing: Concepts of practice* (4th ed.). St. Louis: Mosby.

Orem, D.E. (1995). *Nursing: Concepts of practice* (5th ed.). St. Louis: Mosby.

Parse, R. (1981). *Man-living-health: A theory of nursing.* New York: John Wiley & Sons.

Peplau, H. (1952). *Interpersonal relations in nursing: A conceptual frame of reference for psychodynamic nursing.* New York: G.P. Putnam's Sons. (Reprinted in 1988 by MacMillan and in 1991 by Springer).

Peplau, H. (1992). Interpersonal relations: A theoretical framework for application in nursing practice. *Nursing Science Quarterly, 5,* 13-18.

Rogers, M.E. (1970). *An introduction to the theoretical basis of nursing.* Philadelphia: F.A. Davis.

Rogers, M.E. (1989). Nursing: A science of unitary man. In J.P. Reihl-Sisca (Ed.), *Conceptual models for nursing practice* (3rd ed., pp. 181-188). Norwalk: Appleton & Lange.

Rogers, M.E. (1990). Nursing: Science of unitary, irreducible, human beings: Update 1990. In E.A.M. Barrett, *Visions of Rogers' science-based nursing* (pp. 5-11). New York: National League for Nursing.

Rogers, M.E. (1994). Nursing science evolves. In M.A. Madrid & E.A.M. Barrett (Eds.), *Rogers' scientific art of nursing practice* (NLN Publication No. 15-2610, pp. 3-9). New York: National League for Nursing.

Roy, C., Sr. (1980). The Roy adaptation model. In J.P. Reihl & C. Roy, *Conceptual models for nursing practice* (2nd ed., pp. 179-188). New York: Appleton-Century-Crofts.

Roy, C., Sr. (1984). *Introduction to nursing: An adaptation model* (2nd ed.). Englewood Cliffs, NJ: Prentice-Hall.

Roy, C., Sr. (1989). The Roy Adaptation Model. In J.P. Reihl-Sisca (Ed.), *Conceptual models for nursing practice* (3rd ed., pp. 105-114). Norwalk, CT: Appleton & Lange.

Selye, H. (1974). *Stress without distress.* Philadelphia: J.B. Lippincott.

Selye, H. (1982). History and the present status of the stress concept. In I.A. Goldberger & S. Breznitz (Eds.),

Handbook of stress: Theoretical and clinical aspects. New York: The Free Press.

von Bertalanffy, L. (1956). General systems theory. In B.D. Ruben & J. Kim (Eds.), *General systems theory and human communication* (pp. 7-16). Rochelle Park, NJ: Hayden.

Watson, J. (1979). *Nursing: The philosophy and science of caring.* Boston: Little-Brown.

Watson, J. (1985). *Nursing: Human science and health care.* Norwalk, CT: Appleton-Century-Crofts.

Watson, J. (1988). *Nursing: Human science and human caring—a theory of nursing.* New York: National League for Nursing.

Issues in Health Care Delivery and Nursing

8

Cheryl Bland Jones

Objectives

At the completion of this chapter, the reader will be able to:

- Identify changes in the overall health care system and nursing profession.

- Discuss how the health care environment is responding to escalating costs of care.

- Describe how health care organizations are restructuring nursing and patient care services.

- Discuss the challenges and opportunities that lie ahead for nursing, and how the nursing profession can meet those challenges.

Profile in Practice

Karen Cober, MSN, RN
Administrator, Tennessee Nursing Services,
Morristown, Tennessee

I have assumed a variety of roles since obtaining my associate degree in nursing more than 15 years ago. I was a critical care staff nurse, associate director of nursing education, and, subsequently, director of nursing education in a community hospital. During this time I obtained my BSN and MSN degrees. Although my clinical background is cardiovascular nursing, I was always interested in administration. When the opportunity was presented to me, I accepted the position of director of nursing services in a community hospital. Hospital administration is frustrating during these changing times, and when I accomplished everything I thought I could do in the hospital setting, I looked toward home health for new challenges.

I became an assistant administrator in a proprietary home health agency that ultimately was purchased by the local community hospital. The proprietary agency operated parallel to the hospital-based home health agency for a while, and when they merged, I was asked to assume administrative responsibility for all of home health. This agency covers a geographical area of more than 20 counties, has several offices, and includes three hospice units.

The uncertain direction of the health care system as a whole presents special challenges for home health care. For example, if prospective payment for home health care is introduced, it will require better case management than is currently in place to provide the most cost-effective care possible. Both patients and staff will have to be educated about how to work within a prospective system of reimbursement. In addition, as more hospitals come under capitated contracts, it is anticipated that there will be more and more referrals for home health care. This could be a problem for the financial viability of private home health agencies, since hospitals are more likely to refer to their own home health services.

The greatest challenges of my role are keeping up with changes in health care regulations and trying to outguess the system. It is important to monitor proposed legislation and to use any political ties one might have to influence the system to enact legislation that benefits both patients and providers.

Change and health care delivery are inextricably linked by demographics, government policies, medical technologies, and costs. At the present time, technologies are advancing rapidly, costs are escalating, our population is changing, and government policies are in flux. In an effort to adapt and respond to changing conditions, the health care delivery system is reexamining many economic, allocation, and ethical issues. Changes in health care delivery brought about by these internal and external forces have, and will continue to have, a profound effect on nursing.

In the past, the U.S. health care system has been relatively insensitive to market forces. However, escalating health care costs, societal changes, and reimbursement issues have brought about competition, cost-cutting strategies, downsizing, merging, and organizational restructuring. The full impacts of these organizational responses on access to care, availability and quality of care, and nursing care delivery may not be known for some time.

As health care continues to change and becomes more competitive, individual nurses and the nursing profession will undoubtedly be affected. It therefore becomes imperative that nurses be aware of and anticipate changes in health care, and that nurses welcome the opportunities presented by change. This chapter discusses recent changes in the delivery of health care, issues raised by these changes, and opportunities that these changes present for nursing.

ACCESS, COST, AND QUALITY

Recent health care reform proposals have been introduced to address problems related to access, cost, and quality of health care (see box on p. 170). Nursing's agenda for health care reform, developed by the Tri-Council (a nursing assembly with representa-

The Health Care Reform Debate

Since the late 1980s, health care reform has been a subject of much debate. Some believe that our health care system is in crisis and needs immediate intervention, whereas others believe that our system is working well, as the natural market forces of competition take hold. Regardless of one's view, the sheer fact that "reform" has been discussed widely has pressured health care providers to hold down costs. In fact, earlier health care reform campaigns have had the same effect on health care costs: as awareness and discussions of health care reform intensify, the growth in national health care spending has slowed ("Past Health," 1994). In a similar fashion, as reform discussions abate, health care spending has tended to escalate abruptly.

tion from the National League for Nursing, the American Association of Colleges of Nursing, the American Organization of Nurse Executives, and the American Nurses' Association), articulates the intricate relationship between access, quality, and costs in health care: the escalating cost of health care makes access to health services difficult or impossible for many individuals and potentially jeopardizes the quality of care delivered (American Nurses' Association [ANA] 1991). Given the emphasis on access, cost, and quality, a description of the forces driving these concerns is essential to understanding the changes that are occurring in health care delivery and nursing.

Undoubtedly, the strongest force driving change within health care is cost; the costs of health care are at an all-time high, and we are currently spending more for health care than ever before. Several indicators are frequently used to reflect the escalating costs of health care. Fig. 8-1 illustrates that total national health care expenditures have increased from $27 billion in 1960 to $884.2 billion in 1993 (U.S. Department of Health and Human Services [U.S. DHHS], 1994). This increase represents an 11% average annual growth rate in overall spending during the 33-year period—a doubling every 6½ years. The Congressional Budget Office (CBO) (1993a) predicts that without intervention total national health expenditures will grow to over $2 trillion by the year 2003. This increase in overall spending has been accompanied by an increase in per capita spending for health care—from approximately $204 in 1965 to a projected $3358 in 1993 (CBO, 1993a; U.S. DHHS, 1994). Projections indicate that per capita spending will continue to increase from 1993 levels to over $7000 in 2003 (CBO, 1993a).

A frequently cited indicator of health care costs is the percentage of the U.S. gross domestic product (GDP) that can be attributed to health care. Based on the increase in total and per capita spending, it is not surprising that the percentage of the GDP attributed to health care has increased dramatically over the past 30 years. Fig. 8-2 shows that health care expenditures represented 5.9% of the GDP in 1965 but rose to a level of 13.9% of the GDP in 1993 (U.S. DHHS, 1994). The CBO projects that without intervention national health expenditures will grow to 18% of the GDP by the year 2000 and to over 20% by the year 2003 (CBO, 1993a).

Measures of inflation can also be used to compare increases in health care costs with increases in general costs for all goods and services. For example, in 1993 the consumer

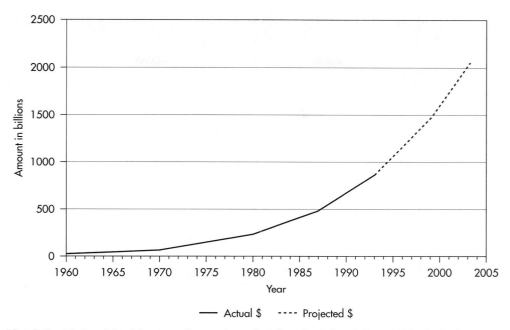

Fig. 8-1   National health expenditures (actual and projected), 1960 to 2023. (Data from Congressional Budget Office. [1993]. *Projections of national health expenditures: 1993 update*. Washington, DC: U.S. Government Printing Office; and U.S. Department of Health and Human Services. [1994]. *National health expenditures for 1993* [Press release]).

price index (CPI) for all items reflected a 3% increase in annual inflation, whereas the costs of physician services and hospital and related services increased 5.9% and 6.7% respectively—approximately twice the general inflation rate (Health Care Financing Administration [HCFA], 1994a). It should be noted that these rates of growth for physician services and hospital and related services actually represent a decline from 1990 rates—10.7% and 10.3% respectively. Nevertheless, these two categories accounted for 63.9% of health care expenditures in 1993 (Levit et al., 1994).

A question that emerges naturally from a discussion of the increasing costs of health care is: Who pays for this increasingly expensive commodity? Not surprisingly, the answer to this question, too, has changed over time (U.S. DHHS, 1994). In 1965, public and private sources funded approximately 25% and 75% of total health care costs, respectively. These percentages have gradually shifted over time. In 1993 approximately 56% of total health expenditures were through private sources, whereas public funding represented approximately 44% of total health expenditures. The CBO projects that public funds will be used to finance approximately 50% of health care spending by 2003 (CBO, 1993a).

The issues of escalating health care costs and how health care is paid for lead directly to concern over access to health care: health care is so expensive that most in-

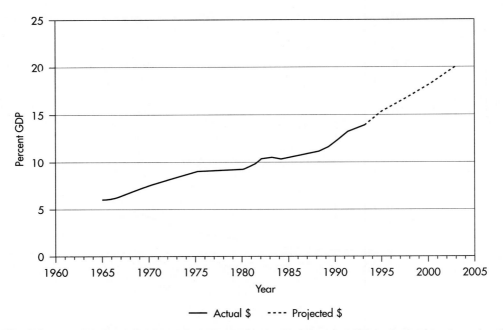

Fig. 8-2 National health expenditures as a percentage of the gross domestic product (actual and projected), 1960 to 2002. (Data from Congressional Budget Office. [1993]. *Projections of national health expenditures: 1993 update.* Washington, DC: U.S. Government Printing Office; and Health Care Financing Administration. [1994]. *1994 HCFA statistics.* Washington, DC: HCFA Press.)

dividuals cannot afford to pay for health care services directly. Overwhelmingly, individuals depend on an outside person or group, (i.e., a third party) to pay for health care. The individual and the health care provider constitute two parties; the term *third party* is used to reflect any institution outside of the individual or health care provider that reimburses for health care services received and/or delivered. Third-party sources include private insurance and the two health care programs financed by state and federal governments: Medicare and Medicaid. Private insurance is obtained either through employer contributions only, a combination of employer and individual contributions, or solely through individual contributions. Medicare is a program funded through the federal government that provides medical care for elderly and/or disabled individuals; Medicaid is a program funded through state and federal governments that provides medical care for the poor. To be eligible for Medicaid, however, one must be practically destitute; hence, there are individuals who do not qualify for this program.

Not all individuals have affordable access to, or qualify for, coverage by third-party payors. Cost-cutting efforts in the business sector have left many full-time employees without employer-based health insurance benefits. Individuals who are employed by small companies or who are self-employed may also lack health insurance benefits because of the prohibitive costs of providing insurance coverage to a small number of enrollees. Hence, without a source to pay for health services, some people effectively may lack access to health care services. In essence, third-party reimbursement for health care providers becomes a proxy for access to care.

Given the increased spending for health care services in recent years, one might anticipate that access to health care would have also increased. Unfortunately, this has not been the case. There are currently more individuals in the United States than ever who, for whatever reason, lack access to third-party payment—that is, they are uninsured—for health services (Office of Technology Assessment [OTA], 1994). As Fig. 8-3 indicates, the number of uninsured has increased from 24.2 million people in 1980 to 37.4 million in 1993, and is projected to grow to over 43 million in the year 2003 (CBO, 1993a). These numbers represent an increase in the proportion of uninsured individuals in the U.S. population from approximately 11% in 1980 to approximately 15% in 1993; if projections are correct, by the year 2003 the percentage of our population without health insurance coverage will grow to approximately 16%.

Locations where health care services are provided also affect access to health care (see box on p. 174). While the bulk of health care is still provided in hospitals, health care delivery is shifting out of inpatient and into outpatient arenas. This shift can be attributed primarily to the cost of health care: inpatient care is generally more costly to provide than outpatient care. According to CBO (1993b) estimates, the number of in-

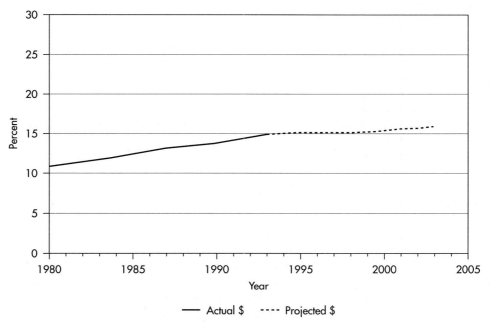

Fig. 8-3 Uninsured percentage of the U.S. population (actual and projected), 1980 to 2003. (Data from Congressional Budget Office. [1993]. *Projections of national health expenditures: 1993 update*. Washington, DC: U.S. Government Printing Office.)

Recent Changes in U.S. Health Care Delivery

- Inpatient hospital beds have decreased from 8.8 to 4.6 per 1000 population between 1960 and 1991.
- Skilled nursing facilities have increased since the mid 1970s, totaling approximately 11,443 in 1994.
- Psychiatric hospital beds have increased since 1975, although the number of beds per 1000 Medicare/Medicaid enrollees has actually dropped from 9.4 in 1975 to 2.8 in 1994.
- Home health agencies have increased from 2254 providers in 1975 to 7000 providers in 1994.
- Ambulatory surgical centers, hospices, and rural health clinics, essentially nonexistent in 1975, numbered 1665, 1445, and 1213, respectively, in 1994.
- Outpatient facilities, such as medical laboratories, end-stage renal disease facilities, outpatient physical therapy facilities, and rehabilitation centers, have also increased dramatically since 1975.

Data from Congressional Budget Office. (1993, June). *Trends in health spending: An update.* Washington, DC, U.S. Government Printing Office; and Health Care Financing Administration. (1994). *1994 data compendium.* Washington, DC: HCFA press.

---

patient hospital beds has decreased from 8.8 per 1000 population in 1960 to 4.6 per 1000 population in 1991. The number of per capita hospital admissions has also declined during that same period, as has the average length of hospital stay. The use of outpatient hospital services, however, has increased (CBO, 1993b). Statistics from the HCFA (1994a) confirm these trends and indicate that the numbers on nonhospital health care facilities have increased significantly during the past two decades.

One might expect that changes in health care delivery sites would have brought about decreased expenditures. However, total health care expenditures have continued to rise (albeit at a lower rate—the rate of growth in 1993 was 7.8%, versus 8.6% in 1992, 8.5% in 1991, and 11.6% in 1990), primarily because of the increasing costs of hospital services. The increasing costs of hospital services can be attributed to three general circumstances (U.S. House of Representatives, 1993). First, hospitals were affected by general inflation in the economy; further, employee wages—including those of nurses—increased faster than other wages because of the increased demand for health care workers. Second, the complexity and intensity of care required to treat patients increased. As less critically ill patients have been shifted to outpatient settings and as the length of hospital stay has decreased, the severity of illness for patients remaining in the inpatient setting has increased. Last, hospital input—that combination of labor and other goods needed to provide health care services—has changed. As the intensity and complexity of inpatient care has increased, the number and types of staff required to provide care have changed, along with the types of goods needed to provide care.

Cost shifting has also influenced the costs of health care. *Cost shifting* refers to the practice by health care providers of charging privately insured patients more than the actual costs of their care to compensate for the loss in revenues realized from treating Medicare, Medicaid, and uninsured patients. Also, because many patients lack access to primary care providers—and in many cases, lack insurance—they show up unnecessarily in emergency rooms, where care is more expensive to provide. Patients with insurance who use emergency room services are charged more for the services received than they would be for the same service in a primary care setting.

Issues of cost and access naturally lead to concerns over quality of care. One might anticipate that with more money being spent on health care than ever before, the quality of care would be increasing. The validity of this expectation, however, remains illusive, given the fact that a universal measure of quality of care is nonexistent.

Satisfaction with care is often equated with consumers' perceptions of quality. In a recent report (Center for Health Economics Research, 1994), the percentage of individuals satisfied with our health system was a low 10%, yet more than 50% of Americans were very satisfied with the medical care they received personally. This incongruence between dissatisfaction with the overall health care system and satisfaction with personal care received makes it difficult to draw any conclusions about consumer perceptions of quality.

Recent concerns over quality stem from the belief that cost-containment efforts implemented by organizations and providers potentially jeopardize the quality of care delivered. There is uncertainty regarding how society will address the issues of cost and access without jeopardizing quality of care. Therefore the actual impact of cost-containment efforts on quality of care is yet to be determined.

In an effort to control the escalating costs of health care, third-party payors have increasingly placed pressure on health care providers to control costs. For example, before 1983, Medicare reimbursement for health care services was made on a retrospective basis, which was dependent on the amounts and types of health care services provided. This retrospective payment system gave providers little or no incentive to control costs or to produce services efficiently. In 1983, however, Medicare implemented a prospective payment system: diagnostic-related groups (DRGs) were introduced whereby predetermined, fixed reimbursement, based on a particular diagnostic category, would be made for hospital care. Private insurance companies have followed suit by rewarding innovative delivery systems that lower costs. These measures have contributed to changes cited earlier in this chapter, such as a decreasing length of hospital stay, a shift from inpatient to outpatient care, and other recent trends in health care delivery.

THE HEALTH CARE ENVIRONMENT

The health care delivery system has become more competitive in response to pressures to control health care costs. This response has led to widespread restructuring of health care organizations and to the development of new health care delivery models. A driving force behind the restructuring of health care and the development of models for care delivery is *managed competition,* a concept that emphasizes value by incorporating economic principles associated with competition (Enthoven, 1993). Managed competition means that providers of health care compete on the basis of price, while at the same time, purchasers (i.e., consumers) are sensitive to the price they pay for a certain level of care (Buerhaus, 1994; Enthoven, 1990). In other words, in a managed competition environment, health care consumers are aware of the type of service they can get for a given amount of money, and based on this information, they make decisions about the level of care they choose to receive and the amount of money they are willing to spend. Managed competition takes into account the notion of the value of health care as a function of cost and quality, since consumers weigh cost and quality in decision making. According to the OTA (1994), "managed competition would attempt to change the incentives faced by consumers, health plans, and providers, and to create new organizations to improve how health insurance markets function" (p. 72).

The "ideal" scenario portrayed by the above description of managed competition has not been realized for two primary reasons. First, given the nature of our insurance system, consumers have been relatively insensitive to the price of health care. Employers or the government typically pay for health care insurance coverage, and individuals' contributions are limited to deductibles and copayments—health care consumers have not had to give up something else in order to purchase health care (Folland, Goodman, & Stano, 1993). In a sense, employers have actually prevented individuals from knowing the price of health care by not providing monetary incentives to individuals for choosing a lower-cost health plan. Tax incentives also make it more attractive for employers, rather than employees, to purchase health care. Subsequently, as employers have chosen, for whatever reason, to pay more to costly health care providers, employees have not enjoyed the real increase in wages that likely would have occurred had employers not agreed to pay the increasing price of health care (Folland, Goodman, & Stano, 1993). It is obvious that the implementation of managed competition would completely change the way health care is bought and sold in the United States.

Second, most individual health care consumers do not have firsthand knowledge of the appropriateness, necessity, or quality of health care services received. It is difficult for consumers to determine the value of the care when they are unaware of the costs and do not have knowledge about quality. On the other hand, providers—as suppliers of health care—have not historically furnished information about the price and quality of their product so that consumers could make informed decisions about the type of care they were willing to purchase. In the past, health care providers have been adverse to advertising because doing so was viewed as unethical, inappropriate, and distasteful. More recently, however, health care firms are engaging in this practice, primarily because of the lifting of regulatory restrictions and the presence of competition in the health care marketplace (Folland, Goodman, & Stano, 1993). Likewise, the implementation of managed competition in the U.S. health care system would require that consumers possess information for making purchasing decisions.

In an effort to remedy these problems and move toward managed competition, new models for health care delivery have evolved. These models provide incentives for the efficient use of resources, attempt to control costs, and, to greater or lesser degrees, involve the consumer in health care decision making (thereby making the consumer more accountable and responsible).

Managed Care

The most prominent of these models is managed care. *Managed care* is a general term that refers to any type of delivery and reimbursement system that monitors or controls the types, quality, utilization, and costs of health care (CBO, 1994; Folland, Goodman, & Stano, 1993). The aim of managed care is to reduce unnecessary or inappropriate care and to reduce costs (CBO, 1994). Managed care usually involves capitation, a payment arrangement whereby a provider will be prepaid a fixed amount of money per person enrolled (usually on a monthly basis) regardless of the amount of services provided or consumed (Folland, Goodman, & Stano, 1993). Other strategies associated with managed care include utilization review, preadmission certification, and second-opinion requirements. Two types of managed care arrangements, health maintenance organizations (HMOs) and preferred provider organizations (PPOs), are discussed here.

Health maintenance organizations. A *health maintenance organization* is a managed care plan wherein a contractual arrangement is made between the providing organization and enrollees: for a prepaid, fixed fee, the organization agrees to provide comprehensive care to enrollees over a specified period of time (Folland, Goodman, & Stano, 1993). There are several types of HMOs (CBO, 1994; Folland, Goodman, & Stano, 1993; OTA, 1994). These are:

Staff model. Individual physicians are employed by the HMO to provide services to members.
Group model. A group practice is contracted by an HMO to provide care to enrollees.
Network model. Several group practices are contracted to provide care to enrollees.
Independent practice association (IPA). Independent practitioners or small-group practices are contracted by an HMO to provide care to enrollees.

The growing popularity of HMOs is evident from the numbers of persons enrolled: HMO enrollment grew from 6 million members in 1976 to approximately 50 million members in 1994 (Inglehart, 1992; "Managed Care," 1995).

Preferred provider organizations. Another type of managed care plan, a *preferred provider organization,* is a plan wherein the payor (i.e., the insurance company) contracts with certain providers (physicians and hospitals) to deliver care to enrollees; the payor then provides financial incentives to enrollees who receive care from those same providers (Folland, Goodman, & Stano, 1993). The types of incentives offered to enrollees may include lower coinsurance and deductibles, increased coverage, and lower premiums (Folland, Goodman, & Stano, 1993). Although payment to providers is made on a fee-for-service basis, payors benefit because contracts for payment are prearranged, and they can often negotiate contracts with providers who discount fees and practice efficiently. Providers who are under contract with payors benefit because the PPO limits enrollees' choices to certain providers unless an enrollee chooses to pay the additional fees associated with a provider who is not under contract with the PPO (Folland, Goodman, & Stano, 1993).

Patient-Focused Care

Traditionally, hospitals and other health care organizations have designed programs and services around the wants, needs, and demands of organizations and professionals. In the competitive marketplace brought about by prospective payment, however, this practice is no longer realistic or feasible. Following the lead of business, hospitals and other health care organizations are currently developing and investing in programs that address the wants, needs, demands, and satisfaction of health care consumers. In essence, health care providers are organizing around consumers and patient outcomes, rather than professional and organizational desires (Strasen, 1991).

Strasen (1991) recognized four major strategies to facilitate the redesign of hospitals around patients: downsizing management, decentralizing ancillary and support services, centralizing the distribution of supplies, and organizing specific ancillary labor around expensive technology. Anecdotally, these types of activities are occurring across the United States (Brider, 1992; Strasen, 1991): the changes involved include increasing the number of employees managed by first-line managers and broadening their span of control; decreasing the number of upper- and middle-level managers while expanding their span of control; moving support services, such as pharmacy, respiratory therapy, and physical therapy, from centralized departments to patient units; cross-training professionals—nurses and other groups—to perform additional tasks; and increasing the number of unlicensed assistive personnel employed on patient care units. In addition, care is provided by teams or "partners" rather than by individuals; the responsibility for maintaining and replenishing supplies is being centralized or contracted to one department; and patients' rooms are being equipped with everything—from charts and medications to computers—needed to care for patients.

In theory, patient-focused care is intuitively appealing. In reality, there are potential drawbacks. For example, at the same time that the use of unlicensed personnel in hospitals is increasing, hospitals are cutting back on the use of registered nurses (RNs) (Cowley, Miller, & Hager, 1995). While this trend is not necessarily bad—in theory, unlicensed personnel could perform "tasks" that do not necessarily require an RN's education—it raises concerns about the amount and quality of training for these personnel and the subsequent quality and costs of patient care (Manuel & Alster, 1994).

Nursing Case Management

Case management, traditionally used by social workers, is a model of care delivery that has become increasingly prevalent in nursing. According to the ANA (1988), *case management* is a system of care that includes health assessment; planning; procurement, delivery, and coordination of services; and monitoring of outcomes to meet the many needs of clients. According to the CBO (1994), case management is a means of reducing the costs and improving the quality of care associated with high-risk cases or high-cost conditions. The goals of case management include enhanced self-care capabilities, improved continuity of care across settings, delivery of high-quality care, and efficient use of resources (ANA, 1988).

Case management can be initiated in a variety of settings—acute care, managed care clinics, or community health—or across settings. Case management services are usually organized around groups or types of patients. For example, case management services might be provided in the acute care setting to patients who have experienced a myocardial infarction (MI), or they might be provided in the community to elderly individuals.

Case management in any setting includes screening of a client by a professional case manager—usually a nurse—to "outline the problem, determine the need for case management services, and determine the client's eligibility for services" (ANA, 1988, p. 4). A thorough assessment of the client is then conducted, and a plan of care is developed with the client's or family's participation. Critical pathways, or detailed outlines of the predictable progression of care, document the types, sequencing, and outcomes of care for typical patients in certain groups. For example, in an acute care setting there might be a critical pathway for MI patients to document and evaluate an individual's progress during and after hospitalization. The individual's progress is compared with the critical pathway, as a benchmark, to determine progress and the relative consumption of resources.

Three outcomes of particular interest to case management professionals and health care organizations are the costs of care, length of stay (or some other measure used to denote the length of case-managed episode), and quality of care. In turn, information related to outcomes of care allows hospitals and other health care organizations to examine system-wide problems in order to control costs and increase the quality of care.

Regardless of the particular model of care delivery, the focus for future health care organizations and health care delivery will be *flexibility*. Those organizations that are adaptable, that anticipate problems, and that quickly respond to changes in the social, economic, and health care environments are apt to survive. Likewise, those models of care delivery that accommodate differences between individuals within groups or types of clients will best meet the needs of our ever-changing society. It is likely that there are new health care models on the horizon, as well as some tried-and-true ones that will be modified and gain favor once again.

THE NURSING PROFESSION

Nursing and the nursing profession, like the overall health care delivery system, have changed and continue to change. Change in nursing has far-reaching consequences given the fact that nurses represent the single largest group of health care professionals in the United States—estimated in 1992 at over 2.2 million licensed RNs, of which an estimated 1.85 million (83%) were employed in nursing (Moses, 1994).

One of the more significant changes in nursing has been that of demographic shifts within the nursing population itself, pointing to real and substantive change in the makeup of the nursing profession. For example, while men constituted only 4% of the employed RN population in 1992 (Moses, 1994), men made up roughly 11% of beginning baccalaureate nursing students that same year (American Association of Colleges of Nursing [AACN], 1993). In addition, racial minorities constituted only 9% of the 1992 employed RN population (Moses, 1994), yet almost 16% of 1992 nursing school enrollments were racial minorities (National League for Nursing [NLN], 1993).

Another interesting trend in the RN population is the "graying" of the nursing profession—the average age of the 1992 RN population was 43 years, up from 40 years in 1980 (Moses, 1994). Since 1980, the number of nurses under 30 years of age has gradually declined to a low of 11%, whereas the number of nurses in all other age groups has steadily increased (Moses, 1994). The average age of the new nursing graduate has also increased, from 25 to 31 years of age between 1982 and 1991 (NLN, 1993). While some of the increase in age of RN graduates can be attributed to the growing proportion of students aged 25 and older in the general student population, a growing number of nurses possessed post-high school degrees before entering nursing (Moses, 1994; NLN, 1993). In essence, nursing represents a second career for many recent nursing school enrollees and graduates.

When nursing educational preparation is considered, approximately 34% of the 1992 RN population possessed a diploma in nursing (down from 55% in 1980), 28% possessed an associate degree in nursing (up from 18% in 1980), and 30% possessed a baccalaureate degree in nursing (up from 22% in 1980) (Moses, 1994). Approximately 8% of the 1992 RN population was prepared with a graduate degree in nursing or a related field (up from 6% in 1984).

Despite recent changes in health care delivery and the nursing profession, certain aspects of the nursing profession have changed little in recent years. First, approximately 66.5% of employed RNs—roughly two thirds of the population—are employed in hospitals (Moses, 1994). Although this proportion has declined slightly from 68% in 1984 and 1988, the actual number of nurses employed in the hospital setting has increased from roughly 1,011,955 RNs in 1984 (Moses, 1986) to 1,104,978 in 1988 (Moses, 1990), and approximately 1,232,717 RNs in 1992 (Moses, 1994). Second, consistent with surveys conducted in 1984 and 1988, approximately two thirds of RNs in all settings hold staff nurse positions (Moses, 1994). Likewise, the actual number of RNs employed in staff nurse positions has increased from an estimated 992,956 RNs in 1984 (Moses, 1986) to an estimated 1,087,878 RNs in 1988 (Moses, 1990) and 1,233,537 RNs in 1992 (Moses, 1994). A summary of 1992 nursing employment date is presented in Tables 8-1 and 8-2.

Given that nurses represent the single largest group of health care professionals, it is not surprising that the nursing personnel budget is often the largest of all departmental personnel budgets in any health care organization. As administrators become increasingly concerned with costs, it is also not surprising that the nursing budget becomes a target for cost savings. To cut costs, hospitals and other health care organizations are training and employing unlicensed assistive personnel to perform certain tasks that need not necessarily be performed by RNs—all at a lesser cost. This type of activity, known in labor economics as substitution, is common during periods of shortage in certain types of personnel and/or to enhance flexibility in the production of goods or services.

At the same time that unlicensed personnel are being substituted for some RNs, nurse practitioners and other advanced practice nurses are being substituted for pri-

Table 8-1   **Settings Where Nurses Work***

Setting	%
Hospitals	67
Community health	15
Ambulatory (including HMOs)	8
Long-term care	7
Other	3

Data from Moses, E. (1994). *The registered nurse population: Findings from the national sample survey of registered nurses, March 1992* (U.S. Department of Health and Human Services, Public Health Service, Health Resources and Services Administration). Washington, DC: U.S. Government Printing Office.
*Based on an estimated 1.85 million employed RNs in 1992.

Table 8-2   **Positions Held by Nurses***

Position	%
Staff nurse	67.0
Administrator	6.2
Supervisor or assistant	5.0
Head nurse or assistant	4.6
Instructor	3.5
Clinical nurse specialist	1.9
Nurse practitioner	1.4
Nurse clinician	1.3
Nurse anesthetist	1.0
Nurse consultant	0.9
Private-duty nurse	0.6
Researcher	0.4
Nurse midwife	0.2
Other	6.5

Data from Moses, E. (1994). *The registered nurse population: Findings from the national sample survey of registered nurses, March 1992* (U.S. Department of Health and Human Services, Public Health Service, Health Resources and Services Administration). Washington, DC: U.S. Government Printing Office.
*Based on an estimated 1.85 million employed RNs in 1992.

mary care physicians. Similar to the case of unlicensed assistive personnel in hospitals, advanced practice nurses are attractive to health care organizations because they can provide many of the same services as physicians at a lower cost.

THE NURSING PRACTICE ENVIRONMENT

Recent changes in the philosophy of employee performance and productivity—employee participation in decision making, concerns about job satisfaction, and employee morale—and the resulting impacts on quality and efficiency have been translated to the nursing practice environment. Some nursing departments have incorporated concepts such as shared governance, career ladders, and professional practice models into their operations to foster the growth and development of individuals and groups, and to ensure their success and survival.

Shared Governance

Shared governance is a governance structure that empowers nursing staff with authority, accountability, and responsibility for decision making within the practice environment. Terms commonly associated with shared governance are *decentralization* (i.e., relinquishing authority to lower hierarchical levels) and *participation* (i.e., involving subordinates in decision making) (Hess, 1994). The central idea behind shared governance is that the individuals closest to patient care situations are best equipped to make decisions about many problems that arise in the practice environment. The success of shared governance is predicated on the notion that such a system makes nurses more invested in the organization and better able to clearly articulate the mission of the organization at the point of service—in the provision of nursing care.

Shared governance structures within nursing organizations tend to take on one of three models (Porter-O'Grady, 1987): the councilar, congressional, or administrative model. The *councilar model* is composed of staff nurses (usually elected) who serve on a variety of councils related to domains of interest (e.g., practice, education, quality of care, and peer relations). These councils have the authority to make decisions according to the defined roles of each individual council. For example, the education council would be responsible for decision making related to nursing education issues within the organization but would not have authority to make practice-related decisions. Management may be represented on these councils, but council chairs are elected. The chair of each council typically represents his or her specific council on some type of oversight council, along with the chief nursing officer, where the efforts of each council are brought forward, integrated, and synthesized into a unified whole for the nursing organization.

In the *congressional model,* officers (i.e., president, vice president, secretary, etc.) are nominated from, and elected by, the nursing staff to oversee the operations of nursing services. This elected group is known as the nursing cabinet. Committees similar to the councils described above address relevant issues (practice, quality of care, education, etc.) and make formal reports and recommendations to the nursing cabinet. The executive group, made up of the chief nursing officer, other members of the organization's management team, and the cabinet, resolve issues related to power and control within the nursing organization. Members of the executive group may sit on the nursing cabinet and vice versa, depending on the beliefs of the organization.

The *administrative model* is a shared governance model wherein authority, roles, functions, and processes are hierarchical and drawn along management and clinical lines. In this model, staff elect a group of representatives to participate in clinical forums that address clinically relevant issues. These clinical forums are similar to the councils and committees described above. The management forum, on the other hand, consists of appointed individuals who deal with systems-related issues, such as human and financial resource allocation. An executive committee consists of members of both the clinical and management forums, who advise the chief nurse executive. In this model, the chief nurse executive usually has ultimate decision-making and veto power, making this the least participative and most traditional of all the shared governance models.

Shared governance has been implemented in a variety of ways, depending on the unique characteristics of the nursing organization. Some organizations have reported implementing shared governance at the unit level, some organizations have started at the unit level and then expanded to the department and division levels, and some organizations have simply implemented the philosophy division-wide from the beginning. *However, to implement shared governance in the truest sense, it must pervade the division and the entire health care organization* (Porter-O'Grady, 1994). Porter-O'Grady advocates "whole-systems" shared governance: moving the concept of shared governance beyond nursing to the whole organization. Whole-systems shared governance "creates a transitional model for ownership at all levels of the organization. It reflects accountability at every level and creates a seamless structural and relational integration of the system . . ." (Porter-O'Grady, 1994, p. 195).

As is obvious from this discussion, it is not possible to implement shared governance in every nursing organization or in every situation. Nursing staff must want to be involved in decision making, they must want to invest time and effort into building the nursing organization, and they must be willing to take responsibility for decisions they make. On the other hand, nursing executives must be willing to pass along a great deal of power and control to subordinates. Nurse executives must also be supportive of the decisions that are made by others, some of which they may not necessarily agree with. Needless to say, it takes a great deal of maturity and leadership by everyone involved to implement a shared governance structure. The rewards of success, however—cost-effectiveness, job satisfaction, and nurse retention—are potentially worth the investment (DeBaca, Jones, & Tornibini, 1993; Jenkins, 1991; Jones et al., 1993; Ludemann & Brown, 1989).

Career Ladders

Career ladders are structures that were developed in the 1970s and 1980s to recognize and reward clinically competent nurses who chose to remain in clinical practice (Hamrick, Whitworth, & Greenfield, 1993). The terms *career ladder* and *clinical ladder* are often used interchangeably. The term *career* is used here to convey the belief that these models should foster growth and development over one's entire career rather than be limited to a short span of time.

The idea behind the development of career ladders was that there were few, if any, advancement or promotional opportunities for nurses who wanted to remain in direct caregiver roles. Before the development of career ladders, if a nurse wanted to advance within a system, generally the only option was to move into a management role. Therefore career ladders were developed to provide more career options for nurses so that nurses who chose to remain clinically active would have a mechanism for being rewarded, recognized, and promoted within an organizational system. Hospitals tend to be the type of health care organizations where career ladders have been implemented.

Depending on the philosophy and values specific to the organization, the theoretical framework, process, and compensation associated with advancement vary (Murray, 1993). Nurses who advance on a career ladder are typically rewarded with an increase in salary, a new job title, and/or other types of nonmonetary rewards (Murray, 1993). The number of levels for advancement on career ladders has been reported to range from as few as one or two to as many as seven or eight, although the majority of organizations have ladders with four levels (Murray, 1993). Advancement is generally based on clinical competence and professional criteria associated with a given level on the ladder. Some organizations have a limited number of slots at each level for which nurses can apply, whereas others do not have these types of quotas.

In most cases individuals who desire to advance up a career ladder generally have to prepare an application for advancement, sometimes called a portfolio, which demonstrates his or her level of practice. A unit, division, department, or some other type of peer review committee usually reviews each applicant's packet. Recommendations for advancement are then made to the appropriate administrative level.

Real benefits have been documented in organizations that have implemented nursing career ladders. Career ladders have been reported to increase nurse job satisfaction, decrease nursing turnover or increase retention, and facilitate recruitment of new nurses to organizations (Corley et al., 1994; Opperwall et al., 1991; Schultz, 1993), and subjective reports indicate a positive impact on patient care (Schultz, 1993).

Professional Practice Models

A *professional practice model* is a framework that reflects the underlying philosophy about the delivery of nursing care within an organization and serves as a guide to nursing care delivery. Hence, a professional practice model is usually unique to a particular organization, although aspects of professional practice models can be shared between organizations. Questions that need to be considered when developing a professional practice model include: What elements are essential to the nurse-patient relationship? What is the best method for delivering care to our patients (i.e., primary, team, functional, modular, or case management)? What is the governance structure that best meets the needs of individual nurses and the nursing organization? What rewards and recognitions should be built into the system? What is the management structure that best meets the needs of individuals, groups, and the nursing organization while at the same time remaining consistent with the overall organizational structure?

Various professional practice models have been reported in the literature. For example, the model in place at Boston's Beth Israel Hospital (Horvath, 1989) is a humanistic model that has the nurse–patient/family relationship as its core. Elements in the model that influence this relationship are nursing practice, the organizational and administrative environment of the organization, and developmental support services. The essential components of nursing practice—accountability, continuity, and collaboration— are achieved through primary nursing care delivery. The organizational/administrative environment is composed of decentralization (to foster participation in decision making), coherence, advancement, recognition, and compensation. Developmental supports include activities that foster evaluation, learning, and inquiry. Horvath (1989) reported increased job satisfaction, staff retention, and positive patient outcomes following the implementation of the professional practice model at Beth Israel Hospital.

The key to successful development of a professional practice model is to find that unique combination of strategies that best meets the needs of a particular nursing organization, build on the organization's strengths, and search for ways to improve other areas. Remember, what works for one nursing organization may not always work for another. As Beth Israel's professional practice model suggests, shared governance, career ladders, delivery models, and any other techniques that facilitate the delivery of nursing care can be built into a nursing organization's professional practice model.

OPPORTUNITIES FOR NURSING

Where does the nursing profession stand, given all of the changes in health care? Actually, many of these changes leave the nursing profession in a very favorable position if it capitalizes on opportunities. The nursing profession can take leadership roles in the delineation of health care policy, in public education, and in the provision of a broad-based education for nursing students to facilitate their movement into a variety of positions and health care settings. Above all, nursing must work for the betterment of health care consumers, both individuals and payors, thereby positioning itself to accomplish several important missions.

First, as the health care delivery system continues to look for more efficiency in the delivery of health care, nurses must be able to document their contribution to the health care delivery system through patient outcomes. Groups have begun to document the cost-effectiveness of care provided by advanced practice nurses (Brown & Grimes, 1993); these activities must continue, and nursing must clearly communicate to consumers and payors the message that nurses can and do provide cost-effective care. The development of methodologies to delineate the revenue-generating aspects of nursing is imperative.

The need to demonstrate nursing's ability to improve the quality of care goes hand in hand with the need to document cost-effectiveness. However, an important distinction between nursing and other professions must be made: nurses provide high-quality patient care by focusing on individual patient needs, expectations, and experiences in an environment that too often emphasizes costs and patient statistics. With this patient-centered focus, nursing is in an exceptionally good position to identify ways of improving quality of care (see box below).

Nursing must also document consumer perceptions of satisfaction with care delivered and perceptions of the quality of care received. The current philosophy in business is that "quality" is defined by the customer, not by the service provider. While health care is moving in this direction, there is still a long way to go. Nurses must embrace this philosophy, document aspects of patients' perceptions of nursing care, and become partners with patients in decision making. The outcome of this effort is likely to enhance nurses' important contributions to health care delivery.

Second, nurses have an opportunity to expand their share of the health care market by serving currently underserved populations. Although nurses already provide a great deal of the care in rural and inner-city areas, we must continue to expand these activities. Nursing must continue to provide care, and even expand the provision of care, to groups that lack access to primary care. It is these groups that experience many of the problems that have such profound effects on our society and on health care costs—lack of basic health care, lack of disease prevention, and violence. Nurses must also realize that many future opportunities will be outside of the hospital environment. Opportunities will exist in agencies and communities that bring the point of service closer to the consumer, rather than closer to the provider.

Third, as a profession, nursing must continue to engage in and expand entrepreneurial activities. As the health care environment becomes more and more competitive, nurses will be in a better position to sell their services in the marketplace. So, too, may be other professionals who embrace this philosophy. As the amount of resources available to pay for health care services becomes increasingly limited, it is likely that other professional groups competing for these resources will become increasingly savvy. Nurses must have the political, economic, and business skills to effectively market their product in this potentially volatile environment.

Fourth, nurses must employ computers and informatics to facilitate the provision of care to clients and to manage the delivery of health care. Computers can facilitate the

Do Magnet Hospitals Make a Difference in Mortality Rate?

Aiken, Smith, and Lake (1994) conducted a study to examine whether hospital mortality rates differed in a sample of magnet and control (i.e., nonmagnet) hospitals. As the name implies, magnet hospitals are those hospitals that "embody a set of organizational attributes that nurses find desirable and that are conducive to better patient care" (p. 771). Aiken and colleagues reported that mortality rates in magnet hospitals were 5% lower than in hospitals in the matched control group. They attributed the difference in hospital mortality rates for the two groups to the organization of nursing care—magnet hospitals provide nurses "more professional autonomy, greater control over the practice environment, and better relationships with physicians" (p. 772).

development of databases, expedite the collection and retrieval of information, allow the integration of new knowledge, and hasten the analysis of large quantities of data to improve efficiency and productivity in health care delivery. Furthermore, informatics can improve diagnostic and consultation capabilities through the use of high-speed computer networks. It is imperative that nurses possess the requisite skills necessary to move forward in a computer-dependent environment.

Finally, nursing education must meet the challenge to better prepare students for the future. In addition to clinical training, nurses of the future will need a broad-based education that encompasses training in informatics, delivery models, economics, data analysis, and management. Future nursing leaders will need more intensive training in these and more diverse topics. A well-trained cadre of nurses will be needed to oversee patient care delivery in a variety of settings. Many health care organizations are restructuring so that all patient care services—including nursing—are provided through multidisciplinary, team efforts. Nurses must be prepared for leadership roles, not just in nursing, but in health care. Nurses in management roles will be called on to document efficiency and effectiveness in the modern health care organization. This requires the knowledge and ability to integrate clinical expertise with business information to oversee the delivery of care to patients.

Key Points

- Many changes are occurring in nursing and health care today. Forces in our society affect access, quality, and cost issues; shape the health care environment; and, in turn, influence nursing and nursing care delivery.

- Total and per capita health care expenditures continue to rise; without intervention, society will no longer be able to afford the care that technology and knowledge provide.

- Increasing numbers within our population have little or no access to affordable health care.

- Questions about health care cost and access lead to concerns about future quality of care.

- Health care organizations have responded to increasing costs by restructuring and moving toward managed competition.

- More and more care is being delivered on an outpatient basis; those who must be treated as inpatients require more complex and intensive care.

- The face of the nursing profession is changing, but nurses remain the single largest group of health care professionals.

- Despite the increasing emphasis on outpatient care, approximately two thirds of nurses continue to work in the hospital setting; two thirds employed in all settings hold the position of staff nurse.

- Increasingly, hospitals are combining nursing and other departments into unified patient care divisions.

- Health care organizations are implementing new and innovative governance models, career ladders, and practice models to facilitate the efficient provision of patient care and to improve the quality of care delivered.

- Nursing can meet the challenges and opportunities that lie ahead by (1) documenting the contribution of nursing through patient outcomes, (2) expanding their share of the health care market by serving currently underserved populations, (3) employing computers and informatics to facilitate and manage the delivery of care, (4) engaging and expanding entrepreneurial activities, and (5) educating nursing students to excel in a rapidly changing and complex health care environment.

 ## Critical Thinking Exercises

1. Considering the changing climate in health care, identify those issues that have changed the manner in which nursing care is provided.

2. Describe recent changes in the numbers of inpatient and outpatient facilities where nurses work.

3. Explain why it has been difficult to move health care toward managed competition.

4. Delineate strategies and specific means by which health care organizations can create a patient-focused environment.

5. Differentiate between shared governance, career ladders, and professional practice models as methods of structuring the nursing practice environment.

6. Forecast changes in health care delivery and the nursing profession in light of escalating costs, decreasing access, and concerns about quality of care.

7. Describe how nurses and the nursing profession might capitalize on opportunities presented by recent changes in health care delivery.

References

Aiken, L.H., Smith, H.L., & Lake, E.T. (1994). Lower medicare mortality among a set of hospitals known for good nursing care. *Medical Care, 32*(8), 771-787.

American Association of Colleges of Nursing. (1993). *1992-1993 enrollments and graduations in baccalaureate and graduate programs in nursing.* Washington, DC: The Association.

American Nurses' Association. (1988). *Nursing case management.* Kansas City, MO: The Association.

American Nurses' Association. (1991). *Nursing's agenda for health care reform.* Washington, DC: The Association.

Brider, P. (1992). The move to patient-focused care. *American Journal of Nursing, 92*(9), 26-33.

Brown, S.A., & Grimes, D.E. (1993). *Nurse practitioners and certified nurse midwives: A metaanalysis of studies on nurses in primary care roles.* Washington, DC: American Nurses Publishing.

Buerhaus, P.I. (1994). Economics of managed competition and consequences to nurses: Pt. I. *Nursing Economics, 12*(1), 10-17.

Center for Health Economics Research. (1994). *The nation's health care bill: Who bears the burden?* Waltham, MA: The Center.

Congressional Budget Office. (1993a, October). *Projections of national health expenditures: 1993 update.* Washington, DC: U.S. Government Printing Office.

Congressional Budget Office. (1993b, June). *Trends in health spending: An update.* Washington, DC: U.S. Government Printing Office.

Congressional Budget Office. (1994, March). *Effects of managed care: An update.* Washington, DC: U.S. Government Printing Office.

Corley, M.C., Farley, B., Geddes, N., Goodloe, L., & Green, P. (1994). The clinical ladder: Impact on nurse satisfaction and turnover. *Journal of Nursing Administration, 24*(2), 42-48.

Cowley, G., Miller, S., & Hager, M. (1995, February 13). Intensive care on a budget. *Newsweek,* p. 86.

DeBaca, V., Jones, K., & Tornibini, J. (1993). A cost-benefit analysis of shared governance. *Journal of Nursing Administration, 23*(7/8), 50-57.

Enthoven, A.C. (1990). Multiple choice health insurance: The lessons and challenges to employers. *Inquiry, 27*(4), 368-373.

Enthoven, A.C. (1993). The history and principles of managed competition. *Health Affairs, 12* (Suppl.), 24-48.

Folland, S., Goodman, A.C., & Stano, M. (1993). *The economics of health and health care.* New York: Macmillan.

Hamrick, A.B., Whitworth, T.R., & Greenfield, A.S. (1993). Implementing a clinically focused advancement system: One institution's experience. *Journal of Nursing Administration, 23*(9), 20-28.

Health Care Financing Administration. (1994a). *1994 HCFA statistics.* Washington, DC: HCFA Press.

Health Care Financing Administration. (1994b). *1994 data compendium.* Washington, DC: HCFA Press.

Hess, R. (1994). Shared governance: Innovation or imitation? *Nursing Economics, 12*(1), 28-34.

Horvath, K.J. (1989). Professional nursing practice model. In G.G. Mayer, M.J. Madden, & E.I. Lawrenz (Eds.), *Patient care delivery models.* Frederick, MD: Aspen.

Inglehart, J.K. (1992). The American health care system: Managed care. *New England Journal of Medicine, 327*(10), 742-747.

Jenkins, J. (1991). Professional governance: the missing link. *Nursing Management, 22*(8), 26-28, 30.

Jones, C.B., Stasiowski, S., Simon, B.J., Boyd, N.J., & Lucas, M.D. (1993). Shared governance and the nursing practice environment. *Nursing Economics, 11*(4), 208-214.

Levit, K.R., Sensenig, A.L., Cowan, C.A., Lazenby, H.C., McDonnell, P.A., Won, D.K., Sivarajan, L., Stiller, J.M., Donham, C.S., & Stewart, M.S. (1994). National health expenditures, 1993. *Health Care Financing Review, 16*(1), 247-294.

Ludemann, R.S., & Brown, C. (1989). Staff perceptions of shared governance. *Nursing Administration Quarterly, 1*(4), 49-56.

Managed care, scarcely heard of a decade ago, becomes the norm. (1995, January). *Washington Post* (Health Suppl.), p. 16.

Manuel, P., & Alster, K. (1994). Unlicensed personnel: No cure for an ailing health care system. *Nursing and Health Care, 51*(1), 18-21.

Moses, E. (1986). *The registered nurse population: Findings from the national sample survey of registered nurses, November 1984* (NTIS Accession No. HRP-0906938). Rockville, MD: Health Resources and Services Administration, Bureau of Health Professions.

Moses, E. (1990). *The registered nurse population: Findings from the national sample survey of registered nurses, March 1988* (NTIS Accession No. PB89-231492). Rockville, MD: Health Resources and Services Administration, Bureau of Health Professions.

Moses, E. (1994). *The registered nurse population: Findings from the national sample survey of registered nurses, March 1992* (U.S. Department of Health and Human Services, Public Health Service, Health Resources and Services Administration). Washington, DC: U.S. Government Printing Office.

Murray, M. (1993). Where are career ladders going in the 90s? *Nursing Management, 24*(6), 46-48.

National League for Nursing. (1993). *Nursing data review 1993.* New York: National League for Nursing Press.

Office of Technology Assessment. (1994, May). *Understanding estimates of national health expenditures under health reform.* Washington, DC: U.S. Government Printing Office.

Opperwall, B.C., Everett, L.N., Altaffer, A.B., Dietrich, J.A., Killen, M.B., Klien, R.M., Libcke, J.M., & Mitchell, M.A. (1991). ADVANCE—A clinical ladder program. *Nursing Management, 22*(5), 67-74.

Past health care reform campaigns brought temporary relief from costs. (1994, January). *Wall Street Journal,* p. A2.

Porter-O'Grady, T. (1987). Shared governance and new organizational models. *Nursing Economics, 5*(6), 281-286.

Porter-O'Grady, T. (1994). Whole systems shared governance: Creating the seamless organization. *Nursing Economics, 12*(4), 187-195.

Schultz, A. (1993). Evaluation of a clinical advancement system. *Journal of Nursing Administration, 23*(2), 13-19.

Strasen, L. (1991). Redesigning hospitals around patients and technology. *Nursing Economics, 9*(4), 233-238.

U.S. Department of Health and Human Services. (1994). *National health expenditures for 1993* [Press release].

U.S. House of Representatives. (1993). *Hearings before the subcommittee on health of the Committee on Ways and Means, House of Representatives.* Washington, DC: U.S. Government Printing Office.

part **II**

DIMENSIONS OF PROFESSIONAL NURSING PRACTICE

Concepts that extend across and influence the full range of nursing activities are referred to as dimensions. In this regard, nursing is a multidimensional discipline because it consists of political, economic, legal, and ethical influences, which have an impact on nursing care delivery and guide nursing practice.

The political dimension of nursing practice reflects the nurse's concern for, and response to, health policy legislation as it affects the health care of individuals, families, and communities. In addition, understanding the short-term and long-term implications of health policy legislation is fundamental to taking a proactive position on issues that positively or adversely influence nursing and health care. The economic dimensions of nursing practice are grounded in the use of scarce resources, which ultimately affects payment for nursing services and the delivery of nursing care. An understanding of the relationship between the economic concepts of the supply of, demand for, and cost of health care services can help the nurse to analyze health care delivery problems, propose solutions, and articulate the nursing role as the health care system is restructured. The legal dimension of nursing practice includes legal concepts, expectations, and consequences that surround the practice of nursing. While it is beyond the scope of this book to examine all of these areas in depth, an overview of the relationships that underlie the practice of nursing (including the nurse-state relationship, the nurse-employer relationship, and the nurse-patient relationship) are presented. As our population becomes more diverse, nurses provide care to clients from varied cultural backgrounds whose value systems may be quite unique. An overview of social and cultural influences and values and beliefs provides the basis on which to plan and implement individualized nursing care to clients from different cultural backgrounds. Finally, the ethical dimension of nursing practice embraces both moral reasoning and ethical decision making. Since nurses are constantly faced with ethical dilemmas, which they are expected to resolve, an awareness of principles and frameworks that guide ethical decision making can facilitate rational and intelligent decisions. These dimensions are further defined and explored in this section.

Political Influences on Health Care and Nursing

9

Donna M. Mahrenholz

 ## Objectives

At the completion of this chapter, the reader will be able to:

- Demonstrate knowledge about terms and processes used in formulating health care policy.

- Use policy-making terms when discussing health care policy.

- Describe the federal budget process.

- Differentiate between categorical health services and entitlements.

- State how nurses have influenced and shaped health care policy.

- Discuss the timing and actions that nurses can use to influence health care policy.

Profile in Practice

Addie Eckardt, MS, RN, CS-P
Maryland House of Delegates (R) and Eastern Shore Hospital Center,
Cambridge, Maryland

I have been a psychiatric–mental health nurse for the past 22 years, 14 of which I practiced as a master's prepared clinical nurse specialist. During my professional career I have seen the delivery of psychiatric–mental health services change a great deal. When I began working at Eastern Shore Hospital Center, there were 500 in-patients; now there are only 77. Changes in psychiatric–mental health care policy and advances in pharmacotherapeutics have been instrumental in returning hospitalized patients back to the community.

I have always been interested in politics but first became involved in the political process as chair of the Legislative Committee of the Maryland Nurses' Association. Because of this experience, I ran for the Republican Central Committee and won on the first try with the third-highest vote out of seven candidates. After serving on the committee and creating a party presence, I ran for the House of

Delegates in 1990. Although this first attempt was unsuccessful, I succeeded the next time and was elected to a 4-year term in the House of Delegates of the Maryland General Assembly. (I am one of five nurses in the Maryland legislature.) I was assigned to the Economic Matters Committee, and although this committee does not deal directly with health issues, it is recognized that a sound business environment contributes to the health of the citizens of the state by providing good health care benefits. My constituents are in a four-county area that includes 22 municipalities and four school boards.

One example of health-related legislation during my term of office includes the Mothers and Infants Security Act of 1994, which states that if a mother and new baby are discharged from the hospital within 48 hours, they must have a home visit by an RN to ensure care according to national pediatric standards. Other legislative issues include who pays for emergency care for patients in managed care systems if preauthorization for care cannot be obtained, and who pays for uncompensated care if the all-payor system is lifted. (In Maryland the all-payor system provides that uncompensated care be spread out among hospitals; if lifted, the burden will be unequally distributed unless a special fund is created to which all providers must contribute.) Medicaid waiver legislation was passed that encourages Medicaid patients to enter into managed care. The legislation frames who can be enrolled and what the business arrangements are.

I will introduce legislation for prescriptive authority for psychiatric–mental health clinical nurse specialists during the upcoming legislative session. I also track health matters through the Maryland Senate. Even though the General Assembly is in session for only 90 days, I am involved in legislative work throughout the entire year. I ran for office on a pro-business stance, and I meet with representatives of business and industry, communities, and special interest groups, as well as individuals, to hear their concerns and respond to their issues. I also give many presentations and speeches, teach some classes, and maintain my position (80% time) at Eastern Shore Hospital Center. My schedule is demanding, but I am enjoying the experience tremendously.

The greatest challenge of my role is how to shape policy. It is necessary to first determine what is important to various constituents and then find the common themes among them. The nursing process has been helpful to me as I gather essential information, devise a plan of action, resolve the issue, and evaluate the effectiveness of the resolution.

Before the twentieth century, health care in the United States was viewed as the responsibility of individuals or private organizations. During the eighteenth and nineteenth centuries, the scourge of epidemics related to impure foods, contaminated water supplies, inadequate sewage disposal, and poor housing conditions forced local governments to respond with measures to protect the health of their citizens. These recurring epidemics also led to the first public health effort by the U.S. federal government: a national port quarantine system. Following the yellow fever epidemic of 1873, Congress established the Marine Hospital Services to regulate and enforce a national port quarantine. Thus the precedent of intervention by the government at the local, state, and federal level was established (Hyman, 1982). Since this initial effort, the government has had increased influence on health care delivery.

Policy decisions are affected by the legislative process, by economics, by individuals, and by special-interest groups. These decisions, in turn, shape the content and form of the legislation and policies regulating health care. Nurses, as the largest group of health care providers, can have an impact on nursing and health care legislation and policies. To have an impact, nurses need to understand the terms and process of health care legislation, past successes and failures, and areas for potential impact.

It is important to first have an understanding of some of the motivations ascribed to changes in health care policies. Feldstein (1988) states that health legislation, especially federal, follows a self-interest paradigm. This paradigm assumes that individuals act according to self-interest, not necessarily the public interest. Individuals, whether they are legislators, voters, or health care providers, act in pursuit of their own self-interests. Individuals who function in organized groups deliver greater political support and have greater political influence than nonorganized or less well organized groups. Feldstein writes that organized groups seek to achieve through legislation what they cannot achieve through the marketplace. Recently, two groups have benefitted from a massive redistribution of wealth in the health care arena: health care providers, especially physicians, whose incomes have risen more than would have occurred otherwise, and the aged, who receive health care services that exceed the value of the payments they have made into the programs. These two well-organized groups have provided the necessary political support to politicians to get legislation enacted in their favor. This chapter explores ways that nurses can have a similar impact on health care legislation.

LEGISLATIVE TERMS AND PROCESS

To understand how the political system influences health care, it is important to understand how health care policies are made. Policies can be either formal or informal. Formal policies are those that are written, such as rules, regulations, and laws. Informal policies are those that result from customs or traditions and are usually more difficult to change. Before any action regarding a policy can be taken, people other than those affected by the issue need to become aware of the issue and its significance. This is called putting the issue on the "public agenda." This action results in gaining the attention of the policymakers and the public.

For example, the elderly have been effective in putting their concerns about costs of health care services for persons with fixed incomes on the public agenda. They have banded together in groups such as the American Association of Retired Persons, the Gray Panthers, and even as groups within condominium complexes to publicize their issues. They endorse and work for political candidates who support their concerns, give newspaper interviews, and contact and inform legislators at local, state, and federal levels. As a result, other segments of the public become aware of their issues and adopt the elderly's concerns. In the past these activities produced changes in the Medicare program. Currently there are attempts to amend Medicare to fully cover health care in nursing homes.

How to Influence Policy

To influence policy, one must know the issue, as well as the players involved, the arena in which the process will occur, and the climate of the times. First and most important, to influence policies, one needs to understand the issue (see box below). This includes not only the questions and problems surrounding the issue, but also some potential solutions to those problems. As nurses, we understand, and are experts about, the issues and health care problems in the areas in which we practice. By knowing how the legislative process works, who the players are, including the opponents and potential opponents, the proponents, and those who will remain neutral, nurses can begin the process of influencing health care policy. Individuals who want to influence policy must identify and become familiar with the arena in which the action will take place, including the socioeconomic climate of the times. For example, financial support from the federal government for nursing education programs will not be a priority in Congress during a stock market crisis or a legislative battle to cut funding in order to balance the budget.

The policy arena includes local, state, and federal levels and may involve the legislature, the courts, or the bureaucracy. Assessment of the players, the arena, and the climate will help the astute nurse know whether the time is appropriate to promote changes to maintain the status quo. The principles apply whether nurses want to influence federal, state, or local policies.

Policies are changed incrementally rather than in one massive step. In the past nurses have accepted these incremental changes without analyzing the additive effect of all the small changes. Alert nurses will recognize the effects of the incremental changes and will support or influence their direction

How to Influence Policies

Understand the Issue
Know the problems
Know the questions
Know the possible solutions

Understand the Legislative and Regulatory Processes
Formal process
Informal process

Identify the Players
Opponents, real and potential
Proponents, real and potential
Neutral players

Identify the Arena
Legislative branch
Executive branch
Judicial branch

Be Familiar With the Climate
Socioeconomic
Political

The Legislative Process

Formal health care policies are created by legislation, by the promulgation of rules and regulations, and by the judicial rulings by courts. For nurses, legislation has become a more visible component of health care policy-making. But frequently after a law has been passed, the rules and regulations developed determine not only the shape of the legislation, but even if the legislation will be implemented.

How a bill becomes law is a similar process in state legislatures and in Congress (Fig. 9-1). This process can be influenced at any time from the formation of the bill to the signing or veto by the executive. The key times to influence the legislative process are at committee hearings, during "markups" of the bills (an activity to reconcile different versions of a bill), and during floor debates and votes.

Since the process of legislation in the 50 states is similar to the federal process (with a few differences, such as the length or the legislative session), discussion of the legislative process will concentrate on Congress and the federal level. Congress is in session for 2 years; thus a bill remains "alive" for the 2 years unless it is passed or killed. The 105th Congress will begin in January 1997 and will end December 31, 1998. The federal fiscal year begins October 1 and ends September 30. A fiscal year is called by the year in which it ends. For example, fiscal year 1997 begins October 1, 1996, and ends September 30, 1997.

TYPES OF LEGISLATION

Two types of bills, authorization bills and appropriation bills, are needed to establish and implement a legislative program. First a program must be authorized by Congress; that is, there must be authority for the program to exist. Authorization bills give broad descriptions of the programs, including the maximum amount of dollars that can be authorized for a fiscal year. Typically, authorization bills are for 2 or 3 fiscal years. Second, appropriation bills must be passed for each authorized program for each fiscal year. Appropriation bills permit federal agencies to incur financial obligations and result in debits from the Treasury for the programs' specified purposes. Thus programs can be authorized without any funds appropriated or with a much lower amount than the maximum authorized.

For example, in 1986 the 99th Congress authorized a program to compensate for injuries resulting from vaccinations. A no-fault compensation program was passed by Congress and signed by President Reagan, but no funds were appropriated from the federal budget, and no other method was established to collect monies to fund the program. The 100th Congress in 1987 approved an excise tax on several child vaccines, ranging from 6 cents to $4.56 per dose, to fund a compensation pool. Thus, even though the authorizing legislation was passed in 1986, the appropriating legislation was not passed until the following year. This type of program whereby money is raised by additional taxes instead of coming out of the operating budget is called a budget-neutral program. In today's economic climate, programs have a better chance of passing if they are deemed to be budget-neutral.

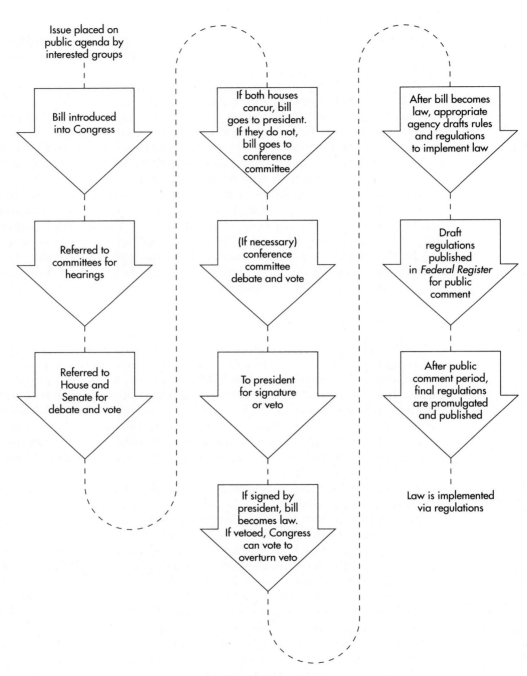

Fig. 9-1   Formal health care policy process.

Fiscal Appropriations

To fund the federal government, including all federal programs, 13 appropriation bills are required for each fiscal year. These bills need to be passed by Congress and signed by the president by the beginning of each fiscal year. These 13 bills represent the amount of monies the 13 cabinet departments (see box below) can spend during that fiscal year. Generally, these appropriation bills are combined into a general appropriation bill called the omnibus spending bill.

Two specialized types of appropriation bills are the continuing resolution and supplemental appropriation bills. A bill called the continuing resolution is needed when a fiscal year begins and Congress has not yet enacted, or the president has not signed, the regular appropriation bills for that year. Congress then has to pass a joint resolution continuing the appropriations for all government agencies at the same levels as the previous year's appropriations. This continuing resolution bill can be a substitute for 1, 2, or all 13 appropriation bills and is in effect until a specific date or until a specific appropriation bill is enacted. Supplemental appropriation bills are passed when unanticipated or emergency funds are needed after the general or regular omnibus appropriation bill has been enacted. Currently the president does not have line item veto and therefore must accept or veto each appropriation bill in its entirety. Therefore, because appropriation or budget bills are required for the functioning of the federal government, other legislation, especially "pet" or specialized programs, are often attached to the budget bills in order to get them enacted. For example, several times during the 1980s the Nurse Education Act's appropriation bills were "tacked-on" to the budget to ensure that they were passed that fiscal year before Congress adjourned.

The budget cycle. The budget cycle is an important part of the federal legislative process (see box on p. 200 for a listing of legislative terms in relation to the budget). The president presents the administration's budget proposal in January. This budget proposal, formulated from all the cabinet departments and prepared by the Office of Management and Budget (OMB), outlines the president's estimates of tax receipts and budget outlays with detailed recommendations for the ensuing fiscal year's appropriations. These estimates are based on the continuation of existing levels of service and are called current service estimates. They reflect the anticipated costs of continuing federal

Cabinet Departments	
Agriculture	Interior
Commerce	Justice
Defense	Labor
Education	State
Energy	Treasury
Health and Human Services	Transportation
Housing and Urban Development	

Legislative (Budget) Terms	
Fiscal year	Budget-neutral programs
Authorization bills	Budget resolution
Appropriation bills	Budget plan or proposal
• General (omnibus spending bill)	Concurrent resolution
• Continuing resolution	Current service estimates
• Supplemental	Entitlements
Balanced budget	*Federal Register*
Budget proposals	Reconciliation bill
• Congressional	
• Presidential	

programs and activities at the current spending levels without policy changes, ignoring all new initiatives, presidential or congressional, that are not yet law. These estimates are accompanied by figures that show the effect of underlying economic and programmatic assumptions, such as the rate of inflation, the rate of the real economic growth, the unemployment rate, program caseloads, and salary increases. The president's budget, with its inherent policy priorities, serves as the starting point for Congress as it begins budget deliberations.

Next, Congress debates the president's budget proposal as it develops its own proposal called a budget resolution. Budget resolutions passed by the Senate and the House of Representatives set forth levels and functional allocations for a fiscal year. If the resolutions from the Senate and the House are different, negotiations occur until an acceptable resolution by both houses is achieved. This concurrent resolution, which must be developed by Congress by April of each year, does not require the president's signature and does not have the force of law. Essentially, the budget resolution is Congress's budget plan, similar to the plan submitted by the president at the beginning of the year. A reconciliation process occurs that enables Congress to bring revenues, expenditures, and entitlements into conformity with the levels set in the budget resolutions. The result of this process is called a reconciliation bill.

TYPES OF HEALTH CARE PROGRAMS

There are two types of federal health care programs, which are classified according to how easily their costs can be controlled: controllable programs and uncontrollable programs. *Controllable health care programs* are subject to annual appropriations by Congress and consist primarily of categorical health services, training, and research programs called discretionary programs. *Categorical health services* are services for relatively narrowly defined categories of problems, such as programs for communicable diseases, family planning, and family planning services. An example of a training program is the Nurse Education Act, and an example of a research program is the National Institute of Nursing at the National Institutes of Health (NIH).

Uncontrollable health care programs are called *entitlements* because enrolled members are entitled to their monetary benefits by law because of age, disability, or economic status. The federal government is obligated to pay these benefits regardless of the total costs. The only way these costs can be controlled is by changing or amending the authorizing legislation. They cannot be limited by simply appropriating less money for expenditures. Social Security, veterans' compensation, and pensions are examples of income entitlement programs. Examples of health care entitlement programs are Medicare and Medicaid.

In the president's budget for fiscal year 1996, 66% of the total federal budget was for mandatory spending. Approximately 76% of the mandatory spending, or 50% of the total federal budget, is for entitlement programs. Also, two thirds of the Department of Health and Human Services' budget is for entitlement programs, which means that only 33% of the amount appropriated by Congress for this department can be controlled.

THE FEDERAL BUDGET DEFICIT

In 1985 Congress passed the Gramm-Rudman-Hollings law (PL 99-177), which required annual deficit reduction targets for the federal budget. This was supposed to result in a balanced budget by 1991. The law was amended in 1988 to extend the time to achieve a balanced budget to 1993. Initially the act contained an automatic mechanism for making across-the-board spending cuts (sequestration) if the deficit targets were not met. This automatic mechanism was struck down in 1986 by the Supreme Court, and thus Congress was mandated to pass a joint resolution making the cuts. This nonmandatory mechanism has not been successful in reducing the deficit because of politics. Each of the major political parties is reluctant to be the one that cuts funding for public programs. In fiscal year 1996 the federal deficit is estimated to reach $197 billion.

During the 104th Congress, the idea of amending the U.S. Constitution to require a balanced federal budget became a reality. If a balanced budget amendment is passed by Congress and signed by the president, it must be ratified by three fourths of the states to become effective. Thirty-eight states must ratify the amendment within 7 years for it to become an official amendment to the U.S. Constitution. If and when this occurs, all entitlement programs will be affected because the federal budget must then be balanced every fiscal year.

IMPLEMENTING LEGISLATION

After a bill is passed and signed into law, rules and regulations to implement that law are written and published for public comment. Initial rules and regulations, as well as any changes, are published by the executive branch of the government at both the federal and state levels. These proposals are published in a government document called the Federal Register at the national level and in similar registers with similar names at the state level. After a period of time for public comment, the rules and regulations are promulgated and are either published as originally proposed or revised based on public comment. Laws are written in broad language; the rules and regulations to implement these laws are written more specifically. Rules and regulations can be revised without changing the original law.

POLITICS, HEALTH, AND NURSING

Nurses are not only the largest group of health professionals in the health care system, but are also the most diverse in terms of education and practice. This "depth and breadth" of the nursing profession give the nurse extraordinary potential to influence the health care delivery system. Nurses can influence health care policy as individuals and as professionals. Nurses as citizens should not abandon their rights to influence legislation and politics. As professionals, nurses are obligated to ensure that the public has access to quality health care at controlled costs. Armed with information on how to influence health care policy, nurses can become advocates for patients and become active participants in the formulation of effective health care policy. Policy decisions regarding financial resources influence the type of nursing staff, the number of nurses, the amount and type of management and support services, and supplies—all of which affect the quality of nursing care.

Economic Influences on Health Care Delivery

The need to control costs of health care without diminishing its quality or accessibility is becoming increasingly important. The public needs to ask continually if its money is being well spent for health care. Nurses are well placed and well equipped to help with this analysis. However, we cannot assume that the public, even local communities or institutions, understands how health care policies are made.

Because 48% of health care monies are spent by state and federal governments (Burner, Waldo & McKusick, 1992), governments control spending, as well as influence the quantity and quality of health care. Most of this spending at the federal level involves the Medicare and Medicaid programs. Thus, government policies are very influential because other third-party payors imitate the "feds." Third-party payors, by setting policies of who will be paid, determine who will deliver care, in what setting, and how much will be paid for it. Although other factors are also at play, third-party payors, by controlling payment, also determine the parameters within which nursing care is delivered, the type of nursing personnel delivering care, and how much nurses are paid to deliver that care.

Health Care Policy Research

Because the policies of the government are important for nursing reimbursement and therefore nursing care, it is important to understand research on health care policy. Health care policy research is essentially any research that affects health care policy. This definition encompasses a broad range of research methodologies and types. The core of health care policy research is research that examines the quality, access, and costs of health care. Nurses are particularly positioned to conduct policy research. Nurses are involved in all areas that impact access, quality, and costs of health care; in addition, the decisions made about access, quality, and costs impact nurses' practices.

Nursing practice is grounded in the values of caring and advocacy, especially for populations who are vulnerable to the impact from these core components of health care policy. Nurses have intimate clinical knowledge of the full spectrum of the delivery of health care services—from minute-to-minute hands-on care, the suffering of the patient and significant others, and the institutional and bureaucratic constraints under which health care is provided, to the practices of a wide array of other health care providers. Nurses are in a strategic position to document and critique the interactional and structural circumstances that impede on the quality, access, and costs of patient care. We need to not only look at the individual patients and their care, but also step back and examine groups or populations of patients and examine their care and the context within which care is delivered.

Access to Health Care

Many of the proposed health care reform packages in the 1990s have called for universal access to health care. Therefore it is important to understand this terminology. One congressman made an analogy about universal access to health care using the concept of everyone having access to Cadillac dealerships. He pointed out that all citizens can walk into a Cadillac car agency, but this does not mean that they have the money to buy a Cadillac or that they need or want to buy one.

What is meant by the term *barriers to universal access?* Does it mean that there are needs but no services? Does it mean that there is no way to pay for care? Does it mean that there are limited numbers of providers available to provide care?

Nurses are in a unique position to gather data to document all components of the access issue. It is becoming increasingly important that we document the nature and frequency of barriers to patients' receipt of care. When we use conclusions based on studies supported by quantitative and qualitative data rather than positions based on subjective or anecdotal reports, we will be effective in influencing policy.

Outcomes as Indicators of Quality

Economic necessity dictates the need to couple access and quality with economical practice. Nurses need to use their practices to identify which outcomes are linked to what strategies and determine which strategies result in the desired outcomes at the least cost.

An important first step is to define desirable outcomes. Many times, providers seek outcomes that only avoid adverse effects of care, or only attempt to return the patient back to "normal" as defined by clinical data, or only reduce or eliminate the patients' signs and symptoms, or only improve the patients' level of functioning. Nurses and physicians generally want to achieve outcomes that improve patients' physiological status, such as achieving a stable blood pressure and "good" blood gas readings or improving the degree of arterial blockage; reduce patients' signs and symptoms, such as lessening shortness of breath or relieving pain; or improve patients' functional status and well-being, such as the ability to climb stairs, work, or care for a family. Are these outcomes defined by patients, or do we as providers do what we think is best?

Outcomes research is needed to determine if the process being used achieves the desired outcomes. We need to identify who is defining the desired outcome, as well as distinguish which individual providers contribute to the outcome. Nurses' practices are independent, interdependent, and dependent on other providers. By measuring the amount and type of each provider's contributions to the achievement of the desired outcomes, we would have data on which policy decisions could be made and on who should provide care to achieve quality outcomes at controlled costs. As nurses, we have been concentrating on the process of delivery of care, and now we need to measure the outcomes in terms of cost, quality, and ability to access care. We need to determine what structural elements and process components lead to the desired outcomes.

Fagin (1990), in a classic article, stated:

> Lack of public access to nursing outcomes, nurses' and nursing's reluctance to make their contributions known, and the method of payment for institutional nursing services all support nursing's low profile in all areas but shortage in hospitals. That invisibility is creating a dangerous situation for the future. Few young people are willing to embark on a career whose practitioners appear underappreciated and unable to practice at their full potential. . . . Nurses have the knowledge and skill to act independently, cost-effectively, and accountably in a vast array of services needed by the American people.

NURSING'S INFLUENCE ON NURSING EDUCATION AND RESEARCH LEGISLATION

Legislation of interest to nurses is of two types: (1) funding bills that provide monies for education, research, innovative projects, or delivery methods, and payment for services that have a direct impact on the nursing profession; and (2) legislation that creates advisory committees, task forces, and commissions that provide opportunities for nurses to become visibly active participants in the deliberations of health care policies.

Nursing Education Legislation

The Nurse Education Act is traditionally the most important piece of federal legislation to nurses. Generally, it is authorized for 3 years, with the amount of appropriations set each year. The present act originated with the Nurse Training Act of 1964.

Nursing is the only health profession to retain a separate funding law with a separate national advisory committee for education. Although no president, regardless of political party, since President Nixon has included nursing education in the budget, Congress, regardless of which political party was in control, at nursing's request, has funded nursing education even over presidential vetoes. This attests to the skill and wisdom of the nursing leaders and the nursing community during these 30 years. Between 1965 and 1971, more than $380 million was spent on nursing education for both students and institutions. Doctoral nursing students and nursing doctoral programs began receiving more emphasis and support during the mid 1970s. Also during this time, advanced practice education programs in the form of nurse practitioner programs were funded by the government (Kalisch & Kalisch, 1982; Scott, 1972).

Nursing Research Legislation

Nursing research funding had been included in most nurse education acts. Although this research was funded by the federal government and was conducted by nurse researchers, nursing leaders argued that nursing research should be "integrated into the mainstream of science if it is to flourish and be better understood by other scientists and the public and that creation of a National Institute of Nursing would help accomplish these goals" (Jacox, 1985, p.78). Jacox also stated that the quality of nursing care would be greatly improved by research and that the promotion of strong nursing research programs could best occur in the mainstream of science. These reasons justified the creation of a separate institute of nursing within the NIH.

Nurses in research coalesced under the guidance of the Cabinet of Nursing Research of the American Nurses' Association (ANA). After the Institute of Medicine (IOM) issued its report on nursing in 1983, acknowledging nursing research and recommending that a federal entity for nursing research be established in the mainstream of science, three organized nursing groups—the ANA, National League for Nursing, and American Association of Colleges of Nursing—agreed in June 1983 to work with nurse researchers to accomplish this goal.

As stated earlier, no administration since Nixon had requested monies for nursing in the president's budget; therefore it was assumed that there would be considerable resistance from the executive branch to the establishment of an institute for nursing in the NIH. In spite of this strong resistance, the nursing organizations relying on the historically strong Congressional support regardless of the political party in the majority were successful in 1983 in getting legislation introduced in the House of Representatives to create a National Institute of Nursing. This bill passed unanimously by voice vote in November 1983. In October 1984, it was successfully considered by the Senate and House Conference Committee and was reported out as part of the NIH reauthorization bill. This bill, passed by both houses, was vetoed by President Reagan, who said in his veto message that this was an example of "unnecessary, expensive new organizational entities" (Reagan, 1984). In January 1985, the secretary of Health and Human Services (HHS) announced the establishment of a Center for Nursing Research in the Division of Nursing, saying that this was the best approach to implementing the IOM's recommendation regarding nursing research. This initiative added 6 new positions, for a total of 12 positions in the Division of Nursing. All this action did was add the additional personnel positions to an already-existing research program within the Division of Nursing. It did nothing to move nursing research into the mainstream of scientific research.

So the nurses tried again. Learning from their experience and initiating actions that would ensure that the "grass roots" of nursing would participate in the legislative process by contacting their legislators, the bill was reintroduced. Opposition to the bill continued, not only from the administration, but also from scientists in other institutes within the NIH. These scientists saw the addition of a nursing institute as taking another slice of the fiscal pie, with a possible reduction in funds for their own research. Nurses working in the Division of Nursing's Center for Nursing Research were also reluctant to support an entity that would take away their work and funding. But with careful planning and enthusiastic support by others in nursing and Congress, the fight was on.

This time, a compromise was worked out because a senator who had consistently supported the idea, but at a center level rather than at an institute level, refused to budge. A center is one level below an institute at the NIH. The sponsor of the original bill and the new bill counseled compromise to the nursing organizations when it became clear that the NIH bill would be vetoed unless it was a center. Republican leaders supporting the bill believed they had reached a compromise with the White House in that there would be no veto if it was a Center for Nursing rather than an Institute of Nursing. Much to their surprise and nursing's, President Reagan vetoed the bill on November 8, 1985. Congress then overwhelmingly voted to override the presidential veto to establish a National Center for Nursing Research (NCNR) ("Nurses Win Battle," 1986).

The NCNR was established in April 1986 with the purpose of providing a strong scientific base for nursing practice. Seven years later, on June 11, 1993, the NCNR became the National Institute of Nursing Research (NINR) and became the seventeenth institute of the NIH. Secretary of Health and Human Services Donna Shalala stated that the establishment of the NINR recognizes that nursing research makes a vital contribution to improving the nation's health.

Nursing Practice Legislation

The most important legislation affecting nursing practice is the nurse practice acts (NPAs) enacted in each state. The United States is governed under the principle of states' rights. This principle derived from the U.S. Constitution, which delineates the powers of the federal government and considers all other powers as belonging to the states. Licensure statutes are designed to protect the public, not to control entry into practice.

Licensure, certification, and registration are all means of labeling the qualifications of individuals. Licensure is the process by which an agency of the government grants permission to persons meeting predetermined qualifications to engage in a given occupation and/or use a particular title. Certification is the process by which a nongovernmental agency or association grants recognition to an individual who has certain predetermined qualifications specified by that agency or association. Registration is the process by which qualified individuals are listed on an official roster maintained by a governmental or nongovernmental agency (Wilson & Neuhauser, 1982).

State legislation. All states have NPAs that license nurses. Some states have NPAs with "sunset" provisions, which automatically terminate a licensure statute after a designated period of time. When this occurs, it is up to the profession to show the state legislature that the profession needs to be licensed to protect the public. This "proving" requires intensive and widespread political effort from nurses within that state to convince the legislators to license nurses (Wilson & Neuhauser, 1982).

Each state, under the practice acts, mandates what qualifications health professionals must possess to be licensed to practice their profession in that state. NPAs define and regulate the entry to nursing practice and are administered by state boards of nursing. These boards are composed of a representative mix of types of nurses within that state (and generally at least one consumer) and are appointed by the governor. Although each state has its own appointment process, generally candidates are nominated by nursing organizations, as well as by other interested organizations, including political parties. These boards of nursing are given the charge to promulgate the rules and regulations necessary to implement the nurse practice statute.

NPAs establish the requirements for licensure, which generally consist of necessary educational experiences, including the requirement of successful completion of an examination. The first practice act for nurses was passed by North Carolina in 1903. By 1923 all states and the District of Columbia had such laws. At first, licensure was not mandatory for the practice of nursing, but it did prohibit any unlicensed person from using the title of "registered nurse."

Federal legislation. Much of the federal legislation affecting nursing practice has centered around payment for services. The first legislation affecting payment to nurses was the Rural Health Clinics Act of 1977 (PL 95-210). This law amended Title XIX (Medicaid) of the Social Security Act to include rural health clinic services by nurse practitioners within the definition of "medical assistance" eligible for payment under the title. It also amended Title XVIII (Medicare) of the Social Security Act to provide payment for rural health clinic services under the supplementary medical insurance program and required the states to establish a plan for medical assistance and payment for rural health services.

This law was the first recognition of nurses as providers receiving third-party payment by the federal government. Senator Barbara Mikulski, a Democrat from Maryland, has stated that because she was a supporter of this bill when she was a congresswoman and because she refused to retract her support for third-party payment for nurse practitioners, she lost financial support from the American Medical Association (AMA) when she campaigned for her Senate seat in 1986 (personal communication, May 1986).

Nurse practitioners have consistently been pioneers in receiving payment for their services from the federal government. Nurse anesthetists and nurse midwives receive payment, though often at a lower percentage rate of the fee for the same service received by the physician. For example, the 1994 Annual Report to Congress by the Physician Payment Review Commission stated that in rural areas, Medicare pays nurse practitioners directly for hospital services up to 75% of the physician fee and, at most, 85% of the physician fee for all other services. For care delivered in nursing homes, the nurse practitioner's employer receives no more than 85% of the physician's payment. Neither nurse practitioners nor physician assistants are paid for services provided in urban areas except when these services are incidental to a physician's care (Physician Payment Review Commission, 1994).

The first session of the 101st Congress flip-flopped over the issue of whether to change Medicare and Medicaid to provide for direct and/or indirect payment for nurse practitioners. This issue has been opposed by organized medicine for the past several years. So Congress compromised and passed legislation in November 1989 that provides direct payments from Medicaid to pediatric and family nurse practitioners for family health services. Specifically, since July 1, 1990, states have been required to cover the services of these two types of nurse practitioners regardless of whether the services are provided under the supervision of, or in association with, a physician. Other restrictions imposed by state laws still apply. As part of nursing home reform, indirect payments for nurse practitioners' services were included, along with the authorization of nurse practitioners to certify and recertify patients in long-term care facilities. These small victories are the result of many years of political lobbying by organized nursing groups and the constant education of legislators and consumers as to the value of nurse practitioners. A report on nurse practitioners and others by the Office of Technology Assessment (OTA) has helped convince government officials of the worth and cost-effectiveness of nonphysician providers (U.S. Congress, OTA, 1986).

POLITICAL INFLUENCES ON HEALTH CARE LEGISLATION

The public is often unaware of the influence of politics on health care legislation. To illustrate this influence, the amendments to the Social Security Act that created Medicare (Title XVIII) and Medicaid (Title XIX) in 1965, as well as a later amendment, the Medicare Catastrophic Protection Act, are presented here as an example.

The law to amend the Social Security Act (PL 89-97) initially established health insurance for the aged and grants to states for medical assistance to the poor. Later amendments to the law added other categories of individuals to be covered: the disabled and end-stage renal patients. This law occurred because of a combination of factors, such as increased medical technology, heightened consumer expectations and use, and rising costs.

Historical Perspective on Health Care Coverage

The United States was the slowest of the Western countries to develop some form of government action regarding the insuring of health care. In 1883 Bismarck in Germany initiated a health insurance plan for industrial workers, and in 1911 England included health insurance for low-income workers in its social security program, which provided pensions. By 1940 no Western European country was without some type of government health insurance program, at least for low-income workers. The benefits of these programs varied widely. The initial restriction to the aged in the U.S. Medicare plan was unlike the European plans, which covered low-income workers.

Although the issue of government-sponsored health insurance was raised during the 1930s, Roosevelt's New Deal programs generally were concerned only with Social Security income proposals. In order to correct the unequal distribution of medical services, a proposal submitted during Truman's administration attempted to remove financial barriers to the accessibility to health care. The underlying belief behind this proposal was that access to health services varied with income, resulting in regions where charity care was not available. Truman's proposal in 1949 to remove the financial barriers to health care through government action failed in Congress. The AMA was not placated by Truman's plan to make physicians' participation voluntary and started a campaign to educate the public that "socialized medicine" was not a good thing for the American people. Truman submitted similar proposals in 1950, 1952, and 1953, all of which failed.

Although these proposals failed, several modifications in the plan were made to streamline it. Truman's staff recommended that he "softpedal the general health issue; push some peripheral programs in the area but not general insurance; or appoint a study commission to go over the whole problem" (Marmor, 1973, p. 14). A commission was established and charged to find the "right people" as well as simultaneously push for "some peripheral programs." The administration attempted to come up with a proposal that would meet one of the major objections to Truman's proposal—that general medical insurance was a "giveaway" program and made no distinction between the "deserving" poor and the "undeserving" poor.

Thus, the focus turned to the aged. The elderly, as a group, could be presumed to be both needy and deserving because it was through no fault of their own that they had a lower earning capacity and higher medical expenses than any other adult age group. Because the proponents wished to avoid an income means test to determine eligibility, believing it would look too much like welfare, they limited eligibility to those over 65 who had contributed to Social Security during their lifetime. A limitation on days in the hospital was added to show that the program was not a complete giveaway program. Physicians' services were excluded in order to reduce their hostility toward the plan.

Different plans, including Truman's compromises, were introduced into Congress at various times throughout the following years. The political climate in Congress remained somewhat opposed to "giving away" monies for health care and provided no opportunity for passage of such proposals. With the election of President Kennedy in 1961, a shift toward a more liberal climate in Congress occurred. Also during this time, several organizations and groups were becoming active supporters or opponents of such a proposal (Table 9-1). Among the supporters was organized labor. Organized labor had been asking for more and more health benefits in collective bargaining agreements for their members.

Even though the political climate in Washington became increasingly liberal, Congress generally responded to the conservative Southern Democratic legislators. However, in 1965 the elections changed this composition of Congress. This shift in Congress, along with Kennedy's assassination and the assumption of the presidency by Johnson resulted in a change in the political climate. The time was ripe for the passage

Table 9-1   **Selected Federal Health Acts of Interest to Nurses**

Year	Public Law Number	Name of Statute	Selected Elements of Statute
1935	74-241	Social Security Act	Provided for the first time grants-in-aid to states for such public health activities as maternal and child care, aid to crippled children, blind persons, the aged, and other health-impaired persons
1939	76-19	Reorganization Act of 1939	Transferred the PHS from the Treasury Department to a new Federal Security Agency
1941	77-146	Nurse Training Appropriations	Assisted schools of nursing in increasing enrollments and improving their programs
1943	78-74	Nurse Training Act	Authorized the creation of the U.S. Nurse Cadet Corps
1944	78-410	Public Health Service Act	Combined all PHS authorities into a single statute (Title 42, U.S. Code)
1946	79-725	Hospital Survey Construction Act (commonly called Hill-Burton Act)	Funded and supported surveys, plans, and new health care facilities
1949	81-380	Amendments to Hospital and Construction Act	Increased funds to promote effective development and utilization of hospital services and facilities
1956	84-911	Health Amendments	Established traineeships for graduate education for nurses
1960	86-788	Social Security Amendments	Authorized grants to states for medical assistance for the aged
1963	88-129	Health Professions Educational Assistance Act	Provided funds for training of physicians, dentists, public health personnel, and others; provided construction grants for schools of nursing
1964	88-581	Nurse Training Act	The beginning of the federal acts for training professional nurses
1965	89-97	Social Security Amendments	Established health insurance for the indigent and grants to states for medical assistance programs called Medicare and Medicaid
1966	89-751	Allied Health Professions Personnel Act	Provided support for training of allied health workers; also provided student loans for health professionals
1968	90-490	Health Manpower Act	Authorized formula institutional grants for training nurses and other health professionals
1970	91-519	Health Training Improvement Act	Provided expanded funds to all allied health professions
1970	91-623	Emergency Health Personnel Act	Provided funds to health manpower shortage areas through the establishment of a National Health Service Corps

Table 9-1　**Selected Federal Health Acts of Interest to Nurses—cont'd**

Year	Public Law Number	Name of Statute	Selected Elements of Statute
1971	92-157	Comprehensive Health Manpower Training Act	Expanded and strengthened federal programs for the development of health manpower
1971	92-158	Nurse Training Act	Expanded and strengthened efforts to support nurse training
1972	92-603	Social Security Amendments	Extended the health insurance program to disabled and to end-stage renal disease patients; established a Professional Standard Review Organization program
1973	93-222	Health Maintenance Organization Act	Assisted in the establishment and expansion of HMOs
1977	95-210	Rural Health Clinics Act	Amended Title XIX, Medicaid, of Social Security Act to include rural health clinic services by nurse practitioners within the definition of medical assistance; also amended Medicare to provide payment for rural health clinic services
1979	96-76	Nurse Training Amendments of 1979	Amended Title VIII of the PHS Act to extend at a reduced authorization the assistance program for nurse training and students
1985	99-158	Health Research Extension Act of 1985	Established a National Center for Nursing Research
1988	100-360	Medicare Catastrophic Protection Act	Mandated unlimited hospital care, limited out-of-pocket expenses, physician bills, and partial payment for prescription drugs; also created the Pepper Commission to study the issue of long-term care for the elderly
1989	101-239	Omnibus Budget Reconciliation Act of 1989	Amendments to Medicaid to provide direct payment for pediatric and family nurse practitioners
1993	103-43	NIH Revitalization Act of 1993	NCNR converted to the National Institute for Nursing Research

of a national health insurance plan. President Johnson took advantage of this, and Medicare was passed and signed into law on July 30, 1965.

Catastrophic Amendments Debacle

In the 1980s, during President Reagan's administration, a debate on the effect that catastrophic illnesses had on the elderly led to a commission to study these effects. This commission developed a plan that was submitted to Congress by President Reagan. Congress debated the issue and proposed several plans of its own. Several areas of debate centered on how to pay for the added benefits. Congress, in an attempt to control the spiraling deficit of the federal budget, attempted to make the added benefits budget neutral by developing a plan that included an income surtax on approximately 40% of the beneficiaries. This surtax would pay for catastrophic benefits for this 40% and for the poorer 60%. Less than 5% of the beneficiaries would pay the full amount, $800, during the first year. This amount would increase every year as new benefits were phased in, with a set maximum rate. This concept had support from many people and a variety of organizations, including the American Association of Retired Persons and the ANA. Several voiced concern that the elderly also needed coverage for nursing home care. However, the cost estimate for an average annual stay in a nursing home in the 1980s was $25,000 and was seen at that time as a prohibitive expense to the federal government.

Several factors delayed the passage of a bill, including the stock market crash in October 1987, the balancing of the budget, and objections from several congressmen. Congressman Claude Pepper, a Democrat from Florida, introduced a proposal to increase coverage of home health care for the elderly and other disabled persons. Since he was chairman of the Rules Committee, he ruled that his bill should go directly to the floor of the House of Representatives for debate, thus bypassing the two health committees with extremely powerful chairmen. These two influential chairmen were angered by Pepper's maneuver and vowed to defeat his bill. This procedural and turf battle defeated Pepper's bill and assisted the passage of the catastrophic amendment bill, which mandated unlimited hospital care, limited out-of-pocket expenses for physician bills, and partial payment for prescription drugs. Because of the respect that the House of Representatives had for Congressman Pepper, however, an addition to the final bill created a commission to examine the problem of long-term care and possible solutions. This commission is commonly referred to as the Pepper Commission and was set up to study the issue of long-term care for the elderly.

The Medicare Catastrophic Protection Act (PL 100-360) was signed into law on July 1, 1988. It was heralded by Congress, the administration, elderly consumer groups, and others, including health care providers. Rules and regulations were written to implement the law, including the precedent-setting financial method of income surtaxes. As the details of the rules and regulations were disseminated to the public, a backlash from the elderly, mainly middle-class elderly, occurred over the surtax. They believed they were being asked to pay more taxes than other, nonelderly citizens for the same benefits they were paying for in private insurance plans called Medigap plans. Their vehement opposition generated such an uproar that in November 1989 Congress repealed most of the measures contained in the catastrophic bill passed the year before. Not only were the catastrophic amendments the largest expansions since the inception of the Medicare program, but this was also the first time that a large health benefit program had been repealed before it was fully implemented. The aftermath of this debacle has been the reluctance of Congress to consider any health insurance plan for the elderly. The final report of the Pepper Commission has not been acted on.

Other health landmark laws passed by Congress before Medicare and Medicaid that had some indirect and direct effects on nursing were the Social Security Act of 1935 (PL

74-241), which for the first time provided grants-in-aid to states for maternal and child care, as well as aid to crippled children, blind persons, the aged, and other health-impaired persons; and the Hospital Survey and Construction Act (PL 79725) enacted in 1946 (commonly called the Hill-Burton Act), which supported surveys, plans, and new facilities such as hospitals and was a turning point in the delivery of health care. During this time, health care delivery shifted into hospitals, with nurses becoming predominantly salaried employees of the institutions.

HEALTH CARE REFORM PROPOSALS

Clinton's Health Care Reform Proposals

In 1993 President Clinton, in response to the mandate that he believed his 1992 election provided him, appointed his wife, Hillary Rodham Clinton, as leader of an enormous Health Care Reform Task Force. This task force tapped about 1000 persons for work and advice on a proposal that eventually was titled the Health Security Act. Working groups were formed around identified health care problems. To avoid ethical problems, the heads of these groups were full-time government employees. This unusual private-public partnership lasted more than a year and produced a plan that was comprehensive in the changes it promoted. The proposals embodied in the Health Security Act are not now as important as the reasons why the act was not enacted and the fallout from this failure.

During the 1992 presidential election the public was very vocal in its concern about many factors that impacted their health care insurance. These factors were (1) the rising costs of health care and, therefore, costs of health insurance; (2) the poor economic climate with high unemployment and the resulting loss of health insurance benefits; (3) an increase in the number of health insurance plans changing from community rating (spreading the costs of insurance across a group of people) to experience rating (increasing the rates when an individual "experiences" illnesses, similarly to automobile insurance); and (4) the approximately 35 million citizens who were underinsured or uninsured.

The amount of time (over 18 months) that elapsed between the first meeting of the task force and the submission of the program to Congress allowed the policymakers to miss the "window of opportunity" for instituting change. The overwhelming amount of details in the plan, the massive changes required to implement the program, and an upturn in the economic climate all coalesced to defeat the Health Security Act.

State Responses to Health Care Reform

Several parts of the proposal, most especially managed care, have surfaced in various proposals subsequently introduced into Congress. Several states, before the Health Security Act and after it, have devised health care reform plans. However, even the most ardent of the states are now pursuing more modest health care reform plans. For example, the state of Washington's health care reform plan (fashioned after Clinton's national reform bill)—a standard, minimum package of health benefits, universal coverage, and a mandate that employers contribute at least half the cost of employee health insurance—was repealed in the spring of 1995. Small reforms were passed by the state legislature to improve access to care by raising insurance subsidies for low-income persons.

Tennessee decided to dump its costly Medicaid program and replaced it with a managed care program called TennCare. This program required a waiver from the federal government and has allowed 400,000 additional low-income persons to receive health coverage. Critics of the program point to the long waiting lines and the financial confusion. Based on the results of Tennessee's program, 10 other states requested and obtained waivers from the federal government to implement similar programs. Florida's managed care program for Medicaid beneficiaries is one of the most ambitious among all the states for uninsured and indigent citizens. Over 17% of the state's gross domestic product is dedicated to health care.

The most original (and some say the most successful) health plan is Oregon's health care rationing plan. The authorities in Oregon held a series of public meetings around the state to determine how to spend their limited resources, and the 13 broad themes that emerged from these encounters were used to set health spending priorities. These themes included such things as the relief of pain and suffering and the right to a quality of life that allows each individual to contribute socially and economically. A commission of health professionals and members of the public took these themes and turned them into a list of fundable treatments. If a treatment is not on this list, the state government will not pay for it. Although this rationing is highly controversial, 17 months after the inception of this plan there was a consensus within the state that this is a permissible way of restricting health care and thereby controlling costs. Oregon has a small, homogeneous population. This plan is untried in states with a large urban, heterogeneous population.

As some states move Medicaid beneficiaries toward managed care in the hope of saving money, the number of privately insured consumers in managed care continues to rise. In 1994 approximately 63% of Americans with employer-sponsored health insurance were in managed care. Thus the revolution in health care policy has been spurred by private market forces rather than state or federal legislation.

Timing of Health Care Reform Proposals

To realistically evaluate if the timing is appropriate for a national health care reform, the climate needs to be assessed. In doing this assessment, several questions need to be asked. The following pertinent questions were posed by a newspaper writer (Priest, 1993, p. 10):

1. Do Americans still believe that private industry can generate solutions such as innovative medical technology or less costly doctor check-ups or, eventually, health everyone can afford? Or should the government guarantee health care to all as an inalienable right, free of the risks and experiments that define the marketplace?

2. Do Americans believe in taking care of those who cannot take care of themselves, and how much are they willing to pay to do it? Is it better to raise more money now to insure the uninsured or to do it gradually over many years, leaving many people uninsured in the interim but keeping the price tag down?
3. Will Americans accept a change that might mean some people will pay more than they are now for health care or have less choice over which [health care provider] they visit? Is this sacrifice worth the gains in curbing the federal deficit or diverting money now spent on health care to other uses?
4. Do Americans believe that government bureaucracy can be trusted to play a role in something as essential as health care?
5. Are Americans willing to take a chance on an untreated new system in the hopes it will avert what most experts agree is a dangerous drain on the national budget and private sector economy?

These questions illustrate in more detail the factors in influencing the policy-making process: know the issues and questions; identify and know the players and arenas; and assess the climate of the times. The answers to these questions, along with the actions or nonactions by Congress and the president, will determine if any national reforms are developed in the future.

SPHERES OF NURSING INFLUENCE

The nurse has the opportunity to make an impact on policies in four spheres of influence as identified by Talbott and Mason (1988). These spheres are (1) government, (2) the workplace, (3) organizations, and (4) communities. Since the community encompasses the other three spheres, only government, organizations, and the workplace are discussed here.

Government

Laws, with their accompanying rules and regulations, impact nursing practice and health care. Nurses have been more involved in federal and state governments, although local governments provide many health care services. Local governments oversee school health programs and local public hospitals, and can impact home and community health care. Several books detail how nurses can influence governments (Archer & Goehner, 1982; Goldwater & Zusy, 1990; Kalisch & Kalisch, 1982; Mason, Talbott, & Leavitt, 1992).

In general, the nurse must first be a registered voter. Nurses can join collective actions by working with political action committees (PACs). These committees support deserving candidates who support nursing and health care issues. The ANA political action committee, called ANA-PAC, supports candidates favorable to nursing issues. The ANA and ANA-PAC depend on nurses at the grass roots level, not only to contribute money, but also to work in endorsed candidates' campaigns for national offices. Goldwater and Zusy (1990) discuss in detail how nurses can participate in campaigns, as well as run for elective offices. Most states have state nurses' association PACs for state and local candidates, and most organizations are set up to instruct novices on how to become involved. Other ways of becoming involved include joining a local branch of a political party and becoming involved in local political clubs. This type of involvement enables nurses to be involved in issues other than health care, as well as developing nonnurse support for health issues.

Another way of becoming involved at the governmental level is to work for an elected official, either as a paid employee or as a volunteer expert consultant. Elected officials have numerous bills or reports to review and respond to; however, a nurse can be influential in molding the official's position on issues. For example, a nurse volunteering in former Mayor Koch's New York City campaign (much to her surprise) was asked to write his position paper on health care. It is also important for nurses to run for elected offices and to assume political appointments. These political appointments can be on task forces, committees, boards of nursing, or positions in the local and state health department.

The Workplace

Since most nurses work in bureaucratic organizations, they can take advantage of the opportunity to influence the policies of their workplace. The workplace is physically changing from the hospital to the home, the clinic, and the office. In the recent past, over 66% of nurses worked in hospitals. Nurses have the potential to influence how quality care is delivered with controlled costs and to ensure that budget cuts do not diminish the amount and type of care needed. Most hospitals currently are reengineering, redesigning, or restructuring their work. This means that they are evaluating many nonnursing and nursing functions and tasks.

The factors that are needed to influence health care policy are the same factors needed to influence organizational policies: know the issues, identify and know the stakeholders and the arenas, and be aware of the climate. By knowing who, where, and how, nurses can influence organizational policies. Nurses can use their interpersonal skills, professional competence, and policy-making knowledge to influence hospital policies. In addition, nurses can serve on interdisciplinary hospital committees and on the board of trustees of the institution. Nurses who successfully practice the politics of change in their place of employment can influence the type and quality of patient care.

Organizations

Nurses can influence policies through professional organizations such as the ANA and the many nursing specialty organizations. ANA members not only have an impact on legislation at the federal and state level, but can also use this forum to make the public aware of nursing issues. The ANA has the capacity to monitor many issues and can alert nurses when to support or oppose issues. Nursing organizations can work in coalition with other health groups to support or oppose issues of interest to all of them. Nursing organizations are often approached to recommend nurses for appointments on task forces and committees. By joining and being active in a professional organization, an individual nurse has access to a wider range of tools and information in order to influence health care policies.

IMPACT OF NURSING RESEARCH ON HEALTH CARE POLICY

Historically, research and reports on nurses and nursing have resulted in policy changes. Studies, such as the 1948 survey entitled "Nursing for the Future," have resulted in legislation to assist the training of nurses by providing funds for nursing scholarships and general support for nursing schools. Selected examples of how nursing research, reports, and studies influenced changes in policy are presented here.

Nursing Practice

The Department of Nursing Resources of the U.S. Public Health Service published its study, "Patients and Personnel: A Method of Studying Patient Care in Hospitals," in 1957. Designed to determine whether satisfaction with nursing care was related to nurse staffing, this exhaustive survey study of some 20,000 patients and staff members was conducted to show hospitals how to incorporate patients' needs into their studies. Studies such as this and others done by the Department of Nursing Resources helped improve the use of nursing resources. For example, Kalisch & Kalisch (1982) reported that in one typical hospital the time spent on nonnursing activities by the nursing staff had been markedly reduced as a result of these studies.

The 1963 study, "Toward Quality in Nursing," recommended an increase in the number of nurses and established goals that resulted in the first nurse training act in 1964. The Department of Nursing has completed several National Sample Surveys of Registered Nurses, which have affected the amounts of monies appropriated by Congress, as well as shaped the types of educational programs that receive these funds.

Nursing Research

To demonstrate the need for a separate entity within the NIH for nursing research, nurses used several studies. Besides the 1983 Institute of Medicine's (IOM) report on nursing, a study sponsored by the ANA Council of Nurse Researchers was used to demonstrate that many nursing studies did not fit into the NIH research programs. This study, conducted by Joanne Stevenson (1983), reviewed 111 draft research proposals written by nurses and submitted to the federal government for funding. Of the 61 directed to the NIH, the NIH determined that 12 were relevant to their mission, 24 were of potential interest, and 25 were clearly outside the research focus of the NIH. These 25 deemed not in the NIH's domain were in the following areas: development of knowledge in the domain of care, rather than cure; studies of the family as the target of health care; studies of interpersonal processes, especially verbal and nonverbal communication, as intervention techniques; and health promotion directed toward chronically ill, as well as healthy, persons. These four areas are the core of nursing research, yet they were deemed not to fit within the scope of research done at the NIH at that time (Jacox, 1985, 1986; Stevenson, 1983). Jacox (1985) cited several studies conducted by the federal government that had implications for finding a place for nursing research within the federal government.

Nursing research studies conducted before the need for the data for policy-making will be more influential than anecdotes or stories. Data gathered from research studies have the potential to influence how health care is financed and delivered in the future.

 ## *Key Points*

- Before the twentieth century, health care was viewed as an individual responsibility.

- Health care legislation is often motivated by influential groups based on their self-interests.

- Nurses, as the largest group of health care professionals, can have a major impact on health care legislation.

- Influencing health policy requires an understanding of the issues involved, as well as the key players, the process, and the climate of the times.

- Legislation includes both authorization bills and appropriation bills.

- Federal health care programs include "controllable" programs and "entitlements."

- Fifty percent of the federal budget is for entitlement programs.

- Since 1985 Congress has attempted, without success, to balance the federal budget.

- Government policies regarding reimbursement for health care services have a major influence on health care delivery.

- Determining desirable patient care outcomes is an important component for health care legislation in the future.

- Nursing is the only health care profession with a separate funding law and national advisory committee for education.

- Nursing leaders worked for years to establish and fund the National Institute of Nursing Research.

- Many states have enacted health care reform in anticipation of federal changes.

- Nurses can exert their political influences in the workplace, government, and community, as well as in organizations.

Critical Thinking Exercises

1. What health care issues are of particular importance in your local community? How can you influence a change in this area? Who are the opponents to this change? What groups could you mobilize to influence this problem?

2. How can nursing research have an impact on particular health care policies? Give an example of a study that would be of interest to legislators.

3. Do you think we will ever be able to decrease the amount of money spent on "entitlement"? Are there any ethical issues to be considered with changes in entitlement?

4. Talk with other health care professionals who have at least 10 years' experience in health care. Ask them to identify how the proposed health care reform has changed practice. Consider their discipline as you analyze their responses.

References

Archer, S.E., & Goehner, P.A. (1982). *Nurses, a political force.* Monterey, CA: Wadsworth Health Sciences Division.

Burner, S.T., Waldo, D.R., & McKusick, D.R. (1992). National health expenditures projection through 2030. *Health Care Financing Review, 14*(10), 1-29.

Fagin, C. (1990). Nursing's value proves itself. *American Journal of Nursing, 90*(10), 17-18, 22-30.

Feldstein, P.J. (1988). *The politics of health legislation.* Ann Arbor, MI: Health Administration Press Perspectives.

Goldwater, M., & Zusy, M.J.L. (1990). *Prescription for nurses: Effective political action.* St. Louis: Mosby.

Hyman, H.H. (1982). *Health planning: A systematic approach.* Rockville, MD: Aspen.

Jacox, A. (1985). Science and politics. *Nursing Outlook 33*(2), 78-84.

Jacox, A. (1986). The coming of age of nursing research. *Nursing Outlook 34*(6), 276-281.

Kalisch, B.J., & Kalisch, P.A. (1982). *Politics of nursing.* Philadelphia: J.B. Lippincott.

Marmor, T.R. (1973). *The politics of Medicare.* Chicago: Aldine.

Mason, D.J., Talbott, S.W., & Leavitt, J.K. (1992). *Policy and politics for nurses: Action and changes in the workplace, government, organization and community* (2nd ed.). Philadelphia: W.B. Saunders.

Nurses win battle for research center at NIH: Congress rebukes Reagan and overides his veto. (1986). *American Journal of Nursing, 86*(1), 75.

Physician Payment Review Commission. (1994). *Annual report to Congress.* Washington, DC: The Commission.

Priest, D. (1993, July 13). Framework for health reform plan is set. *Washington Post Health Magazine,* p.10.

Reagan, R. (1984, October 30). *Memorandum of disapproval.* Washington, DC: Office of the Press Secretary, White House.

Scott, J.M. (1972). Federal support for nursing education 1964-1972. *American Journal of Nursing, 72*(10), 1855-1861.

Stevenson, J. (1983). *New investigator federal sector grantsmanship project* (Final report ANA Publication No. D-75). Kansas City, MO: American Nurses' Association.

Talbott, S.W., & Mason, D.J. (1988). Power and professional influence. In B. Kozier and G. Erb, *Concepts and issues in nursing practice.* Menlo Park, CA: Addison-Wesley.

U.S. Congress, Office of Technology Assessment. (1986). *Nurse practitioners, physicians' assistants, and certified nurse-midwives: Policy analysis.* Washington, DC: U.S. Government Printing Office.

Wilson, F.A., & Neuhauser, D. (1982). *Health services in the United States* (2nd ed.). Cambridge, MA: Ballinger.

Economic Issues in Health Care 10

Karen MacDonald Thompson

 ## Objectives

At the completion of this chapter, the reader will be able to:

- Define the economic principles of supply, demand, and cost.

- Describe how the economic concepts of opportunity costs, price elasticity, complements and substitutes, competition, and marginal utility apply to the health care environment and specifically to nursing.

- Define and differentiate the two methods of cost evaluation discussed in this chapter.

- Discuss the interrelatedness of costs of care and quality of care.

Profile in Practice

Judith W. Ryan, PhD, RN, CRNP
Nurse Practitioner,
Clinical Director, EverCare,
Baltimore, Maryland

Economic issues are becoming increasingly important in the delivery of health care. As a nurse practitioner, I have had to be alert, not only to the cost-effectiveness of this provider role, but also to the realities of whether a patient had money to pay for a prescription I was writing. Could the patient pay for the full prescription, or would I need to write two prescriptions so that the patient could buy the rest of the medication after his or her next paycheck? Quality-of-care issues and economic realities are constantly interacting, and the health care provider who is not attentive to both will be ineffective.

With EverCare, we are providing a unique, cost-effective method of caring for the long-term residents in nursing homes. Our program uses a collaborative model of care with nurse practitioners and physicians, with a care- and cost-shifting emphasis on early detection and treatment in the nursing home environ-

---

ment. The nurse practitioner makes rounds and follows the patient more closely, and when a medical problem arises, it is addressed directly. This can often save the cost and trauma of transporting the patient to the emergency department of a local hospital, where the nursing home resident is often not a priority. Keeping patients in familiar surroundings and bringing the services to them can be much more cost-effective and also have more positive quality-of-care outcomes. Working closely with the patient's family is an important component of this program and promotes having clearly defined advance directives and a good flow of communication. Our nurse practitioners carry note cards to write a few sentences to the responsible family members who may not be able to visit and for whom a telephone contact is not needed. This way, they stay in contact about the health status of their loved one (without having to initiate it), and peace of mind or consumer satisfaction is the usual outcome.

The challenge to today's nurse is to become and stay informed. It is not prudent for a nurse to think that just because he or she gives high-quality clinical care that there will be continuing employment. The health care system is changing too rapidly. The relevant and employable nurse is one who knows the marketplace, who can provide outcomed-based care that is cost-effective and satisfying to the consumer.

PROBLEMS OF COST AND ACCESS

Economics is the study of the distribution of scarce resources across a population. Similarly, *health economics* is the study of the distribution of health care. The study of health economics is increasingly of interest and necessity, not only to economists, health administrators, government policy formulators, and financiers of health care, but also to providers of health care services (including physicians and nurses) and to consumers of health care. This widespread concern in relation to the economic environment of the current health care system is justified and results from current problems of health care costs and access.

U.S. health care expenditures continue on a historic escalation and represent an increasing share of the gross domestic product (GDP). Not only have health care expenditures as a percentage of the GDP grown at alarming rates as illustrated in Fig. 10-1, but the growth in health care spending has outpaced the growth in the GDP (Fig. 10-2). The GDP grew 2.8% in 1991, whereas national health care expenditures increased by 11.4%, four times that of the GDP (Letsch, 1993). The rate of growth of health care spending has exceeded the rate of growth of the overall economy over the past three decades. Health care expenditures in 1991 represented 13.2% of the GDP and totaled $751.8 billion. Barring widespread health care reform, national health care expenditures are expected to top the $1 trillion mark by 1995 (Standard & Poor's Corporation, 1992). The United States spends a larger percentage of its GDP on health care than do other industrialized nations (Fig. 10-3).

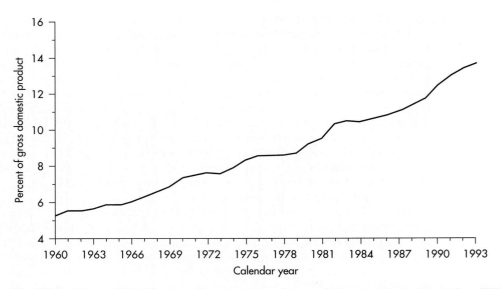

Fig. 10-1 National health expenditures as a percentage of the gross domestic product (GDP), 1960 to 1993. (Redrawn from Levit, K.R., et al. [1994]. National health expenditures, 1993. *Health Care Financing Review, 16*[1], 247-294; data from the Office of National Health Statistics.)

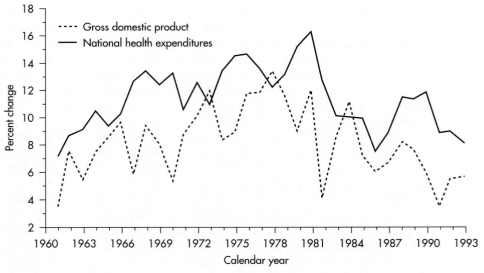

Fig. 10-2 Percentage of growth in national health expenditures and the GDP, 1960 to 1993. (Redrawn from Levit, K.R., et al. [1994]. National health expenditures, 1993. *Health Care Financing Review, 16*[1], 247-294; data from the Office of National Health Statistics.)

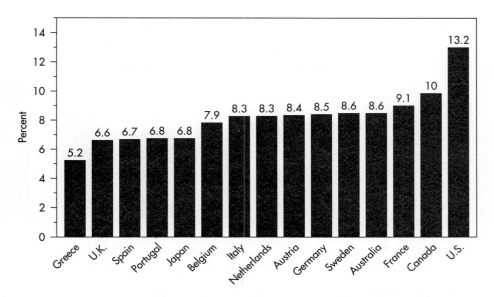

Fig. 10-3   Percentage of the GDP spent on health care in 1991: comparison of the United States with other industrialized nations. (Redrawn from U.S. Congress, Joint Economic Committee. [1994]. *Report of the Joint Economic Committee, Congress of the United States, on the 1994 economic report of the President* [Report 103-496]. Washington, DC: U.S. Government Printing Office; data from the Organization for Economic Cooperation and Development.)

Individual Americans are spending a greater percentage of their annual income on health services than in the past. Personal health care expenditures are third only to food and housing expenditures in household budgets (Folland, Goodman, & Stano, 1993). Personal health care expenditures have grown from $143 in 1960 to $346 in 1970, $1064 in 1980, and $2601 in 1990 (Letsch, 1993).

In addition to cost, issues of access to care are a growing concern. A rise in personal health care expenditures has caused an increase in the number of uninsured Americans (who do not receive health coverage through their employer, do not purchase private insurance out-of-pocket, and do not qualify for Medicare or Medicaid) and an increase in the number of underinsured Americans. The total number of individuals under age 65 without health insurance is now over 37 million and represents about 17% of the population under age 65 (almost all Americans aged 65 and over are covered under Medicare) (U.S. Congress, Joint Economic Committee, 1994). Fig. 10-4 illustrates the growth in the number of uninsured since 1988. Many either do not get the health care they need or cannot pay for the costs of the health care they receive. Of all the uninsured under 65 years of age in 1990, 60% were employed (Fig. 10-5).

Guaranteed access to care is one of the guiding principles of the Canadian health care system, as are universality, portability, comprehensiveness, and public administration of the plan on a nonprofit basis (Spence-Laschinger & McWilliam, 1992). The Canadian system, implemented in 1968 by the National Medicare Act, is a public in-

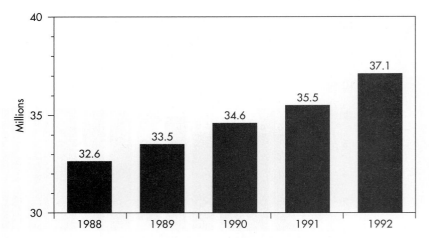

Fig. 10-4   Number of individuals under age 65 without health insurance, 1988 to 1992. (Redrawn from U.S. Congress, Joint Economic Committee. [1994]. *Report of the Joint Economic Committee, Congress of the United States, on the 1994 economic report of the President* [Report 103-496]. Washington, DC: U.S. Government Printing Office; data from the Urban Institute analysis of the 1993 Current Population Survey.)

surance model, as opposed to a government delivered services model, as in the United Kingdom. As in the United States, the Canadian system is undergoing economic constraints, and the majority of health care expenditures goes to illness care in acute care settings. Canadian nurse advocates are calling for resource commitment to wellness and primary care services and for improved access to, and reimbursement of, nurse provider services (Spence-Laschinger & McWilliam, 1992).

Less than 5% of the total annual health care budget in the United States goes toward preventive health care services (Centers for Disease Control, 1992), despite the fact that approximately half of all deaths in the United States are attributed to lifestyle and behavior (McGinnis & Foege, 1993). The lack of resource commitment to primary care and wellness services results in higher-cost, reactive care for illness rather than proactive care for the promotion of health and prevention of illness. Historically, nurses have served as health promotion/illness prevention advocates in the community, in outpatient settings, and even in acute care settings, educating patients about health promotion, illness prevention, and chronic disease management. Like their Canadian counterparts, American nurses are calling for increased resources for preventive services and for improved access to, and reimbursement of, nurse provider services (American Nurses' Association [ANA], 1992).

There are currently over 2,200,000 registered nurses in the United States, and nursing constitutes the largest single category of the health care workforce (Moses, 1994). Health economic concerns now permeate every aspect of nursing, and an understanding of basic economic issues has become essential, not only to the nurse administrator, but also to the nurse educator, the nurse researcher, and the practicing clinician. In an

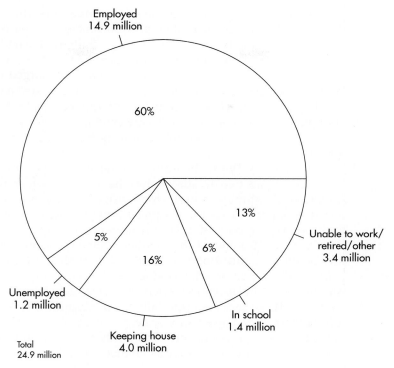

Fig. 10-5 Adults aged 18 to 64 without health insurance by labor force status, 1990. (Redrawn from U.S. Congress, House of Representatives. [1993]. *Hearings before the Subcommittee on Health of the Committee on Ways and Means* [Vol. 1, Report 103-5]. Washington, DC: U.S. Government Printing Office; data from the 1990 Current Population Survey, courtesy of the Congressional Budget Office.)

era of cost containment, health care providers must be able to incorporate economic principles into their administrative and clinical decision making. After an introduction to principles of economics and how they relate to health care and nursing, the interplay between economics and current health care issues are discussed.

PRINCIPLES OF ECONOMICS

Supply

Supply of health care refers to the availability of resources for delivery of health services. Resources include (1) health care facilities, (2) human resources, and (3) financing. Substantial changes have occurred within the past 10 to 15 years in relation to each type of resource:

1. *Health care facilities.* While hospitals continue to be the primary facility for delivery of health care, economic pressures have resulted in the closure of many traditional hospitals and the emergence of alternative delivery facilities, such as managed care organizations, ambulatory care centers, and home health units (Stoline & Weiner, 1993). Patients are being discharged from hospitals earlier, and the length of stay is declining. The "quicker-sicker" patient population is requiring greater quantities of home health services. Table 10-1 demonstrates actual and projected changes in health care expenditures for selected services. Note the large actual and projected increase in home health care expenditures as compared with hospital care.

2. *Human resources.* While the number of health care personnel has grown substantially in the past two decades, as has the health provider–to–consumer ratio, distributional inequities continue to persist, especially in rural areas. Such inequities provide opportunities for advanced practice nurses to practice in areas where there are large groups of medically underserved individuals.

3. *Financing.* Unlike many other markets where consumers pay directly for a product or service, consumers of health care predominantly purchase insurance, which in turn pays for the products and services, or they rely on subsidized insurance. It is the exception when the consumer of health care services pays directly for those services (especially hospitalization). Financing of health care is primarily provided by either private, commercial insurance companies or by public entitlement programs, predominantly Medicare and Medicaid (Fig. 10-6). In 1991, 81% of all health care was financed by third parties (Letsch, 1993). Rising

Table 10-1   **Change in Actual and Projected National Health Expenditures for Selected Services, 1991 to 1995**

	Expenditures (In Billions)			Average Annual Change (%)	
	1990	1991	1995	1990-1991	1991-1995
National health expenditures	$675	$752	$1124	11.3	10.6
Hospital care	258	289	447	13.7	11.5
Physician services	129	142	212	9.9	10.5
Dental services	34	37	47	5.5	6.1
Other professional services	31	36	55	12.0	11.4
Nursing home care	53	60	94	11.5	11.8
Home health care	8	10	19	21.5	17.8

From U.S. Congress, House of Representatives. (1993). *Hearings before the Subcommittee on Health of the Committee on Ways and Means* (Vol. 1, Report 103-5). Washington, DC: U.S. Government Printing Office; data from ProPAC estimates based on unpublished Health Care Financing Administration data.

costs of health care are passed on in part to consumers, however, in the form of higher insurance premiums, deductibles, and copayments (Fig. 10-7).

Financing of health care, whether by public or private third parties, changed dramatically in 1983 when Medicare introduced the prospective payment system. The former retrospective payment system allowed hospitals to recover their costs regardless of how excessive or efficient the costs and services were, and thus hospitals had no incentives to contain costs. In contrast, under the prospective payment system, payment rates are set before the provision of care and are based on diagnostic-related groups (DRGs). The hospital receives a fixed amount for an admission based on diagnosis and thus has the incentive to contain costs (conserve resources) (Dougherty, 1989).

Changes in the availability of health care facilities, health care providers, and funding for health care all affect the supply of health care services. Without available resources to provide services, the supply of health care is not able to meet the demand for health care.

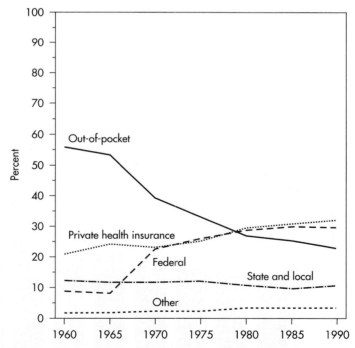

Fig. 10-6   Distribution of spending for personal health care by source of payment, 1960 to 1990. NOTE: Personal health care expenditures are equal to national health expenditures less spending for public health, research, construction, and administrative costs. The "other" category includes philanthropy and industrial in-plant spending for health. (Redrawn from U.S. Congress, House of Representatives. [1993]. *Hearings before the Subcommittee on Health of the Committee on Ways and Means* [Vol. 1, Report 103-5]. Washington, DC: U.S. Government Printing Office; data from Congressional Budget Office calculations based on data from the Health Care Financing Administration, Office of the Actuary, 1992.)

Demand

Demand is the amount of a product or service that consumers are willing and able to purchase. When dealing with the health care market, however, the concept of demand is somewhat tenuous to understand. When a consumer purchases a dress or a car, it is the dress or the car that they want. In the health care market, however, a consumer purchases health care but really desires, with a few exceptions, health. Thus the demand for health care "is derived from the more basic demand for health" (Feldstein, 1983, p. 81). Consumers' purchase of health care is dependent on their perceptions of the impact of the care on their health (McMenamin, 1990). The decision to purchase health care is also dependent on the cost of the care to the consumer. Total consumer costs of health care include monetary costs (copayment, deductibles, insurance premiums, out-of-pocket expenses, and lost time and wages from work) and nonmonetary costs (risk, pain, inconvenience, etc.). The demand for health care depends on the willingness of consumers to purchase services after weighing the expected benefits of the care with the costs of the care. If consumers carry insurance, their direct out-of-pocket expenses for the care will be less than if they are uninsured (Feldstein, 1983). Therefore the insurance status of consumers

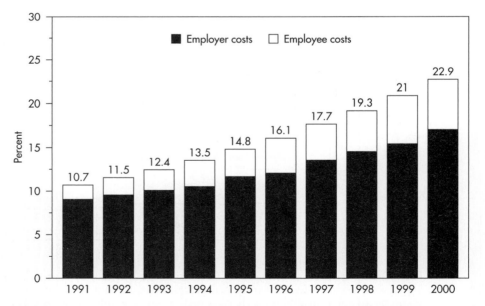

Fig. 10-7   Health insurance premiums as a percentage of payroll are rising. (Redrawn from U.S. Congress, Joint Economic Committee. [1994]. *Report of the Joint Economic Committee, Congress of the United States, on the 1994 economic report of the President* [Report 103-496]. Washington, DC: U.S. Government Printing Office; data from Johns Hopkins University, 1992.)

impacts the costs of care (to the consumers) and thus their demand for care. This separation of consumers from the price of health care resulting from health insurance coverage (either private or public) has dramatically increased demand for health care services. However, since demand is based on willingness and ability to purchase, demand for health care does not necessarily correlate with need for health care.

Demand for health care services changes over time as societal demographics and morbidity patterns change. As the "baby boomers" of the post–World War II era enter middle and old age in the coming decades, their demands for health care will only contribute to the already-expanding demands of an ever-growing elderly population. Cures for heart disease and cancer remain elusive, whereas the incidence of these diseases in the elderly remains significant. The incidence of AIDS has changed the types of health care services demanded and has led to the development of new treatments through research and development.

Demand for specific services is also influenced by the recommendations and decisions of health care providers (Feldstein, 1983). Because providers of care possess more knowledge regarding treatment options than consumers, the personal practice styles of providers, as well as how much information they share with consumers, can greatly impact the demand and consumption of services (Rice & Labelle, 1989). Similarly, the risk of litigation by consumers can result in a "defensive practice" style by providers. Fear of litigation can lead to overprescription of (often unnecessary) diagnostic tests and/or therapeutic interventions and ultimately result in higher health care costs.

Cost

Costs are resources required by the provider of services to produce health care products and services, as well as the amount a consumer pays to purchase the products and services. Costs to produce health care are the actual costs of inputs incurred for production, whereas costs to purchase health care services are what the health care economy will bear (i.e., what the consumers and financiers are able and willing to pay). Thus costs are dependent on supply and demand. Costs may be monetary (pecuniary) or intangible (nonpecuniary). *Pecuniary costs* of care include salaries of health care providers, insurance premiums, supplies and equipment used during care, administrative overhead, pharmaceuticals, transportation, and lost salary of the consumer, as well as construction and maintenance, and research. *Nonpecuniary costs* are those associated with the personal loss, pain, suffering, and other consequences associated with the consumption of health care services.

Costs of health care are affected by multiple factors, including supply of services, demand for services, and use of medical technology. An increase in the input costs of providing a service increases health care expenditures while the quantity and quality remain constant. Efforts are focused on reducing health care expenditures through reducing input costs of care without sacrificing quantity and quality of services.

Opportunity Cost

The resources consumed to produce or purchase a product or service are no longer available for the production or purchase of an alternative product or service. The value of the alternative product or service that is forgone is known as the *opportunity cost* (Pauly, 1993). The opportunity cost is therefore what is given up in order to obtain some good or service. A hospital that can afford to purchase only one of two diagnostic/therapeutic technologies must, in choosing one, give up known benefits of the other. The value of the forgone benefits (revenue generated, lives saved) is the opportunity cost.

Price Elasticity

Price elasticity is the change in demand for a product or service in response to a 1% change in its price. Remember, the price or cost that a person pays for health care is not only the monetary expense, but also the person's inconvenience of waiting for and receiving services and the physical and psychological costs of care, including risk, pain, and discomfort. In deciding whether to purchase a health care service or procedure (e.g., an elective surgical procedure), an individual will weigh the expected benefits of the procedure against the expected costs of the procedure (price in dollars, necessary time off work, anticipated pain and complications). A change in the costs associated with the procedure, such as a less-invasive technique that reduces price, length of stay, and associated pain, will influence the demand for that service. Fig. 10-8 illustrates the relationship between the price of a product or service and demand. The degree of change (elasticity) of demand is dependent on the necessity of the product, the availability of alternative products (substitutes), and the percentage of income spent on the product (Cleland, 1990).

Complements and Substitutes

Complements are products or services that are usually consumed jointly, such that an increase in the price of one decreases the demand for both. An example of complements in health care is intravenous fluids and tubing. If nursing services are complements to physician services, then an increase in the price of physician services will decrease demand for both physician and nursing services (Griffith, 1984).

Substitutes, on the other hand, are goods or services that satisfy the same want or need, so that an increase in the price of one will increase the demand for the other. One example of substitutes in health care is two pharmaceuticals that have the same therapeutic effect. Another example is an obstetrician and a nurse midwife. If nursing services are substitutes for physician services, then an increase in the cost of physician services will increase the demand for nursing services (Griffith, 1984).

In the physician arena there is an imbalance between generalists and specialists and a shortage of primary care physicians (Bocchino, 1993). This disparity between consumer demand and physician supply creates favorable opportunities for advanced practice nurses to practice in primary care capacities as physician substitutes. Nurses are

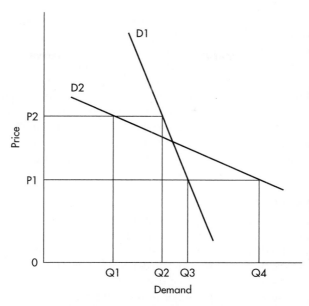

Fig. 10-8   Price elasticity of demand. The demand curves illustrate price elasticity: a change in demand results from a change in price. Demand for product 2 (D2) is more elastic (or responsive to a change in price) than product 1 (D1); a change in price from P1 to P2 results in a large change in demand for D2 (from Q1 to Q4), whereas the change in demand for D1 is small (from Q2 to Q3). *D,* Demand; *P,* price; *Q,* quantity.

making arguments for their use as substitutes for more expensive providers of care for services that they have been formally trained to provide. Similarly, hospitals, in an effort to reduce input costs, are incorporating the use of unlicensed personnel as substitutes for nurses for those activities that do not require licensure. Thus nurses are both substituting for some types of providers and being substituted by other types of providers.

Competition

In a truly competitive market, the market structure consists of numerous buyers and sellers each with no power over price, perfect information by all concerned, free entry and exit into the market, and a homogeneous product (Folland, Goodman, & Stano, 1993). The health care market violates these assumptions of competition in several ways. First, providers of services are often so few that they possess monopoly power, and information asymmetry often exists between provider and consumer and between consumer and insurer. Second, barriers to entry into the health care field exist in the form of licensure and practice laws, and the services provided vary in type and quality.

In addition, since most Americans rely predominantly on third-party reimbursement, consumers are insulated from the true costs of health care. Many consumers (whose insurance is paid by the government or by their employers) believe that health care does not cost them anything. Or consumers feel that they have already paid their share through insurance premiums and that they ought to get their money's worth (Stoline & Weiner, 1993). Thus consumers have no incentive to "shop around" for the best price. The separation of the consumer from costs has compromised the "ability of the marketplace to set prices that reflect societal value" (Letsch, 1993, p. 108). An effort to move the health care market to a more competitive market has been debated for the past decade and is discussed in more detail later under managed competition.

Marginal Utility

Marginal utility is the extra utility (satisfaction, welfare, or well-being) gained from consuming one more unit of a good or service. In other words, it is the benefit obtained by purchasing more of a product (Folland, Goodman, & Stano, 1993). When the marginal utility of a product or service is low, the resources consumed by the purchase of the additional amount of that good or service are not used to their fullest potential. Thus the opportunity cost of purchasing one more unit of the good or service is high, since other goods or services that may have resulted in greater benefit or well-being were foregone. There are many examples in health care of use of resources for services that have at best a questionable marginal utility. Many health care reformers argue that the resources consumed by high-cost, life-sustaining technologies could be better used for lower-cost, highly effective primary care services, such as immunizations.

EVALUATION OF COSTS

Cost-Benefit Analysis

Cost-benefit analysis (CBA) is an analytical technique for evaluation of resource consumption and benefit production of a project, program, or technique. CBA requires assessment and evaluation of the costs and benefits of a program to determine if the benefits of a project outweigh its costs. In a CBA all costs and benefits undergo valuation and are stated in monetary terms. This process places monetary terms on both pecuniary and nonpecuniary costs and benefits so that a comparison can be made. In doing so, value or worth is assigned or placed on nonmonetary aspects of the project's costs and benefits. While this may be an attractive feature of the analysis and may aid in determining the "worthiness" of a project, it is also a pitfall and a drawback. The valuation of such intangible costs as pain or grief or premature loss of life not only varies from case to case but differs among analysts assigning the values. Specific criteria and arithmetic maneuvers have been suggested for determining the value of intangible costs and benefits but are controversial at best (Klarman, 1982; Pruitt & Jacox, 1991). CBA is therefore difficult in health care settings, which are wrought with such emotional and subjective outcomes.

Cost-Effectiveness Analysis

Cost-effectiveness analysis (CEA) is an analytical technique of comparing resource consumption between two or more alternatives that meet a particular objective (such as minimum quality of a product or production of a specific patient outcome). CEA measures the costs involved with each alternative and determines the most cost-effective, or least costly (Kristein, 1983). In a CEA only monetary costs of inputs into each alternative are considered. Since the objective (or outcome) of the alternatives is assumed to be the same, the valuation of benefits is not considered (Folland, Goodman, & Stano, 1993). Thus CEA avoids making valuations while providing empirical evaluation of costs of alternative health care interventions. An example of CEA in nursing research is provided in the box below.

MANAGED COMPETITION AND HEALTH ECONOMICS

The health care reform debate of the 1992 presidential election and the proposed health care reform strategies of the administrative and congressional offices since the election have brought the issue of health care expenditures into physicians' offices, nursing organizations, and living rooms across the country. The difficulty in structuring an equitable and efficient system and obtaining support for such proposals is the

---

An Example of Cost-Effectiveness Analysis in Nursing Research

Chappell and Dickey (1993) conducted a cost-effectiveness analysis of intermittent consultative nurse visits in reducing hospital readmission for nursing home patients who used a Veterans Affairs (VA) medical center. The study, reported in the March 1993 *Journal of Nursing Administration,* compared a group of nursing home patients who received VA nurse visits after discharge with a group of nursing home patients who did not receive VA nurse visits after discharge. The researchers found that the visiting VA nurses enhanced stability of nursing home patients (through nursing consultation, using nursing assessment, early detection of potential problems, and making recommendations for problem solving to the nursing home staff), which resulted in reduced hospital readmission. To evaluate expenditures and savings related to the visiting nurse program, financial data were categorized into:

- Rehospitalization (ambulance transfer to and from the medical center, per diem rates on number of days readmitted)
- Emergency room visits (ambulance transfer to and from the medical center, cost of emergency room visit)
- The nursing intervention (salaries of nurses and clerks, travel expenses)
- Costs not incurred (nursing home costs during readmission to the acute care facility)

The annual cost of care for the group receiving VA nurse visits (hospital readmission costs plus costs of emergency room visits plus cost of nurse visits minus nursing home cost) was $70,395 less than the corresponding costs for the group that did not receive nurse visits. Thus the $7000 nursing intervention resulted in annual savings of $70,000 to the medical center, as well as improved patient outcomes.

inability to satisfy all involved (i.e., providers of services, financiers, and consumers). With the goal of any strategy being expenditure minimization, providers (physicians, hospitals, etc.) and insurance companies fear loss of profits, whereas consumers fear loss of benefits.

The primary element of concern in proposed strategies for alternative health care delivery systems is cost. Most proposals for health care delivery structure changes are based on a managed competition model, which is a combined government-regulated and market-driven model (Joint Commission on Health Care, 1993). Under such a model, costs are controlled through market-based mechanisms in that multiple provider groups compete for contracts from consumers through bargaining pools composed of individuals and small business employers. Members of consumer groups pool their purchasing power, thus achieving economies of scale to get lower-priced coverage. Competition between provider groups should occur on the basis of each plan's prices, measures of quality of care, and level of enrollee satisfaction. Thus consumers "shop" among the provider groups for the best deal. Theoretically, such competition will increase choice, drive costs down, and improve quality. With the failure of health care reform in the U.S. Congress, the regulation component of managed competition (through federally mandated reporting of provider price and quality) has not been realized. It is hoped that a purely market-based competition will emerge, however, despite the failure of national health care reform.

Many of the health care reform proposals of the early 1990s included a national cap on expenditures (all U.S. health care expenditures would be held to growth no more than the growth of the GDP), whereas others had no federal budget restrictions. It is doubtful that without some other cost-containment measure (like global expenditure limits), competition alone will be sufficient to keep costs from escalating further (Aaron & Schwartz, 1993; Altman & Cohen, 1993; Rogal, Gauthier, & Barrand, 1993; Starr & Zelman, 1993).

Physicians have traditionally held a monopolistic power as primary care providers, since regulations prevented others from "practicing medicine." As alternative providers of health care services demonstrate their ability to provide comparable services, regulations are being changed to allow these substitutes to enter the market and compete with physicians. Such changes in regulation have only come about since societal demands for more cost-effective providers have escalated while organized physician interests have lost political power. With the use of advanced practice nurses as physician substitutes, competition between these two providers can occur on the basis of cost-effectiveness. Studies have demonstrated that the use of advanced practice nurses as primary care providers can reduce costs of outpatient care, including laboratory costs, per visit costs, per episode costs, and long-term management costs (Brown & Grimes, 1993; U.S. Congress, Office of Technology Assessment [OTA], 1986). Nurse-managed care, when compared with physician-managed care, has been documented to reduce the frequency of hospitalizations, reduce the acuity of those admitted, reduce the length of stay, and reduce the cost of hospitalization (Michaels, 1992; Rogers, Riordan, & Swindle, 1991).

HEALTH CARE TECHNOLOGY AND ECONOMICS

The expansion of health insurance since World War II has led to an interdependent relationship between health care technology and insurance and has dramatically impacted today's soaring health care costs (Garber, 1994; Weisbrod, 1991). As individuals shifted financing of services received from themselves to insurance companies, individuals became removed from, and insensitive to, the actual costs of health care technologies. Because of the retrospective payment system in which all services rendered were reimbursed, health care providers (namely, physicians and hospitals) had financial incentives to use any and all technologies available regardless of cost. Research and development markets also had the financial incentives of reimbursement to continue to produce new health care technologies at any cost (Weisbrod, 1991). Consequently, there has been heightened and widespread patient and provider demand for greater technology (Callahan, 1990) and soaring health care expenditures. Today, however, payors are willing to pay only for what is cost-effective and medically appropriate.

Technology assessment and outcomes research are intended to help decision makers deal with the development, acquisition, and utilization of health care practices and technologies. The goal is to improve patient health, efficiency, and value. Technology assessment, as a form of policy research, evaluates the safety, effectiveness, and costs of technologies to provide the basis for clinical and social policies, including resource allocation. A comprehensive technology assessment encompasses four aspects of the technology: safety, efficacy/effectiveness, costs/benefits, and social impact (Pillar, Jacox, & Redman, 1990).

Technology assessment and outcomes research are time consuming and costly. Traditional health care markets provide little incentive for the investment in the process. Under managed competition, however, health care providers would be competing for contracts from consumers, since consumers would "shop" among the providers on the basis of reported price, quality indicators, and level of enrollee satisfaction. Providers would be accountable for quality and would stand to lose consumers if quality fell below the level of competitors. The managed competition approach would therefore provide an environment and the incentives for the generation of cost-effectiveness and quality outcomes data of health care technologies, since providers of care would "compete" on the basis of quality and cost.

Nursing practice, education, and administration are directly affected by the application of new medical and health care practices and technologies. However, there is little participation in technology research by nursing despite nursing's contribution to the implementation and assessment of technology in the clinical setting (Pillar, Jacox, & Redman, 1990). Nurses directly witness the individual, as well as societal, benefits and burdens that various practices and technologies bring and possess a wealth of clinical knowledge and expertise that could advance technology assessment. Nurses must become involved in multidisciplinary technology assessment and participate in the development of clinical practice guidelines, as well as social policy regarding health care technologies.

Rationing Health Care Technology

Opportunity costs of health care, the diversion of scarce and finite resources from other purposes (education, law enforcement, roads and highways, defense, etc.), generated largely by high-cost technology, are now under intense scrutiny. Since demands for health care are insatiable, whereas resources are finite, and since society cannot afford to do everything that is now technically possible for every member of society, the necessity to explicitly ration health care resources has emerged. Oregon's Basic Health Services Act has used a priority system incorporating outcomes of treatment to establish a state Medicaid benefits package. The plan is based on the utilitarian principle of doing the greatest good for the greatest number of people. Therefore, high-cost technologies with marginal outcomes are not provided under the plan, whereas lower-cost, highly effective technologies are funded (Dougherty, 1991). Oregon has essentially reduced growth in health care expenditures while delivering quality care by eliminating the use of technologies that are not effective or are only marginally effective. The responsibility of prioritizing health services for inclusion or exclusion for coverage was placed on a Health Services commission. In addition to five primary care physicians, a social worker, and four consumers, the commission contained one public health nurse (Southard, 1992). Such inclusion of nursing expertise in the policy-making process can greatly impact not only resource allocation, but also patient outcomes.

QUALITY OF CARE AND ECONOMICS

The idea that high-quality care equals high-cost care has emerged with the use of high-cost technologies. However, high cost does not always ensure high quality, and high quality does not have to be high cost. Consider the concept of marginal utility. There comes a point in the course of care when the investment for any additional treatment will make little difference and will not further improve the outcome. In fact, the quality of care many actually deteriorate by the continued input of services if the additional services have high risks of adverse effects (Davis, et al., 1990).

In the era of cost containment and cutbacks, there are increased pressures and incentives to provide only those services that provide actual benefits to patients and to eliminate those services with marginal outcomes. From this economic force comes the need to determine the impact of care on the lives of patients. Such information regarding outcomes of care must become a propelling component in the decisions that affect resource allocation between competing services. To assess, evaluate, and document quality, data must be generated that provide indicators of quality of care. Outcomes research and technology assessment are attempting to move from evaluation of biometric measures (blood pressure, mortality) toward measurements of functioning, well-being, and quality of life in an effort to assess treatment effectiveness more comprehensively. The challenge of evaluating care is in balancing results from quality assessment of outcomes research with results from the efficiency assessment of a cost-effectiveness analysis. While the idea of incorporating cost research with quality research is logical (and necessary in the current economic environment), such methodologies and data collection tools are relatively undeveloped and not standardized (Buerhaus, 1992). Already clinical experts in evaluating responses to care, nurses must also become experts in quality and cost research as the field of outcomes research develops and grows.

The ANA's *Nursing's Agenda for Health Care Reform* (1992) advocates universal access in response to the overwhelming number of Americans who are unable to enter the health care system. The inability to access care and subsequent delay in treatment exacerbate health problems and escalate the costs of health care. Studies have shown that nurse practitioners enhance access to, and delivery of, basic health care in a wide variety of geographic and practice settings, including school-based clinics, long-term care facilities, correctional institutions, industrial health clinics, community health clinics, and community birthing centers, as well as in the more traditional settings of hospital ambulatory and inpatient departments and private practice offices (Safriet, 1992; U.S. Congress, OTA, 1986). The OTA's assessment of studies on care provided by nurse practitioners versus that provided by physicians found that nurse practitioners provide care equivalent to, or superior to care provided by physicians in regard to assessment competency, patient compliance, resolution of acute problems, and improvement in the patients' physical, emotional, and social functional status. Brown and Grimes' (1993) meta-analysis of 38 studies found that, compared with physicians, nurse practitioners provided more health promotion activities, scored higher on quality-of-care measures, achieved higher scores on resolution of pathological conditions and on functional status of their patients, and achieved higher scores on patient satisfaction and patient compliance. In addition, they found that patient knowledge was equivalent between patients of nurse practitioners and those of physicians, and that nurse practitioners' patients experienced fewer hospitalizations. As mentioned under managed competition, these studies also showed that care provided by nurse practitioners was more cost-effective than that provided by physicians (Brown & Grimes, 1993; Michaels, 1992; Rogers, Riordan, & Swindle, 1991; U.S. Congress, OTA, 1986). The role of the nurse practitioner as an accessible, cost-effective, and high-quality provider of primary care services has been validated, and nurse practitioners have demonstrated that quality does not have to be sacrificed to cost-containment.

ECONOMICS AND THE FUTURE OF NURSING

Peter Buerhaus (1992) has identified several changes that nurses can anticipate in lieu of the shift in the economic climate in health care to a more competitive marketplace:

- Intensifying pressure to provide nursing care in the least costly manner
- Increased demand by licensed practical nurses (LPNs), clinical pharmacists, physicians, and other economic competitors for regulations that either protect or expand their practice "turfs," coupled with actions by employers to change both state nurse practice acts and institutional traditions that restrict them from achieving productivity gains and lowering labor-related costs
- Developing opportunities to advance the value of nursing practice in all health care settings if the profession's research and management communities can successfully orchestrate a multifaceted quality assessment effort

- Struggling to balance the tensions, costs, and benefits of pursuing a narrowly focused nursing quality assessment strategy with finding ways to integrate nursing's quality assessment concepts and methods into quality assessment systems and management initiatives that are controlled largely by non-nurses
- Having to seriously consider what it is that purchasers and consumers want from nursing and taking steps to satisfy these wants

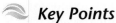

Key Points

- Economics in health care represents a strong relationship among the supply, demand, and costs of health care.

- Supply of health care refers to the amount of health care facilities, personnel, and financing available to consumers. Supply levels are impacted by technological discoveries, costs for services, consumer demands, the level of competition in the marketplace, and the effect of government regulations.

- Demand for health care indicates what health care the consumer is willing to purchase. The demand level revolves around consumer needs and desires, costs of health care, treatment selections ordered by health care providers, and general societal needs.

- Costs for health care reflect any financial expenditures contributed by providers or consumers to deliver and receive health care, as well as intangible costs of receiving care. Factors influencing the cost of health care are numerous, ranging from consumer demands to advancements in medical technology to the status of the nation's economy.

- Economic concepts relevant to nursing practice include opportunity cost, elasticity, complements and substitutes, competition, and marginal utility. Nurses must be able to incorporate these economic concepts into their administrative, as well as clinical decision-making, processes.

- Cost-containment pressures require that nurse researchers be able to incorporate economic methodologies such as cost-effectiveness analysis and/or cost-benefit analysis into clinical and administrative research programs. Such economically, as well as clinically, based research can serve as the basis for policy decision making regarding regulatory reform, prioritization and rationing of health care technologies and services, and reimbursement for advanced practice nurses.

- Nurses can bring a unique perspective to the economic analysis of health care that can impact health care delivery systems, health policy, and, most important, patient care.

- Rising costs of health care necessitate the provision of more cost-effective ways to provide comparable services. Nurses must continue to demonstrate their accessibility, quality of services, and cost-effectiveness in order to validate existing and expanding roles, to broaden reimbursement policies for services that nurses are trained to render and are capable of providing, and to effectively compete with physicians and other providers of care.

 Critical Thinking Exercises

1. Discuss the economic concepts of supply, demand, and costs of health care as they relate to your nursing practice.

2. What are the implications for the nursing profession of the issues of:
   a. Access to health care
   b. Cost containment
   c. Quality of care

3. How can nurses in clinical practice become involved in decisions regarding the rationing of health care resources and services? How can nurses become involved in formulation and evaluation of social policies regarding health care?

4. What suggestions do you have for restructuring the health care delivery system to address problems associated with access to care, cost, reimbursement, and quality of care?

5. In his book, *Not All of Us Are Saints: A Doctor's Journey With the Poor,* David Hilfiker, M.D. (1994), tells a story of a homeless man and reveals an extreme example of the economic consequences of health care:

> After breaking his jaw several weeks earlier, Mr. McRae had gone to an emergency room, had his jaw wired shut to heal, and then been discharged back to the streets. Most likely, he had found it impossible to eat and drink enough to keep himself going, and so it was that the police found him severely dehydrated, unconscious, and close to death. [Subsequently,] Mr. McRae had been hospitalized for weeks at a cost of tens of thousands of dollars; attended to by teams of nurses, physicians, and social workers; and fed three carefully prepared meals a day. He was now about to be discharged to the streets, where he would sleep in a shelter, forage for food during the day, and wait in line in the evening in the hope of getting a bed for the night. (pp. 171-173)

What characteristics of our current health care system contributed to the outcome? What actions could have been taken, and by whom, to prevent the costly rehospitalization? What are some of the broader societal implications of this scenario?

References

Aaron, H.J, & Schwartz, W.B. (1993). Managed competition: Little cost containment without budget limits. *Health Affairs, 12*(Suppl.), 204-215.

Altman, S.H., & Cohen, A.B. (1993). The need for a national global budget. *Health Affairs, 12*(Suppl.), 194-203.

American Nurses' Association. (1992). *Nursing's agenda for health care reform.* Washington, DC: American Nurses Publishing.

Bocchino, C.A. (1993). A new accountability in health care: Providers, insurers, and patients. *Nursing Economics, 11*(1), 44, 51.

Brown, S.A. & Grimes, D.E. (1993). *Nurse practitioners and certified nurse-midwives: A meta-analysis of studies on nurses in primary care roles.* Washington, DC: American Nurses Publishing.

Buerhaus, P.I. (1992). Nursing competition and quality. In M. Johnson & J. McCloskey (Eds.), *The delivery of quality health care.* St. Louis: Mosby.

Callahan, D. (1990). *What kind of life: The limits of medical progress.* New York: Simon & Schuster.

Centers for Disease Control. (1992). Estimated national spending on prevention: United States, 1988. *Morbidity and Mortality Weekly Report, 41,* 529-531.

Chappell, H., & Dickey, C. (1993). Decreased rehospitalization costs through intermittent nursing visits to nursing home patients. *JONA, 23*(3), 49-52.

Cleland, V.S. (1990). *The economics of nursing.* Norwalk, CT: Appleton & Lange.

Davis, K., Anderson, G.F., Rowland, D., & Steinberg, E.P. (1990). The impact of cost containment efforts on the quality of care. In *Health care cost containment* (pp. 200-217). Baltimore, MD: Johns Hopkins University Press.

Dougherty, C.J. (1989). Ethical perspectives on prospective payment. *Hastings Center Report, 19*(1), 5-11.

Dougherty, C.J. (1991). Setting health care priorities: Oregon's next step. *Hastings Center Report, 21*(3), 1-16.

Feldstein, P.J. (1983). *Health care economics* (2nd ed.). New York: John Wiley & Sons.

Folland, S., Goodman, A.C., & Stano, M. (1993). *The economics of health and health care.* New York: Macmillan.

Garber, A.M. (1994). Can technology assessment control health spending? *Health Affairs, 13*(3), 115-126.

Griffith, H. (1984). Nursing practice: Substitute or compliment according to economic theory. *Nursing Economics, 2*(2), 16-23.

Hilfiker, D. (1994). *Not all of us are saints: A doctor's journey with the poor.* New York: Hill & Wang.

Joint Commission on Health Care. (1993, September 22). *Comparison of major federal health care reform proposals,* 1-7.

Klarman, H.E. (1982). Application of cost-benefit analysis to the health services and the special case of technological innovation. In R.D. Luke & J.C. Bauer (Eds.), *Issues in health economics.* Rockville, MD: Aspen.

Kristein, M.M. (1983). Using cost-effectiveness and cost/benefit analysis for health care policy making. In R.M. Scheffler & L.F. Rossiter (Eds.), *Advances in health economics and health services research.* Greenwich, CT: JAI Press.

Letsch, S.W. (1993). National health care spending in 1991. *Health Affairs, 12*(1), 94-110.

Levit, K.R., Sensenig, A.L., Cowan, C.A., Lanzenby, H.C., McDonnell, P.A., Won, D.K., Sivarajan, L., Stiller, J.M., Donham, C.S., & Stewart, M.S. (1994). National health expenditures, 1993. *Health Care Financing Review, 16*(1), 247-294.

McGinnis J.M. & Foege, W.H. (1993). Actual causes of death in the United States. *JAMA, 270*(18), 2207-2212.

McMenamin, P. (1990). What do economists think people want? *Health Affairs, 9*(4), 112-119.

Michaels, C. (1992). Carondelet St. Mary's nursing enterprise. *Nursing Clinics of North America, 27*(1), 77-85.

Moses, E.B. (1994). *The registered nurse population: Findings from the national sample survey of registered nurses, March 1992.* Rockville, MD: Health Resources & Services Administration, Bureau of Health Professions.

Pauly, M.V. (1993). U.S. health care costs: The untold true story. *Health Affairs, 12*(3), 152-159.

Pillar, B., Jacox, A.K., & Redman, B.K. (1990). Technology, its assessment, and nursing. *Nursing Outlook, 38*(1),16-19.

Pruitt, R.H., & Jacox, A.K. (1991). Looking above the bottom line: Decisions in economic evaluation. *Nursing Economics, 9*(2), 87-91.

Rice, T.H., & Labelle, R.J. (1989). Do physicians induce demand for medical services? *Journal of Health Politics, Policy and Law, 14*(3), 587-600.

Rogal, D.L., Gauthier, A.K., & Barrand, N.L. (1993). Managing the health care system under a global expenditure limit: A workshop summary. *Inquiry, 30*(3), 318-322.

Rogers, M., Riordan, J., & Swindle, D. (1991). Community-based nursing case management pays off. *Nursing Management, 22*(3), 30-34.

Safriet, B.J. (1992). Health care dollars and regulatory sense: The role of advanced practice nursing. *The Yale Journal on Regulation, 9*(2), 417-488.

Southard, P. (1992). The Oregon Health Plan. *Journal of Emergency Nursing, 18*(5), 471-473.

Spence-Laschinger, H.K., & McWilliam, C.L. (1992). Health care in Canada: The presumption of care. *Nursing and Health Care, 13*(4), 204-207.

Standard & Poor's Corporation. (1992). *U.S. grapples with health care crisis.* Health Care Industry Surveys, H15-H17.

Starr, P., & Zelman, W.A. (1993). A bridge to compromise: Competition under a budget. *Health Affairs, 12*(Suppl.), 7-23.

Stoline, A.M., & Weiner, J.P. (1993). *The new medical marketplace* (rev. ed.). Baltimore, MD: Johns Hopkins University Press.

U.S. Congress, House of Representatives. (1993). *Hearings before the Subcommittee on Health of the Committee on Ways and Means* (Vol. 1, Report 103-5). Washington, DC: U.S. Government Printing Office.

U.S. Congress, Joint Economic Committee. (1994). *Report of the Joint Economic Committee, Congress of the United States, on the 1994 economic report of the President* (Report 103-496). Washington, DC: U.S. Government Printing Office.

U.S. Congress, Office of Technology Assessment. (1986). *Nurse practitioners, physician assistants, and certified nurse midwives: A policy analysis* (Health Technology Case Study 37; OTA-HCS-37). Washington, DC: U.S. Government Printing Office.

Weisbrod, B.A. (1991). The health care quadrilemma: An essay on technological change, insurance, quality of care, and cost containment. *Journal of Economic Literature, 29,* 523-552.

Legal Aspects of Nursing Practice   11

Patricia McMullen and Nayna Philipsen

 Objectives

At the completion of this chapter, the reader will be able to:

- Describe the constitutional and administrative principles foundational to nursing practice.

- Analyze contract law and its effect on the nurse's employment relationships.

- Differentiate between torts of relevance to nursing practice.

- Discuss strategies the nurse can use to reduce legal exposure.

Profile in Practice

Ann Mech, JD, RN
School of Nursing, University of Maryland,
Baltimore, Maryland

My decision to become an attorney was based on my experiences as a nursing supervisor on the evening shift. Questions requiring a legal opinion would frequently arise, and there was not a lawyer around who could be consulted as needed. I also had a personal experience with a member of my family involving a decision to terminate treatment, which sparked an interest in living wills and right-to-die issues. I believed that law school would enable me to find the answers to some of these questions.

After law school, I remained at the University of Maryland Medical Center. My legal responsibilities included staff education and preparation for upcoming malpractice cases (although actual litigation was handled by outside defense counsel). I developed nursing policies, reviewed contracts with affiliating schools of nursing, monitored incident reports involving the nursing staff, and had overall responsibilities for meeting regulations imposed on the department of nursing by outside agencies (e.g., Joint Commission on Accreditation of Healthcare Organizations, Board of Nursing).

After several years, I moved from the hospital setting to the academic setting. Responsibilities at the University of Maryland, School of Nursing, include initiating clinical affiliation contracts; monitoring state and federal regulatory requirements related to clinical placements and faculty credentialing; reviewing and implementing university policies related to the Americans with Disabilities Act and Affirmative Action as needed; and drafting contractual arrangements for the nurse-managed clinics operated by the school.

Many nurse-attorneys have combined their nursing and legal backgrounds in their careers. Most work as either plaintiff or defense counsel in personal injury cases, which include medical malpractice. Some serve as in-house counsel for large hospitals or health care systems. Others are risk managers for health care insurers. And a few, like me, are faculty members at schools of nursing.

Nurses confront legal principles on a daily basis. Legal concepts, legal expectations, and legal consequences surround the practice of nursing. An informed and safe nurse must be aware of the effect these legal principles have on nursing practice to reduce exposure to adverse legal consequences.

Law is defined as the sum total of man-made rules and regulations designed to assist people to order their society, organize their affairs, and settle their problems. *Statutory law* is established through the legislative process and expands each time Congress or state legislatures pass new legislation. *Common law* is decisional and expands each time a judge makes a legal decision.

The function of law is to create and interpret legal relationships. *Public law* defines and interprets relationships between individuals and the government. The major categories of public law are constitutional law, administrative law, and criminal law. *Private law* defines and interprets the relationship between individuals and includes contract law and tort law.

These areas of law have an effect on the practice of nursing. The clients' and nurses' constitutional rights and remedies are defined by *constitutional law*. *Administrative law* determines the licensing and regulation of nursing practice, as well as areas such as collective bargaining. *Criminal law* usually involves the nurse as a witness. However, it can also involve the nurse as a defendant who is accused of a criminal offense. *Contract law* identifies the common types of employer-employee relationships and determines the risks and protections inherent in each type of relationship. *Tort law* is concerned with the reparation of wrongs or injuries inflicted by one person on another. It defines the legal liability for the practice of nursing and identifies the elements that are essential for each tort. This chapter describes the interaction between law and nursing in three major areas: administrative law, employment law, and civil (or tort) law.

ADMINISTRATIVE LAW IN NURSING

Nurses become aware of their board of nursing (the "board") and state nurse practice acts (NPAs) when they finish school and seek to acquire a license, if not before. Nurses are licensed under state NPAs. NPAs establish entry requirements into the profession, set definitions of nursing practice, and establish guidelines for professional discipline when a nurse fails to obey state laws or becomes incompetent. For most nurses, licensing will be their only direct contact with the board; however, many will find themselves tangentially involved with the board through some level of conflict about the definition of nursing. Few nurses will have direct contact with the board's disciplinary unit.

The power of the state to license nurses and other health care professionals originates in the U.S. Constitution (*Dent v. West Virginia*, 1889). The Tenth Amendment allows the states to enact legislation that is not preempted or prohibited by federal law. All states have a "police power" to enact legislation to protect the health, safety, and welfare of their citizens. Each state constitution has a health and welfare clause allowing it to pass such legislation.

Licensing

Licensing is an exercise of the state's police power, which is employed by the legislature to protect the health, safety, and welfare of its citizens. Through state licensing statutes, the nursing profession controls entry into the profession, the discipline of colleagues, and the nursing activities of nonnurses. Nurses themselves implement these controls because they are best qualified by their specialized knowledge to evaluate and oversee nursing practice.

Regulations controlling the licensing and practice of nursing have been enacted by all of the states, the District of Columbia, and the U.S. territories. National guidelines exist and serve as useful references for nurses in proposing and implementing state laws. For example, the American Nurses' Association and other professional groups promulgate definitions and standards of nursing education and practice that are often incorporated into state NPAs. These NPAs are implemented through a state agency, called the health professions board, nursing board, or a similar title. Rules and regulations promulgated by the board give meaning to the NPA.

The most visible function of NPAs is the control over entry of new members into the nursing profession. Nursing and other professions have been criticized for entry requirements that discriminate against minorities and the poor and discourage diversity. Thus nursing boards must continually examine their criteria for admission to the profession for bias. Some licensure questions facing the nursing profession include the following: Is licensing perhaps too restrictive by limiting entry into the profession? Do the tests and criteria used really identify the individuals who are good nurses, or do they shut out good nurses who are different from a homogenized stereotype? Does licensing protect the public, or does it really protect nursing professionals by eliminating competition?

Control Over Practice

The power to control entry and the power to discipline licensed and unlicensed practitioners give the profession an ability to exert control on the nursing market. Nurses are granted a privileged place in the occupational hierarchy, but it is a position challenged both by the public and by other professions who fear the surrender of power. Nurses control the quality and standards of nursing care in the state because they control the disciplinary process of nurses through the NPAs. Thus, as in many other professions, NPAs leave public consumers of nursing care dependent to a large degree on members of the profession to control access to nursing services and maintain the quality of nursing care. The result is that nurses have the duty to advocate for patients, not only at the bedside, but also to the licensing board for high-quality care from competent licensed practitioners. The ability of nurses to meet this great responsibility is challenged by members of the public who fear competing professional incentives. There has also been an argument that this is too much power to give any profession, since professionals are reluctant to discipline their own colleagues.

This power is also challenged by other professionals, from physicians to wound care specialists and lay midwives, who are afraid that nursing's scope of practice will compete with their own professional and financial incentives. NPAs permit nurses to function under a broad definition of nursing while restricting the practice of nonnursing personnel who might otherwise deliver many services provided by nurses.

Enforcement of the prohibition against the unauthorized practice of nursing is exemplified by the practice of lay midwifery. In many states, lay midwives have been absorbed into an area of nursing practice rather than being established as a separate profession. Practicing lay midwives who are not registered by the board of nursing may be served with cease and desist orders. Boards may also file criminal charges for misrepresentation against lay midwives with the local office of the state's attorney (*People of the State of Illinois v. Margaret Jihan,* 1989). Some boards have administrative fining powers for "unlicensed practitioners," which they can impose on lay midwives. These powers are invoked regardless of client satisfaction and often in spite of great public protest. Boards argue that a threat to the public safety and welfare is inherent whenever there is unlicensed practice, regardless of the specific fact situation. Similar processes have prevented nursing from taking over functions that have been absorbed into medical specialties.

Jurisdictions may overlap with other professions that perform some of the same functions as nursing. For example, the expanded role of the nurse has resulted in clashes with physicians at the regulatory level (*Sermchief v. Gonzalez,* 1983). While nursing boards move to limit the practice of unlicensed lay midwives, medical organizations have moved to limit the practice of certified nurse midwives (CNMs) by such actions as denying CNMs the hospital privileges that they need to care for their patients and defining the delivery of a baby to be the practice of medicine and therefore a prohibited practice for a nurse (Shimberg & Roederer, 1994; U.S. Congress, OTA, 1986).

The above arguments illustrate the restrictive nature of licensing by limiting entry and practice. Is licensing too restrictive, or is licensing really too permissive by granting "blanket" licenses? Does licensing today permit nurses to practice beyond their actual competence? It is likely that no one nurse can competently perform *all* services that nurses are licensed to deliver. While most nurses practice only in a limited field (e.g., surgery, obstetrics, or oncology), a nursing license permits a nurse to practice in all areas of nursing. In addition, after initial licensure, there is little or no demonstration of performance competency. Initial credentials do not guarantee competency into the indefinite future. For this reason, some states and health care agencies are requiring mandatory continuing education or advanced certification as an indicator of ongoing competency.

External Regulation of Nursing Practice

Policy-makers debate how to regulate professional practice. Other external forces, such as health care legislation, managed care models, and financing of health care, also affect how nursing is practiced. Although it failed to pass in 1994, the *Clinton Health Security Act* (HSA) reflects prominent policy concerns. The HSA incorporated state law credentialing requirements for health care professions. Section 1161 provided for the override of state laws that restrict the practice of any class of health professions beyond what is justified by the skills and training of such professions. Section 3071(e) established funding for a program for advanced practice nurses and physicians assistants. Legislative proposals, such as the HSA, put nurses on notice that federal trends and federal laws are likely to have more impact on licensing in the future than in the past. Currently, all professional self-regulation is under attack. Consumers often do not perceive the professions as being the best ones to protect consumer interests.

If licensing is seen as a barrier to developing a free market in health care and a contributor to rising costs, it may be redefined in terms of a cost-to-performance ratio. An example of this principle is found in Title V of the HSA, which required periodic evaluation of actual performance of specific functions of licensed professionals. Licensing is supposed to protect the public from incompetence. Does a blanket license accomplish that purpose? Further, do requalification tests scrutinize actual competence? These issues have yet to be resolved.

Disciplinary and Administrative Procedures

A board of nursing practice usually has both regulatory and adjudicatory power (Fig. 11-1). The *regulatory power* authorizes the board to develop rules and regulations for nursing licensure, nursing education, and nursing practice. The *adjudicatory power* authorizes the board to investigate, hear, and decide complaints that involve violations of the act of the rules and regulations promulgated by the board. As mandated by the NPA, the board must ensure that a licensed nurse continues to practice within the standard of care, behaves professionally and ethically, and obeys all state laws. The NPA contains or incorporates a number of grounds to achieve this. The disciplinary action is on the license of the nurse, and that license may be suspended or revoked.

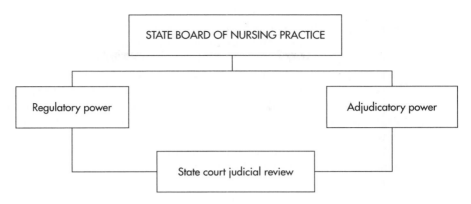

Fig. 11-1   Enforcement of state law by the board of nursing.

Boards are state administrative agencies. Their delegated powers are to protect the public from unfit nurses. It is important to understand the responsibility of state boards to protect the safety of the public. Boards can only limit or deny a nursing license. They cannot incarcerate a nurse, nor can they require a nurse to compensate a patient for damages, financial or otherwise. Most board actions cannot be used in a lawsuit against a nurse. If an injured patient does seek monetary damages, he or she must file a civil lawsuit against the nurse. If a party thinks a nurse has acted criminally, that party must contact the state's attorney's office.

A professional license is property protected by the U.S. Constitution. This means that it cannot be limited or taken away without "due process." Each state has an *Administrative Procedure Act,* which guides state agencies in their dealings in order to guarantee this due process right. Each state agency has its own regulations that describe how the agency implements the law. These regulations can vary greatly from state to state, and even among professional boards within a state. A board of nursing in one state may hear all arguments concerning nursing issues. The board in a neighboring state may delegate this to an administrative law judge or a hearing officer. Within a state, a board of nursing may hear its own cases, whereas another professional board in the same state may have its cases heard by an outside hearing officer.

Due process requires a right to be heard, and it also includes "notice." A licensed nurse has a duty to be aware of the state's NPA. The NPA is notice to nurses in that state about the grounds for which they may lose their license to practice. Further notice comes when a nurse receives a charging document. This paper advises the nurse that the board has probable cause to believe that the nurse is violating the NPA. It has to be specific enough to give the nurse notice about what any defense could be and about the time and place of the hearing.

Due process further requires that a nurse have the right to appeal any decision made by the board that seems improper. This appeal is usually to the state civil courts. In some states, the nurse may reargue the facts of the case, but in many states appeal is limited to such issues as whether the board had a right to hear the case and whether the board gave the nurse proper "due process" rights.

Although there are commonalities among all NPAs, each state has its own unique legislation. The nurse who moves from one state to another should obtain a copy of the new state's NPA. A convenient time to do this is during the process of applying for a license. The differences in state NPAs can be significant. For example, one state may impose no legal duty on a nurse to report the incompetence of a physician. In the next state, the nurse may find that failure to report such a physician can result in the loss of the nurse's license. The nurse needs to be familiar with the local NPA's requirements to obtain a license, boundaries and definitions of the practice, areas of discipline on the practice, and procedures in place to protect the nurse when the license is challenged by the board.

The Americans With Disabilities Act

A relatively new law affecting board action is the 1990 *Americans With Disabilities Act* (ADA). This is a federal law, and like the Constitutional right to due process, it applies to all state boards.

Formerly, disabled nurses could be handled by the boards the same as any other nurse. Now, disabled nurses, such as those with a drug dependence who are *in treatment,* are granted special confidentiality. This is meant to encourage nurses to seek treatment, to report nurses who need treatment, and to ensure that the disabled are not the object of discrimination. Some boards have responded to this mandate by creating their own internal methods to comply with the ADA, such as a rehabilitation committee. Others have made arrangements with external groups, such as rehabilitation services that are provided privately or by a professional organization. A nurse in treatment for a protected disability does not have a public record connected with that disability.

The ADA also requires the board to make any special arrangements to facilitate access to practice by nurses. Examples are special communication services for the sensory impaired and handicapped access to the site of examinations or hearings.

NURSING AND EMPLOYMENT LAW

Most nurses work as employees, rather than as independent practitioners. Nurse employees deal daily with the tension of being professionally independent and responsible for their actions in practice, while being simultaneously constrained by the standards and requirements of their employer. How can nurses' voices be heard and valued in creating work environments that promote the delivery of high-quality care? What avenues of redress do nurses have if they experience employee-management problems such as hospital downsizing or cross-training of nonprofessionals to carry out nursing functions under their supervision? How can nurses tell whether they are employees or part of management for bargaining purposes?

Contract Law

Nurses who are employed work under some form of contract. A *contract* is a promissory agreement between two or more parties that creates (or modifies or destroys) a legal relationship (Prosser, 1984). A contract can be either in writing or in spoken language with specific terms, in which case it is called an *express contract*. A contract can also be based solely on the conduct of the parties. These contracts are referred to as *implied contracts*.

An enforceable contract must first be for the performance of legal goods or services. A nurse cannot contract to practice medicine, for example. Second, the parties must have legal capability to make the contract. This means, for example, that they must all have the mental ability to understand their actions and all be old enough to make a legal agreement. Third, all parties at the time of the contract must agree to do something, and they must agree on what that something is. Finally, there must be "consideration" (i.e., some kind of trade in which each party gets something from the contract). In a typical nurse employment situation, the employer gets nursing services, and the employee gets financial reimbursement.

All states have a *statute of frauds* that limits the enforcement of some contracts that are not written. These vary and are usually not significant to a nurse employee situation. It is obvious, however, that a nurse who wants to prove the specific terms of a contract will have difficulty with an oral contract.

Of more significance is the state *parole evidence rule*. This rule provides that if oral agreements are made that are different from the written contract, the courts will not allow them to add to or change the written contract. It will be difficult for a nurse to overcome a written contract (though it can be done), for example, by showing fraud or duress by the employer. When nurses agree to an employment position, they should be familiar with their employment contracts, should get them in writing, and should not rely on oral agreements that are not part of that written contract.

What about the role of the contract when the nurse is being terminated from employment or wants to leave that employment? A contract can be legally terminated when it has been completely performed, its terms have been met, both parties agree to a change, it becomes impossible (e.g., the death of a party or the destruction of the subject matter), or both parties agree to annul the contract. A contract can also be terminated by a *breach,* which means that one of the parties fails to meet the terms of the agreement. When that happens, the other party can sue in civil court for any damages. For instance, an employee could sue for lost wages, and an employer could sue for lost profits. A nurse employee in a private setting could also file a grievance with the National Labor Relations Board. Of utmost importance for nurses is that most employment contracts are not individual contracts but are "at will." The next section clarifies this concept.

Employment at Will

Employment at will means that the employee has the right to quit employment anytime for any reason, or "at will." The employer has the parallel right to terminate the employee anytime for any reason, also at will.

The law of *Employment at Will* considers the employee and employer to have equal power, an assumption that nurse employees know does not reflect employee-employer realities. For this reason, it is a harsh legal doctrine. An example is an employee who is terminated for reasons that are against the public good, such as for joining a union or serving on a jury. Courts have found ways to restrict this doctrine, but they are limited to (1) public policy, (2) implied contract, and (3) good faith. Employees terminated against an implied contract are those who can show that this contract included hospital procedural manuals and personnel handbooks, employer's conduct or policy, or sometimes oral promises. An informed nurse employee must be familiar with such manuals and handbooks, document any oral promises, and get them in writing as soon as possible. What else can nurses do to enhance their protection as employees?

Labor Law

Approximately 20% of nurses employed in hospital settings are currently represented by unions (McMullen & Campbell-Philipsen, 1994). This means that they have formed a collective bargaining unit and can bargain with the employer as a group, in good faith, to make an agreement regarding similar interests in wages, hours, and working conditions. Collective bargaining agreements contain grievance procedures guaranteed to all employees. Furthermore, they usually contain a clause protecting the nurse employee from discharge except for "good cause." Nurses who work in a unionized facility cannot bargain individually with the employer. The employer must bargain with the union, which must represent all employees, whether or not they join the union (McMullen & Campbell-Philipsen, 1994).

Nurse employees can enforce employment agreements under the *National Labor Relations Act* (NLRA) enacted on July 5, 1935 (29 U.S.C. 141-178). The provisions of the NLRA are enforced through the National Labor Relations Board (NLRB) and various federal courts. The NLRB is a federal agency charged with implementing the NLRA, much in the same way that the nursing board implements the NPA. Its protections apply in all states.

Only nurses who are employees can participate in collective bargaining with the union. The NLRA also has a special provision allowing "professionals" to bargain collectively. In the past, many nurses who supervised health care workers, such as nursing assistants, were able to participate in collective bargaining under the "professional exemption." Nurse supervisors, however, were, and still are, excluded from collective bargaining participation and protection. In May 1994, the Supreme Court narrowed the NLRA coverage of professional nurses. In a split decision, the Court found that nurses who supervised others in a nursing home were part of management because such activities were "in the interest of the employer" (*NLRB v. Health Care and Retirement Corporation of America,* 1994). The scope of this ruling for nurses is not yet clear; however, every nurse has to ask whether supervision of other employees might be interpreted as "management," therefore depriving the nurse of the right to bargain collectively and of its protections (Ketter, 1994).

Government Employees

The NLRA applies only to privately employed nurses. Federal employees, such as nurses who work for the Veterans Administration, are covered under the *Civil Service Reform Act* of 1978. The employment rights of state employees are governed by each state's public employee statutes.

TORT LAW IN NURSING

Another area of the legal system of particular importance to nurses is that of tort law. *Torts* are private civil wrongs, as contrasted with *crimes,* which are wrongs committed against the state (Aiken & Catalano, 1994). The plaintiff, or person filing the law suit, files a tort action to recover damages for personal injury or property damage occurring from negligent conduct or unintentional misconduct (Prosser, 1984). *Unintentional torts* are those where persons suffer harm or injury as a consequence of an unintended, wrongful act by another person. Negligence and the related legal concept of malpractice are examples of unintentional torts (Aiken & Catalano, 1994). Several types of torts are often encountered in legal actions against nurses. These include negligence, assault, battery, false imprisonment, lack of informed consent, and breach of confidentiality. A brief discussion of each of these types of torts follows.

Negligence and Malpractice

Negligence occurs when a person fails to act in a reasonable manner under a given set of circumstances (Prosser, 1984). For example, if a person drinks excessively at a party, drives down the highway, and injures another motorist, the injured motorist could file a tort suit for negligence. Driving a car under the influence of alcohol or drugs is not typically considered reasonable conduct. Consequently, in addition to possible criminal action by the state where the accident happened, a negligence lawsuit would probably also result.

Unreasonable conduct by a nurse or other professional is a specific type of negligence, one referred to as *malpractice.* The nurse has the legal duty to provide the patient with a reasonable *standard of care.* This is usually referred to as "what the reasonably prudent nurse would do under the same or similar circumstances." In malpractice lawsuits, the issue is whether or not the conduct of the nurse is below the standard established by law for the protection of others or whether the care given by the nurse involves an unreasonable risk of causing damage to another (Hoffman, 1991; Simpson, 1994). The courts, based on long-established legal precedent, usually place the responsibility on the injured patient of establishing that the nurse acted wrongly. Initially, it is assumed that the nurse is innocent of the malpractice charge. Consequently, the plaintiff has the responsibility of establishing that the nurse's conduct was unreasonable. To accomplish this, the plaintiff must provide evidence related to four elements:

1. *Duty.* A duty is a legal obligation toward the patient (Aiken & Catalano, 1994). In health care settings, this legal obligation is usually based on express or implied

types of health care service contracts (Dornette, 1991). For instance, in prepayment health care systems, such as health maintenance organizations (HMOs), there is usually a written (express) contract between the HMO and the patient. The patient, through a health insurance plan or personal payment, pays a set fee for health care. In exchange, the HMO agrees to render certain health care services in a reasonable manner.

In other circumstances, the duty element may be based on a nonwritten (implied) contract (Dornette, 1991). For example, if the patient is seen in the emergency room and signs an admission sheet guaranteeing payment of a reasonable fee for all services in the emergency room, there is an implied contract that the services received will be reasonable. For purposes of establishing the element of duty in a malpractice case against a nurse, the question at issue is "Did the nurse have a legal obligation toward the patient?"

2. *Breach of duty.* This element of negligence and malpractice considers whether the nurse's conduct violated his or her duty to the patient (Danzon, 1985). To determine whether or not there was a breach of duty, the plaintiff must show that the nurse's conduct did not comply with reasonable standards of care rendered by an average, like-specialty provider under similar circumstances (Prosser, 1984). There are a number of methods used to determine whether the nurse's care was reasonable. Expert witness testimony, nursing texts, professional journals, standards developed by professional organizations, institutional procedures and protocols, and equipment guidelines developed by manufacturers can all be used to decide whether the nurse's care complied with reasonable care (Aiken & Catalano, 1994; Danzon, 1985; Prosser, 1984). Use of detailed documentation techniques, such as those specified in the documentation guidelines (see box on p. 253), will help the nurse to establish that the care delivered was reasonable.

3. *Causation.* This element really addresses two issues: whether the nurse's action or inaction caused the patient's injury and whether the patient's injury was foreseeable (Aiken & Catalano, 1994; Danzon, 1985; Prosser, 1984). To determine whether the nurse's actions or inaction caused the injury to the patient, lawyers frequently use the "but for" test (Prosser, 1984), which asks, "But for the acts or inaction of the nurse, would the injury to the patient still have occurred?" If the answer to this question is yes, then the first causation consideration is satisfied. The second part of the causation element looks at whether or not the nurse could have reasonably anticipated that his or her conduct might lead to patient harm (Aiken & Catalano, 1994; Bernzweig, 1990; Hoffman, 1991).

4. *Damage.* For a patient to recover from a nurse in a malpractice suit, he or she must have suffered some type of damage (i.e., injury or harm [Dornette, 1991; Prosser, 1984]). For example, if the nurse gave the patient the wrong medication but the patient did not experience any adverse effects, the damage element would be missing and the malpractice suit would be unsuccessful.

If sufficient evidence is established concerning all four of these elements and the defendant does not provide an adequate defense, the plaintiff can recover damages for

Charting Basics

Documentation is always the big stickler for nurses. Knowledge of a few basic rules can help you protect yourself in the event of a lawsuit. And, these rules can really help you communicate what great nursing care you deliver. So, let's examine some tips that should prove helpful:

- *Never alter or falsify a record.* You will lose all of your credibility if it is discovered that you altered or falsified a record.

- *If you make an error, draw one line through it and explain why (e.g., wrong chart). Never use correction fluid or a sticker over an error.* You want others to clearly see what you have changed so that you maintain your credibility and your client goals.

- *Know and adhere to your agency's policies and guidelines.* Policies and guidelines help convey what the expectations are in your facility. They are frequently evaluated in lawsuits to determine whether what the nurse did or did not do complies with reasonable standards of care. Consequently, the policies and guidelines need to delineate what the reasonable expectations are. But, they should not be so stringent that they cannot reasonably be accomplished.

- *Document in clear and chronological order. If you need to go back, chart a "late note." If there is a lengthy delay in charting, explain why.* It's important to keep orderly records. Remember to always date and time all notations. Nurses often leave blank spaces in the chart so that others can come back and make their additions. However, blank spaces leave room for a sanitized record. So, it's a good idea to avoid gaps in charting. Incidently, no one expects you to prolong a code to make a timely nursing entry. So, if you code a patient at 0900 and your adrenaline finally becomes manageable at 1100, just make a late entry note. This will make perfect sense to attorneys, judges, and other health team members.

- *Record accurate and complete information. If there is an abnormality, chart your appropriate actions.* Complete information is that data that another member of the health care team would need to reasonably care for that particular patient. If you fill your charting with irrelevant details, other providers will have a hard time locating the important facts. Part of your nursing role is to separate the critical information from the filler.

  If you identify a patient abnormality, don't forget to chart your appropriate nursing actions. And, remember to record what the physician's response to your concerns was. An unsatisfactory response (or no response) from a physician warrants a call to your nursing superior.

- *State objective, factual information. Avoid conclusory statements like "well," "good," "fine," and "normal".*

- *Sign your legal name and title. And, always make your charting legible.* A plaintiff's attorney can have a field day with illegible charting. If there is any way black could be interpreted as white, it will be.

- *Keep records in a safe and confidential manner.* Institutions and professionals are charged with the responsibility of maintaining a patient's privacy.

One last tip: Unusual circumstances warrant an incident report. But, do not refer to the incident report in your notes. Incident reports are designed to improve the quality of care rendered in an institution. They are not designed to communicate the needs of a particular patient. Generally, incident reports are not discoverable during a lawsuit. After all, courts want to promote quality care in institutions. However, if you refer to the incident report in your patient's chart, a little known legal doctrine may be applied. That doctrine is the doctrine of incorporation by reference. Under this doctrine, the incident report becomes part of the patient's record and not just the institution's quality assurance program, and is consequently discoverable.

Modified from McMullen, P., & Philipsen, N. (1993). Charting basics 101. *Nursing Connections* 6(3), 62-64.

pecuniary (monetary) and nonpecuniary (pain and suffering) injuries (Danzon, 1985). The defendant nurse usually tries to ward off an adverse verdict by producing evidence that the nursing care was reasonable, that the patient's conduct contributed to the injury, that the time for filing the lawsuit (stature of limitations) has expired, or that he or she is immune from the lawsuit (Prosser, 1984). If, however, a defendant nurse is called to give testimony in a legal action, the strategies for giving oral testimony presented in the box below could prove very useful.

Assault and Battery

An *assault* is a deliberate act wherein one person threatens to harm another person without his or her consent and has the ability to carry out the threat (Prosser, 1984). A *battery* is an unconsented touching, even if the touching may be of benefit to the patient (Prosser, 1984). For example, a lawsuit for assault could result when a nurse threatens to medicate a competent person against his or her will. Battery would occur when the nurse actually administers the medication to the unwilling, competent patient.

In some circumstances, such as restraint situations, the law allows providers to touch patients without their consent. However, special circumstances and safeguards must be adhered to in order to excuse the battery. Initially, courts will look at whether the battery was needed to protect the patient, health care team members, or the property

---

Giving Oral Testimony

- Bring your own attorney with you to review any records, for depositions or trials, to answer interrogatories, or for other legal requests if you are a party to a lawsuit.
- Never go to a deposition or a trial after working an off-shift; your brain will be mush!
- Thoroughly prepare for your testimony.
- Bring a recent, thoroughly updated copy of your resumé or curriculum vitae with you to the deposition or trial.
- During your testimony, always tell the truth.
- Dress professionally for your trial or deposition.
- If you're asked a question that is lengthy or convoluted, ask that it be restated and then rephrase it in your own words.
- Do not testify as to the medical standard of care.
- If you become fatigued during your testimony, ask for a brief break.
- Try to remain calm throughout the testimony.
- If asked if a source is "authoritative" or a "classic," you will almost always answer no.
- Maintain eye contact during your testimony.
- Do not waive your signature.

Modified from McMullen, P., & Pepper, J. (1992). Surviving the legal hot seat. *Nursing Connections, 5*(2), 33-36.

of others, such as those circumstances where the patient threatens to set a fire in an emergency room. Next, courts will examine whether restraining the patient was the least intrusive method to control the patient. For example, could the patient have been placed in a quiet room rather than being placed in a restraint? Finally, courts typically inquire as to whether the health care team regularly reassessed the need to continue using the restraint. If the health care team can demonstrate that they have complied with these requirements, an unconsented touching will be excused. Consequently, nurses need to be sure that they provide detailed documentation to indicate that (1) the patient was a threat to self, others, or the property of others; (2) the restraint was the least intrusive means to control the patient; (3) there was regular reassessment of the need to continue the restraint; and (4) the restraint was discontinued as soon as practicable. It is also important to note that many hospitals and clinical facilities have specific procedures and protocols dealing with the application of restraints. Every nurse needs to be familiar with applicable agency policies.

Informed Consent

Informed consent lawsuits focus on whether or not the patient was given enough information before a treatment in order to make an informed, intelligent decision. In these types of cases, the focus will be on whether the patient was given adequate information concerning the nature of the proposed treatment, material risks, benefits of the proposed treatment, alternative therapies, and potential consequences if the patient decides against the treatment. In other words, did the patient get enough information so that he or she was the ultimate decision maker when a decision was made to pursue or abandon the proposed treatment?

In many states lack of informed consent is a separate tort action. In other states the plaintiff files a battery action alleging that the failure to give adequate treatment information constituted an unconsented touching.

It is important to note that there are a few pertinent exceptions to the doctrine of informed consent. An emergency situation is one example of an informed consent exception. If a patient were admitted to an emergency department with a severe hemorrhaging abdominal injury that required the immediate removal of his spleen, there could be an exception to the normal explanation of the splenectomy procedure and informed consent. Furthermore, not all patients desire information about a proposed treatment or procedure. In these situations, patients can waive their consent. Finally, some courts have allowed a provider to avoid full disclosure to a patient if disclosure of information might lead to further harm to the patient. This type of exception to informed consent is known as *therapeutic privilege*. For example, if the provider thought a patient's knowledge of terminal cancer would lead the patient to commit suicide, the provider might exert therapeutic privilege and not reveal the cancer to the patient.

Typically, the consent procedure rests in the hands of the physician who will be performing the treatment, and the nurse serves as a witness. When the nurse signs the "witness" portion of the consent form, he or she is attesting that the signature on the consent form is the patient's. If the nurse witnesses the physician giving the pertinent information regarding the treatment or procedure, the nurse may want to place "consent procedure witnessed" below his or her signature. If a lawsuit later develops concerning whether the provider gave the patient information concerning the procedure or treatment, the "consent procedure witnessed" statement can furnish powerful evidence that the patient did receive adequate information.

Today's advanced practice nurses often perform procedures and treatments that require consent, such as suturing, obstetrical care, and prescription of medications. In these circumstances, the advanced practice nurse must ensure that the patient has enough information to make an informed decision with respect to a proposed treatment.

Even if the patient does not sign a consent form expressly consenting to a proposed treatment or procedure, courts sometimes find that the patient gave implied consent to the treatment or procedure by coming to the health care facility and submitting to the treatment or procedure.

False Imprisonment

False imprisonment occurs when a person is unlawfully confined within a fixed area. The confined person must be aware of the confinement or harmed as a result of the confinement. To prevail in a false imprisonment action, the patient must prove that he or she was physically restrained or restrained by threat or intimidation and that he or she did not consent to the restraint (Prosser, 1984). False imprisonment suits may involve situations wherein a patient was kept in a mental health facility against his or her will and without a judicial order, or a restraint device was applied to a patient against his or her will.

The laws on false imprisonment vary from state to state. Most states allow some degree of patient confinement if the patient poses a serious threat of harm to self, others, or the property of others. In deciding whether a valid confinement occurred, judges and juries often look at the reasonableness of the decision to confine the patient, how long the patient was confined, whether the need for the confinement was regularly reassessed, and whether the least restrictive methods for detention of the patient were employed.

Breach of Confidentiality

Confidentiality is the duty of health care providers to protect the secrecy of a patient's information, no matter how it is obtained. Until recently, patients had few legal remedies when the privacy of their medical records was breached. Today, state and federal laws provide patients with legal remedies to compensate them for confidentiality breaches.

Several cases demonstrate why there are valid concerns about medical record confidentiality. In *Doe v. Roe* (1993), a flight attendant asked her treating physician not to reveal her HIV status to her insurer or her employer. The physician verbally promised not to reveal her HIV status. Several months later, the flight attendant found that her entire chart, complete with HIV information, had been forwarded to her employer. The attendant recovered damages against the physician for his breach of confidentiality and for breaching his expressed oral promise not to disclose her HIV status. Breach-of-confidentiality lawsuits have resulted wherein psychiatric, drug, and alcohol treatment information was released.

Typically, there is a very strict level of confidentiality for patients receiving drug or alcohol abuse treatment. Providers are usually prohibited from even disclosing information on whether a certain person is a patient. If a member of a health care team discloses confidential information, there may be federal statute violations (*Code of Federal Regulations* [CFR]). In addition, state laws may exist that dictate who has authority to control access to medical records of patients who are incapacitated, incompetent, minors, or deceased. Information concerning these types of special situations is available through the state's attorney's office and through the employer's legal counsel.

● ● ●

A basic understanding of the impact of legal principles on nursing practice is essential to safe and effective performance as a nurse. It is also important to understand the role of the state board of nursing in the control and regulation of nursing practice. A thorough knowledge of employment right and responsibilities when nurses enter into employment contracts can make nurses better negotiators. Knowledge of tort law is mandatory, not only to prevent being sued, but also to serve as both a professional and patient care advocate.

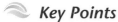

Key Points

- The power of the state to license nurses is derived from the Constitution.

- Licensing of health professionals is intended to protect the health, safety, and welfare of the public.

- Nurse practice acts define the practice of nursing, identify the scope of nursing practice, set the requirements for licensure, and proved guidelines for disciplinary action.

- A nurse who is charged with a violation of a state's nurse practice act has a right to "due process" in the investigation, hearing, and decision of the charge.

- The Americans With Disabilities Act grants special confidentiality to nurses who are in treatment for protected disabilities.

- Nurses work under a contract, which is an express or implied agreement with an employer that creates a legal relationship.

- A collective bargaining agreement establishes a contractual relationship between the union and the employer.

- Torts are private civil wrongs, in contrast to crimes, which are wrongs against the state.

- Negligence occurs when a person fails to act in a reasonable manner.

- Malpractice occurs when the conduct of a nurse or other professional is below the established standard.

- Assault is a threat to touch or harm another person.

- Battery is an unconsented touching, even if the touching is beneficial to the patient.

- The principle of informed consent requires that the patient be given enough information before treatment to make an informed, intelligent decision about whether to pursue or abandon treatment.

- False imprisonment occurs when a person is unlawfully confined within a fixed area.

- The health care provider is duty bound to keep information about a patient confidential, no matter how it was obtained.

 ## Critical Thinking Exercises

1. Review your state nurse practice act and delineate the definition and scope of nursing practice. Evaluate its relevance for today's health care environment.

2. Discuss the administrative and disciplinary functions of state boards of nursing.

3. How does the right of "due process" protect the nurse? How does it protect the public?

4. What must a plaintiff prove in order to recover damages in the following situation?

   An IV was left in place for 5 days although the hospital policy specified 2 days. As a result, the patient sustained a thrombosis and inflammation at the site.

5. Discuss the concepts of employment law as they relate to your employment situation.

6. Apply knowledge of tort law to formulate risk reduction strategies that could protect the nurse against legal action.

References

Aiken, T.D., & Catalano, J.T. (1994). *Legal, ethical and political issues in nursing.* Philadelphia: F.A. Davis.

Bernzweig, E.P. (1990). *The nurse's liability for malpractice: A programmed course* (5th ed.). St. Louis: Mosby.

Code of Federal Regulations, Title 42, Part 2.

Danzon, P.M. (1985). *Medical malpractice: Theory, evidence and public policy.* Boston, MA: Harvard University Press.

Dent v. West Virginia, 129 U.S. 114, 9 S. Ct. 231, 32 L. Ed. 623 (1889).

Doe v. Roe, No. 0369 (N.Y. App. Div., 4th Jud. Dept. May 28, 1993).

Dornette, W.H.L. (1991). Nonnegligent intentional torts. In W.H.L. Dornette (Ed.), *Legal issues in anesthesia practice.* Philadelphia: F.A. Davis.

Hoffman, A.C. (1991). Torts. In American College of Legal Medicine (Ed.), *Legal medicine: Legal dynamics of medical encounters* (2nd ed.). St. Louis: Mosby.

Ketter, J. (1994). Employers use Supreme Court decision against RNs: ANA devises legal, legislative strategies. *The American Nurse, 1,* 7.

McMullen, P., & Campbell-Philipsen, N.D. (1994). The end of collective bargaining for nurses? NLRB v. Health Care and Retirement Corp. *Nursing Policy Forum, 1* (1).

McMullen, P., & Pepper, J. (1992). Surviving the legal hot seat. *Nursing Connections, 5*(2), 33-36.

McMullen, P., & Philipsen, N. (1993a). Charting basic 101. *Nursing Connections, 6*(3), 62-64.

McMullen, P., & Philipsen, N. (1993b). Medical records: Promoting patient confidentiality. *Nursing Connections, 6*(4).

NLRB v. Health Care & Retirement Corp. of America, 114 S.C.1778, 18 L.Ed. 586, 6 U.S.L.W. 4371, 146 L.R.R.M. (B.N.A.) 31, 18 Lab.Cas. 11,090 (May 3, 1994).

People of the State of Illinois v. Margaret Jihan, 537 N.E.2d 751m 127 Ill.2d 379, 130 Ill. Dec. 422 (1989).

Prosser, W. (1984). *Handbook of the law of torts* (4th ed.). St. Paul, MN: West Publishing.

Sermchief v. Gonzalez, 660 S.W.2d 683 (Mo. 1983).

Shimberg, B., & Roederer, D. (1994). *Occupational licensing: Questions a legislator should ask.* (2nd ed.). Lexington, KY: Council on Licensure, Enforcement and Regulation.

Simpson, J.M. (1994). Understanding malpractice litigation. In American Association of Nurse Anesthetists (Ed.), *Professional aspects of nurse anesthesia practice* (pp. 225-250). Philadelphia: F.A. Davis.

United States Congress, Office of Technology Assessment. (1986). *Nurse practictioners, physician's assistants, and certified nurse-midwives.* Washington, DC: U.S. Government Printing Office.

Ethical Dimensions of Nursing and Health Care

12

Sara T. Fry

 Objectives

At the completion of this chapter, the reader will be able to:

- Describe how the subject matters of ethics and methods of ethics are used to investigate morality.

- Apply a representative framework for case study analysis to ethical questions in nursing practice.

- Comprehend how personal values and beliefs, professional moral standards, moral concepts of nursing, and ethical principles influence the nurse's ethical decisions and actions in providing patient care.

Profile in Practice

Mitzi W. Davis, PhD, RN
College of Nursing, University of Tennessee,
Knoxville, Tennessee

I became interested in ethical issues and decision making as a result of both personal and professional experiences. My clinical speciality is maternal child nursing, an area in which technology and limited resources have added to the multiple conflicts inherent in pregnancy, childbearing, and child rearing. My practice forces me to confront such issues as maternal versus fetal rights, the concept of personhood as applied to the ancephalic infant, surrogacy, the right to reproduction or to sterilization for the mentally retarded client, and so forth. In addition, as a parent I once faced the possibility of having to decide how aggressively to treat a child whose capacity for meaningful interaction was questionable. Ethical questions are part of everyday life.

I am a member of the ethics committee of the medical center where I practice. The committee is composed of physicians, nurses, social workers, attorneys, clergy, and faculty from the University of Tennessee, Knoxville, medical ethics department. The issues we address are varied but most often relate to withholding or withdrawing life-prolonging medical treatment. Any interested person—client, family member, or staff—may seek consultation with the ethics committee. The committee does not make decisions on behalf of care providers, but provides a forum for discussion so that all points of view may be considered and involved parties may fully evaluate the choices available. An attempt is made to honor the client's wishes whenever possible and to help the client and/or family to determine and express preferences.

The challenges of this role have changed as I have become more experienced. I can now see the ethical questions and underlying values more clearly and find it easier to support the decisions of the client or family, even when resultant emotions are painful. The era of limited resources presents new challenges. A decision to provide expensive treatment for one individual may now negatively impact on the ability of the organization to provide for others. I am challenged to see that institutional responsibility and court review play the appropriate secondary role in decision making. I consider the opportunity to serve on this committee a privilege.

The term *ethics* has several meanings. The term is sometimes used to refer to the practices or beliefs of a particular group of individuals, as in Christian ethics, physician ethics, or nursing ethics. *Ethics* also refers to the expected standards and behavior of a group as described in the group's code of professional conduct. Nurses and physicians are expected to maintain certain standards of ethical conduct as described by their professional codes of ethics (i.e., The American Nurses' Association [ANA] *Code for Nurses* [1985] and the American Medical Association [AMA] *Principles of Medical Ethics* [1986]). The term *ethics* is also used to refer to a philosophical mode of inquiry that helps us understand the moral dimensions of human conduct. In this sense, ethics is an activity, a particular method of investigation, that one undertakes to respond to particular types of questions about human behavior.

Throughout this chapter, the term *ethics* is used in all of the senses described above. *Ethics* refers here to the moral practices and beliefs of professionals who work together in the delivery of health care, the particular moral standards of a single group of professionals (nurses, physicians, and others), and inquiry about the principles of morality. Ethics is a mode of inquiry that helps us understand the moral dimensions of human conduct. To engage in or to *do* ethics is to undertake a particular method of investigation into matters of human concern (Fry, 1986).

SUBJECT MATTERS OF ETHICS

Ethics has several subject matters or areas of inquiry (Fig. 12-1). *Descriptive ethics* investigates the phenomena of morality and then describes and explains the phenomena in order to construct a theory of human nature that responds to ethical questions

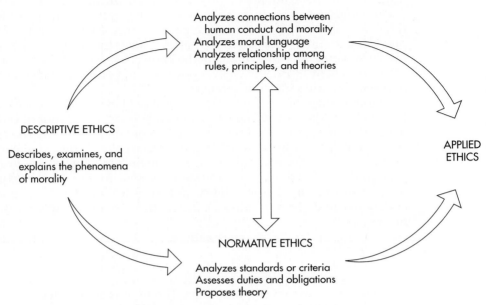

Fig. 12-1   The subject matters of ethics.

(Frankena, 1973). Those who investigate the moral-reasoning patterns and moral judgments of nurses (Chrisham, 1981; Ketefian, 1981a, 1981b) are usually engaged in descriptive ethics. Other investigators have described how nurses make clinical decisions (Prescott, Dennis, & Jacox, 1987).

Normative ethics is an area of inquiry that investigates standards or criteria for right or wrong conduct (Frankena, 1973). It usually begins with the question, "What ought I to do?" and examines various ethical principles, rules, or standards of right or wrong commonly associated with moral behavior. The moral weight of the perceived duties and obligations in human interaction are assessed, and theories for moral human conduct are often used to support one ethical judgment or action rather than another. Common moral theories used in normative ethics are utilitarianism, natural law, formalism, and pragmatism.

Metaethics is a secondary level of inquiry that examines the nature of ethical inquiry itself (Frankena, 1973). It gives us theories *about* ethics rather than theories *for* ethical conduct. Typical metaethical investigations consider the connections between human conduct and morality, the connections between ethical beliefs (values) and the facts of the real world, and the relationships among ethical theories, principles, rules, and human conduct. Inquiry about the moral language of nursing (e.g., advocacy, accountability, cooperation, caring) falls within the area of metaethics as well.

The subject matters of ethics are closely related. One might start by engaging in descriptive ethics to describe moral phenomena (such as the protection of patients from harm), then engage in normative ethics to argue for the moral accountability of the nurse in patient care, and then engage in metaethics to explicate the meaning of accountability within a particular patient care situation. Sometimes it is not possible to engage in normative ethics without prior knowledge from metaethics, and vice versa. For example, the meaning of a moral concept (such as accountability) needs to be clearly understood before it is applied to a specific situation. Both normative ethics and metaethics depend on descriptive ethics for the moral phenomena of human conduct. All three subject matters of ethics are particularly helpful in understanding the nature of the increasingly difficult ethical problems experienced by health professionals in the past decade.

VALUES

A *value* is a worthwhile or desirable standard or quality. Values can easily be identified in the everyday life experiences of any person. They can be expressed in language, behaviors, or standards of conduct that a person endorses or tries to maintain (Omery, 1989). Values are organized into a system that has meaning to the individual. This system of values represents the individual's set of beliefs about what he or she believes to be true. Some values are more important than others and are given higher priority within an individual's value system. This hierarchy is usually fairly stable over time, but other values can and do replace higher values based on life experiences and an individual's reassessment of his or her values (Rokeach, 1968).

Once part of the person's value system, any value can have motivational power and guide that person's choices. Unfortunately, individuals are often unaware of the values that motivate their choices and decisions (Fry, 1994).

Personal values are beliefs and attitudes held by an individual that form a basis for behavior and a basis for how each of us experiences life. For example, one nurse may personally value both cleanliness and honesty. These values are important to the nurse and either allow or prevent making certain judgments and carrying out specific actions. Personal value systems vary widely from person to person. One can never assume that another's personal value system is similar to one's own (Burnard & Chapman, 1988).

Each nurse has a personal value system influenced by family, religious and political beliefs, culture, education, and life experiences. Identifying the personal values in one's value system through introspection and self-reflection is the first step in making ethical decisions. The second step is understanding what values are important to other individuals and the reasons why they are important. Each person prioritizes his or her values differently, based on his or her belief system and hierarchy of values. Someone else's value system is equally as valid as one's own value system.

Cultural values are values that are indigenous to a culture or people. They often influence our beliefs about health, illness, and what is morally required behavior in providing health care. Some cultures, typified by Western culture, value individual choice more than obedience to authority. Some cultures, such as some Asian cultures, value the elderly in the community more than other cultures do. One culture may value health-promoting behaviors, such as physical exercise, more than another culture. One's culture reinforces personal values.

Since nursing is practiced in many different cultural systems, any discussion of ethics must consider the values expressed by the culture of the population cared for and how those values relate to proposed nursing interventions. Many cultural values stem from religious beliefs and may be acted out unconsciously by individuals. These values are deeply embedded in the background and experience of the person and cannot be called into question without questioning that person's very self-concept (Burnard & Chapman, 1988).

Professional values are general attributes prized by a professional group. Professional values in nursing are those promoted by the professional code of ethics and the practice standards of nursing. Nurses learn about professional values, both from formal instruction and from informal observation of practicing nurses, and gradually incorporate professional values into their personal value system (Fry, 1994).

Some traditional professional values of nursing are based on preferences or taste: cleanliness, efficiency, organization, to name a few. Other professional values are based on moral norms: honesty, competence, compassion, and the like. Some of the professional values in nursing have a rich historical background, constituting "nursing etiquette" over the years (see box below).

Historical Note: Early Nursing Ethics and Etiquette

Early interpretations of nursing ethics tend to be associated with the image of the nurse as a chaste, good woman in service to others and as an obedient, dutiful servant. Florence Nightingale's good nurse was committed to the ideal of doing what was right. She was disciplined by moral training and could be relied on to do her duty in service to others. This view of the good nurse as a good woman pervaded early textbooks on nursing ethics. In addition to being physically and morally strong, the nurse was required to be dignified, cultured, courteous, well educated, and a reserved woman of good breeding. Moral virtue, moral duty, and service to others were thus established as important foundations on which later interpretations of nursing ethics would be built.

At first, the practice of nursing ethics was virtually indistinguishable from nursing etiquette and the performance of duty. Nursing *etiquette* included forms of polite behavior, such as neatness, punctuality, courtesy, and quiet attendance on the physician. The nurse demonstrated her acceptance of her duties by following rules of etiquette and by being loyal and obedient to the physician (Robb, 1921).

Some important distinctions were made between etiquette and ethics. Nurses learned proper ward etiquette in order to promote professional harmony in patient care—such etiquette became the foundation for all other nursing behaviors. Ethics, however, was taught to promote moral excellence and technical competence on the part of the nurse. Ethics was viewed as a science, the knowledge of which would enable the nurse to carry out prescribed duties with moral skill and technical perfection.

Values Conflicts

Values can easily conflict with one another and with individual rights and professional duties. Personal values may conflict with professional values, which in turn might conflict with cultural values. The nurse's value of providing good care for the patient might conflict with the nurse's value of honoring the patient's choices or right to make such choices. The nurse's value of giving safe medication dosages might conflict with the patient's value of relief from pain and the perceived professional duty to relieve suffering. The elderly patient's value of personal liberty or being able to get out of bed whenever he or she wants might conflict with the institution's value of patient safety, achieved by having patients wait for nursing assistance during the night. In each of these situations, the nurse must first identify the values involved, the value of relevant rights and duties, and where a conflict between values, rights, and/or duties is occurring. Then the nurse must make a decision based on which values are most important. When moral values, rights, and duties are involved, resolving values conflicts becomes a complex ethical decision-making process (Fry, 1994).

MORAL CONCEPTS IN NURSING PRACTICE

Advocacy, accountability, cooperation, and caring are moral concepts that constitute part of the foundation for nursing ethics. These concepts seem to have enjoyed a special place of honor among nursing standards and statements over the years.

Advocacy

Advocacy is the active support of an important cause (Fry, 1987a). It is sometimes used in a legal context to refer to the defense of basic human rights on behalf of those who cannot speak for themselves. For example, many institutions employ patient advocates who are expected to defend and speak for patients who cannot, by virtue of hospitalization or diminished autonomy as a result of illness, voice their own concerns or choices, or assert their rights. The role of the advocate is to assert the patient's choices or desires on his or her behalf in the same way that a lawyer presents the case of a client, pleads for an interpretation of the case, and defends the client's rights.

There are several interpretations of the advocacy concept (Fry, 1987a). One interpretation (the *rights protection model*) views the nurse as the defender of patient rights against an impersonal health care system. The nurse informs the patient of his or her rights, makes sure that the patient understands these rights, reports infringements of these rights, and is expected to prevent further violations of rights.

A second interpretation *(values-based decision model)* views the nurse as the person who helps the patient to discuss his or her needs, interests, and choices consistent with values, lifestyle, or personal plan of action (Fry, 1987a). The nurse does not impose decisions or values on the patient but helps the patient explore the benefits and burdens of available options in order to make decisions most consistent with the patient's own beliefs and values.

A third interpretation *(respect-for-persons model)* views the patient as possessing certain human characteristics that require respect (Fry, 1987a). The patient's human dignity is respected and advocated regardless of whether or not the patient is self-determining or autonomous. As advocate, the nurse keeps the basic human values of the patient foremost among his or her considerations and acts to protect the patient's human dignity, privacy, and choices (when applicable). When the patient is not self-determining, the nurse advocates the patient's welfare as defined by the patient while he or she was self-determining, or as defined by the patient's surrogate decision maker. When no other person defines the welfare of the patient, the nurse promotes the best interests of the patient to the best of his or her nursing ability. In this role, the nurse assumes responsibility for the manner in which the patient's human dignity and other significant human values have been protected during his or her illness and is accountable to society and other members of the nursing profession for how this important advocate role has been carried out.

This last model of advocacy seems to be consistent with the values in the ANA *Code for Nurses* (see box below). Indeed, the code describes advocacy as acting so as "to safe-

---

American Nurses' Association Code for Nurses

1. The nurse provides services with respect for human dignity and the uniqueness of the client, unrestricted by considerations of social or economic status, personal attributes, or the nature of health problems.
2. The nurse safeguards the client's right to privacy by judiciously protecting information of a confidential nature.
3. The nurse acts to safeguard the client and the public when health care and safety are affected by the incompetent, unethical, or illegal practice of any person.
4. The nurse assumes responsibility and accountability for individual nursing judgments and actions.
5. The nurse maintains competence in nursing.
6. The nurse exercises informed judgment and uses individual competence and qualifications as criteria in seeking consultation, accepting responsibilities, and delegating nursing activities to others.
7. The nurse participates in activities that contribute to the ongoing development of the profession's body of knowledge.
8. The nurse participates in the profession's efforts to implement and improve standards of nursing.
9. The nurse participates in the profession's efforts to establish and maintain conditions of employment conducive to high-quality nursing care.
10. The nurse participates in the profession's effort to protect the public from misinformation and misrepresentation and to maintain the integrity of nursing.
11. The nurse collaborates with members of the health professions and other citizens in promoting community and national efforts to meet the health needs of the public.

From The American Nurses' Association (1985). *Code for nurses with interpretive statements*. Kansas City, MO: The Association.

guard the client and the public when health care and safety are affected by incompetent, unethical, or illegal practice by any person" (ANA, 1985). This means that the advocate role of the nurse has important long-range implications for the quality of patient care and the role of the nurse in the health care system. It is an important role that cannot be underestimated in today's world.

Accountability

The concept of *accountability* has two major attributes: answerability and responsibility (Fry, 1987a). Accountability can be defined in terms of either of these attributes, but answerability is the preferred one for the *Code for Nurses,* which defines accountability as answerability for how one has promoted, protected, and met the health needs of the patient. It means to justify or to "give an account" according to accepted moral standards or norms for choices and actions that the nurse has made and carried out (Fry, 1989c). It involves a relationship between the nurse and other parties and is contractual. The nurse is a professional who enters into an agreement to perform services and who can be held accountable for performing them according to agreed-on terms and standards of practice.

The terms of *legal accountability* are contained in licensing procedures and state nurse practice acts. The terms of *moral accountability* are contained in the *Code for Nurses* and other standards of nursing practice in the form of norms set by the members of the profession. In the *Code for Nurses,* it is noted that accountability means "providing an explanation or rationale for what has been done in the nursing role" (ANA, 1985, p. 8). This is a very important concept of professional nursing practice and should be emphasized in the educational process. It is a concept from which important values are derived and principles are frequently formulated. Along with advocacy, cooperation, and caring, accountability forms the conceptual framework for the moral dimensions of nursing practice and helps sustain the tradition of nursing by providing both the practice of nursing and the social role of nursing with a necessary historical content.

Cooperation

Cooperation is a concept that includes *active participation* with others to obtain quality care for patients, *collaboration* in designing approaches to nursing care, and *reciprocity* with those with whom nurses identify professionally. It means to consider the values and goals of those with whom one works as one's own values and goals. The ANA *Code for Nurses* (1985) indicates support for cooperation as a moral value by its statement, "The nurse collaborates with members of the health professions and other citizens . . . to meet the health needs of the public" (p. 3).

Cooperation fosters networks of mutual support and close working relationships. The concept of cooperation supports such nursing actions as working with others toward shared goals, keeping promises, making mutual concerns a priority, and sacrificing personal interests to the long-term maintenance of the professional relationship.

All of these actions express feelings traditionally valued by all human beings and support professional collaboration in designing patient care (Jameton, 1984).

Nursing's historical documents and professional statements have often emphasized different aspects of professional cooperation. For example, Isabel Hampton Robb (1921), an early nurse leader and scholar in the United States, linked cooperation to a special loyalty shared by members of the professional group.

The concept of cooperation has also been expressed as the power that enables professionals to work together. Nightingale (Nutting & Dock, 1907) emphasized this aspect of cooperation as maintaining and strengthening a community of nurses working toward a common goal. Cooperation does not mean that conflicts will not occur, or that the good of patients should be sacrificed for the maintenance of the nurse's relationships with colleagues or with the employing institution. It does mean, however, that individual goals and interests might need to be ethically compromised in order to achieve organizational and policy changes that will improve the quality of patient care.

Cooperation is also an altruistic concept because it expresses the human bonds that grow from working together and spending time together. It can threaten patient care if one's relationships with members of the profession or co-workers become more important than the quality of patient care. The appropriate role for cooperation, however, is the maintenance of working relationships and conditions that express obligations toward the patient and are mutually agreed on. Cooperation can help unite nurses and other health care workers toward the shared goal of improved patient care. Along with advocacy and accountability, cooperation helps form a strong conceptual framework that enables nurses to meet the requirements of professional practice.

Caring

The ethical concept of caring is valued in the nurse-patient relationship, and caring behaviors are often considered fundamental to the nursing role. Leininger (1984), for example, argues that caring has a direct relationship with human health and that all cultures and communities practice caring behaviors that serve to reduce intercultural stresses and conflicts. Caring behaviors also protect human survival.

Nurse caring is specifically directed toward the protection of the health and welfare of patients. To some, *caring* is defined as a moral obligation or duty in special relationships (Pellegrino, 1985). This means that the nurse, for example, is obligated to promote the patient's good because the nurse and patient share a relationship that is created by the patient's need for nursing care. The nurse is obligated to show caring behaviors toward those in need of health care because doing so promotes their good.

Caring can also be defined as a form of involvement with others that creates concern about how other individuals experience their world (Benner & Wrubel, 1989). Caring therefore involves being there for the patient, respecting the patient, feeling with and for the patient, and closeness with the patient (Forrest, 1989).

The degree to which caring behaviors can be implemented in nursing practice is influenced by several factors. Nurse-related factors include such things as individual beliefs, educational experiences about caring, feeling good about nursing work, and one's own experiences in caring for others or in being cared for (Forrest, 1989). Patient-related factors include whether or not the patient is hard to care for or confirms the nurse's caring behaviors. Other factors that influence nurse caring include time to care, administrative support for caring behaviors, and the physical environment where care takes place (Forrest, 1989).

Some nurses have expressed concern about the extent to which nurses are expected to care for patients. For example, some believe that too much caring may result in nurses becoming physically and emotionally drained, resulting in "burnout" and unresolved nurse stress. There is a potential personal cost to caring on the part of the nurse that has not been adequately understood or investigated. Yet, caring behaviors on the part of the nurse continue to be expected and valued by the profession and the public because caring is universally considered fundamental to the nursing role where human health is concerned (see Chapter 14). Perhaps burnout could be reduced by changing the physical environment where care takes place or changing administrative support for nurses.

ETHICAL PRINCIPLES

Ethical principles are action guides to moral decision making and are an important element in the formation of moral judgments in professional practice (Beauchamp & Childress, 1994). They generally assert that actions of a certain kind ought (or ought not) to be performed and serve to justify the rules that are often applied to patient care and the context of professional practice. The ethical principles important in nursing practice are beneficence, justice, autonomy, veracity, sanctity of human life and fidelity (Veatch & Fry, 1987).

Beneficence

The obligation to do good and to avoid doing harm is understood as the ethical principle of *beneficence* (Frankena, 1973). Acting on this principle means to help others gain what is of benefit to them, to reduce risks of harm to patients, and to provide positive benefits to patients in terms of goods or assets.

Applying the principle in nursing practice often poses difficult problems for the nurse. For example, it is uncertain whether or not the nurse is obligated to take into consideration all of the ways in which the patient might be benefited. The *Code for Nurses* seems to imply that the nurse should do this when it states that the "nurse's primary commitment is to the health, welfare, and safety of the client" (ANA, 1985, p. 6). This is a substantial obligation and, if literally interpreted, would entail multiple obligations toward the patient, some of which may actually lie outside the expertise or competency of the nurse.

A second problem in applying the principle is deciding whether the obligation to provide benefit has greater priority over the obligation to avoid harm. Some ethicists claim that the duty to avoid harm is a stronger obligation in health care relationships than the obligation to benefit (Beauchamp & Childress, 1994; Ross, 1939). If this is the case in nursing practice, nurses could fulfill the obligation to avoid harm by simply doing nothing for patients. Yet, we would hardly call doing nothing for patients acceptable nursing care. The avoidance of harm must be balanced by the provision of benefit, and acceptable ranges of both benefit and risks of harm need to be established.

A third problem in applying this principle in nursing practice concerns the limits of providing benefit to patients. At what point do benefits to other parties (one's own family, the employing institution, co-workers) take priority over the benefits to the patient? Is the nurse obliged to provide benefits rather broadly or simply to the identified patient? Nurses need to be very clear about the boundaries of their obligation to provide benefits and avoid harm in patient care.

Justice

Once the boundaries of the obligation to benefit and avoid harm are determined, nurses should be concerned about how benefits and burdens ought to be distributed among patient populations (Veatch & Fry, 1987). In other words, the nurse must decide what is a just or fair allocation of resources among patients under his or her care.

The formal principle of *justice* states that equals should be treated equally and that those who are unequal should be treated differently according to their needs (Beauchamp & Childress, 1994). This means that those equal in health needs should receive the same amount of health care resources. When some people have greater health needs, a principle of justice allows that they should receive a greater amount of health resources. This type of allocation is just because it distributes health resources according to need in a fair manner. While it is not possible to provide equal amounts of health care goods and resources for everyone in society, it is possible to provide for equal access to health care resources according to individual need. The focus on need allows for the just distribution of resources among patients and forgoes the distribution of resources outside of need.

Autonomy

The principle of *autonomy* ensures that individuals are permitted personal liberty to determine their own actions according to plans that they have chosen (Veatch & Fry, 1987). To respect persons as autonomous individuals is to acknowledge their personal choices.

One of the problems that arises in applying a principle of autonomy to nursing care is that persons appear to be autonomous in varying degrees. Patients cannot make choices about their care entirely free from internal and external constraints. Internal constraints on patient autonomy are mental ability, level of consciousness, age, and disease states. External constraints on patient autonomy are the health care agency environment, nursing resources, information for making informed choices, and financial resources.

The principle of autonomy may also be difficult to apply in patient care when there is a strong conviction on the part of the nurse or other members of the health care team that respecting self-determined choice is not really in the best interests of the patient. In this type of situation, the nurse may need to consider the limits of individual patient autonomy and the criteria for justified paternalism on the part of the nurse. *Paternalism* is defined as the overriding of patient choices or intentional actions in order to benefit the patient (Beauchamp & Childress, 1994). Although paternalism is seldom justified in the care of patients, there is reason to believe that some situations warrant overriding patient autonomy when the benefits to be realized are great and the harms that will be avoided are significant (Childress, 1982).

Heeding the principle of autonomy means that nurses should also respect a patient's choice to refuse treatments. The basic human right of all patients to refuse treatment was formally legislated by the Omnibus Budget Reconciliation Act (1990). The Patient Self-Determination Act became effective December 1, 1991, and requires all health care institutions receiving Medicare or Medicaid funds to inform patients that they have the right to refuse medical and surgical care and the right to initiate a written *advance directive* (i.e., a written or oral statement by which a competent person makes known his or her treatment preferences and/or designates a surrogate decision maker in the event he or she should become unable to make medical decisions on his or her own behalf) (see box below). Hospitals, home health care agencies, and managed care organizations are required to make this information available, in writing, at the time the patient comes under an agency's care.

In some situations the nurse may need to assess whether an advance directive is an accurate statement of what the patient wants. Other nursing assessments might include whether a patient has fully taken into account the consequences of a treatment decision before completing an advance directive, and whether a surrogate decision maker is inappropriately making decisions for a patient with intact decision-making capacity (Mezey, et al., 1994).

Requirements of the Patient Self-Determination Act

- Provide written information to adult patients about their rights to make medical decisions, including the right to accept or refuse treatment and the right to formulate advance directives.
- Document in each patient's record whether the patient has previously executed an advance directive.
- Implement written policies regarding the various types of advance directives.
- Ensure compliance with state laws regarding medical treatment decisions and advance directives.
- Refrain from discrimination against individuals regarding their treatment decisions via an advance directive.
- Provide education for staff and the community on issues and the law concerning advance directives.

From Omnibus Reconciliation Act of 1990, Sections 4206 and 4751, Public Law 101-508, November 5, 1990.

Veracity

The principle of *veracity* is defined as the obligation to tell the truth and to not lie or deceive others. Truthfulness has long been regarded as fundamental to the existence of trust among individuals and has special significance in health care relationships.

Truthfulness is expected because it is part of the respect that we owe people. Individuals have the right to be told the truth and to not be lied to or deceived. Truthfulness also supports the relationship of trust that exists in special relationships. Nurses are obliged to be truthful because to not do so will undermine the effectiveness of the nurse's role with the patient and may, in the long run, bring about undesirable consequences for future relationships with patients.

When patients are seriously ill, nurses may sometimes withhold information from the patient because they think that the patient may not really want to know the truth about their condition. Studies of terminally ill patients, however, have indicated that despite illness, patients want to know the full truth about their conditions (Veatch, 1978). The *Code for Nurses* points out that "truth telling and the process of reaching informed choice underlie the exercise of self-determination, which is basic to respect for persons" (ANA, 1985, p. 2). This means that the nurse is obliged to respect and follow a principle of veracity in providing nursing care to patients.

Sanctity of Human Life

The issue of taking human life arises in a number of patient care situations and especially in decisions to withhold or withdraw life-sustaining treatments. It can also occur in situations of assisted suicide and whenever patients are suffering from a life-threatening disease or illness. The principle of *sanctity of human life* is defined as the obligation to not infringe on the sacredness of human life, or the obligation to not take human life (Veatch & Fry, 1987).

The taking of human life may be contemplated by the nurse whenever a patient is suffering. Someone might consider assisting the patient's death as an act of mercy. He or she might feel that the patient would be better off dead (or family members would be better off if the patient were dead). Should the nurse relieve a patient's misery by hastening his or her death in some manner? Is this a role for the nurse? Are nurses expected to make these types of judgments, especially when patients are no longer capable of making their own decisions or of carrying out such an action on their own? Is there a difference between assisting a patient's death for reasons of mercy and withholding or withdrawing treatments for reasons of medical futility? Both actions will surely hasten the death of the patient, although with the latter action the patient will continue to live a while longer.

Some ethicists claim that these questions can be answered by applying the principles already discussed. In other words, the principles of beneficence, justice, and autonomy already provide arguments that will support sanctity of human life on the part of the nurse. Yet each of these principles has been demonstrated to be insufficient for questions about assisted dying in patient care. A principle of sanctity for human life is needed to support nurses' ethical reasoning for these situations.

The *Code for Nurses* seems to address this issue when it states, "Nursing care is directed toward the prevention and relief of the suffering commonly associated with the dying process. The nurse may provide interventions to relieve symptoms in the dying client even when the interventions entail substantial risks of hastening death" (ANA, 1985, p. 4). Yet the *Code for Nurses* also prohibits assisting the death of a patient when it states, "Nurses are morally obligated to respect human existence and . . . therefore they must take all reasonable means to protect and preserve human life when there is hope of recovery or reasonable hope of benefit from life-prolonging treatment" (ANA, 1985, p. 2).

Is withholding nutrition and hydration from a patient assisting that patient's death? This question is at the center of some of the most controversial patient care issues confronting nurses today (Fry, 1988). Several philosophers (Lynn & Childress, 1983; Paris & Fletcher, 1983) and some legal cases (*in re* Conroy, 1983; Cruzan, 1990; *in re* Hier, 1984) have come to the conclusion that nutrition and hydration can be withheld for the same reasons that other treatments are withheld, as long as there is clear and convincing evidence that this would be the patient's wish. Others, however, have been reluctant to accept the withholding of nutrition and hydration even when the patient has formally requested that this be done. Some scholars, for example, have expressed concern that the provision of food and fluids is a basic caring function that should always be required in the care of patients (Callahan, 1983). One reason given for this view is that provision of food and fluids is symbolic of our care for the hungry and thirsty among us. If patients in terminally ill states, however, do not experience hunger and thirst, does this mean that food and water should not be administered? The difficult nature of these questions is obvious.

In situations of doubt, the nurse must resort to the weight and importance of the obligation to respect human life in nursing practice. A principle of sanctity for human life is needed because nurses may often be uncertain whether or not their actions will contribute to the patient's death and whether or not such actions are morally wrong. Assisting a patient's death by facilitating his or her suicide or by acts of active euthanasia is simply not an option for the nurse.

Fidelity

Fidelity is defined as the obligation to remain faithful to one's commitments (Veatch & Fry, 1987). Commitments that usually fall within the scope of fidelity are obligations generic to the trust relationship between patient and nurse. These obligations are keeping promises, maintaining confidentiality, and caring.

Individuals tend to expect that promises will be kept in human relationships. We also expect that promises will not be broken unless there is a good reason. The same expectations concern the obligation of confidentiality, which is one of the most basic ethical requirements of professional health care ethics. However, exceptions to both obligations can sometimes be made. For example, some individuals maintain that it is morally acceptable to break promises when the breaking of the promise produces more good than if the promise is kept. Confidences are often broken for the same reasons.

It is also argued that breaking promises and confidences is morally acceptable when the welfare of a third party is jeopardized by the keeping of the confidence or promise. In the *Code for Nurses,* it is stated that the obligation of confidentiality "is not absolute when innocent parties are in direct jeopardy" (ANA, 1985, p. 4). Some form of this reason is usually given when confidences or promises are broken in order to report child abuse or the laboratory results of a serious communicable disease.

Others, however, argue against the breaking of confidences, in particular, on the basis of benefit to other parties. They claim that keeping information confidential is a right independent of consequences to others. While there may be good moral reasons to break promises to provide benefit to others, it is not morally acceptable to break confidences for the same reason (Veatch & Fry, 1987).

One way to understand the conceptual nature of the moral commitments surrounding confidentiality and promise keeping is to ground these obligations within an independent principle of fidelity. Thus, to maintain fidelity with the patient, nurses should carefully consider the information that should be kept confidential and when promise keeping is a legitimate expectation in the nurse-patient relationship. The duty to keep one's commitments thus becomes the focus of these obligations and not just the keeping of promises or confidentiality.

The duty to care is also included in aspects of the principle of fidelity. In fact, caring is consistently mentioned as one of the most important components of nursing practice, especially in the care of the terminally ill patient (Fleming, Scanlon, & D'Agostino, 1987; Larson, 1986; Mayer, 1987). Individualized caring, affective behaviors, comforting, and nursing competence have all been mentioned by nurses and patients as important to caring and feeling cared for.

In summary, making moral decisions and carrying out moral actions are strongly influenced by the extent to which nurses incorporate ethical principles into their actions and relationships with patients. How do the principles of ethics apply to patient care, and how do nurses resolve conflicts of values in patient care?

APPLICATION OF ETHICS TO NURSING PRACTICE

No one denies that ethical decision-making ability is a requirement of professional nursing practice (Fry, 1989a). Evidence of this ability is generally regarded as a desirable outcome of nursing education. Indeed, the majority of educational programs in nursing in the United States offer some course content in ethics. The goal is to assist the student in integrating his or her personal values and beliefs, the professional code of ethics, moral concepts of nursing practice, and ethical principles into a decision-making framework for making moral decisions and taking moral action (Fig. 12-2).

A national study of nursing education, however, has demonstrated that significant numbers of senior nursing students do not feel that they can apply knowledge of ethics to resolve ethical problems in nursing practice (American Association of Colleges of Nursing, 1986). Few of the basic baccalaureate students surveyed (under 40%) consciously used the ANA *Code for Nurses* to guide their actions, and only a minority (23%) reported that they used an ethical framework or model to assist them in the assess-

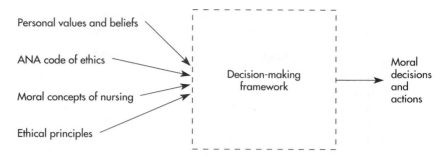

Fig. 12-2   Essentials of moral decisions and actions in nursing practice.

ment and resolution of an ethical problem. A survey of RN baccalaureate students revealed a perceived increase in their abilities to use ethical frameworks or models to address ethical problems when the educational process included this type of content (American Association of Colleges of Nursing, 1988).

Are ethical decision-making frameworks really useful in nursing practice? If so, how does one choose such a framework?

Decision-Making Frameworks

Ethicists recognize that there are many components and variables in decision making. No one decision-making method is appropriate or useful for everyone. However, *ethical* decision making can be enhanced by an orderly process of ethical analysis (Fry, 1989a, 1994). Frameworks represent the process of analysis that one might employ in making an ethical decision. They are useful in helping the nurse examine (1) the values involved, (2) the context within which the decision will be made, and (3) the nature of the nurse's responsibilities in the situation. They do not provide a foolproof formula for arriving at the "right" decision. There is no recipe for ethical decision making in nursing practice. Each decision maker must supply his or her own values, cognitive ability, reasoning abilities, and moral intuitions to the process of arriving at an ethical decision. Frameworks for ethical decision making simply help the individual to analyze the value dimensions of a situation and use his or her abilities to arrive at an ethical decision.

Since ethical decision making is a cognitive and moral ability that can be taught in the educational process and learned by anyone with a moral conscience, course content in ethics often includes ethical decision-making frameworks and their application in patient care situations. Used in conjunction with knowledge of the discipline of ethics, frameworks promote development of the abilities required for nursing practice.

A number of ethical decision-making frameworks for nursing practice have been proposed. All of them provide an orderly approach to analyzing the value dimensions involved in ethical conflicts and offer a systematic approach to implementing ethical decisions in patient care. Some are skeletal guidelines; others offer a more detailed approach to ethical decision making. Some frameworks proposed by nurses have been derived from physicians' models of ethical decision making (Murphy & Murphy, 1976). A few apply contemporary philosophical positions to nursing practice (Aroskar, 1980; Benjamin & Curtis, 1986), whereas others closely resemble the problem-solving or nursing process approach taught in nursing education (Bergman, 1973; Curtin, 1978; Jameton, 1984; Stanley, 1980). One other framework combines the problem-solving process in nursing with a theological perspective (Shelly, 1980).

Choice of a framework should be guided by the implicit values of the framework and their importance to the decision maker. Some frameworks clearly support the application of traditional theories of ethics and ethical principles to the patient care situation. Other frameworks help the nurse explore and analyze the context within which the value conflict has arisen and the views of the key parties to the decision. Nurses should not believe that one and only one framework works best in all situations.

The majority of ethical problems faced by the nurse are important but not necessarily complex. They are situations involving conflicts of values in fairly routine patient care situations. They become interesting and morally complex, however, when the values involved arise from strongly held cultural, religious, and moral beliefs. Because of the nature of values, a framework for case study analysis is offered here that can be used in conjunction with other models or alone.

Representative Framework for Case Study Analysis

The following framework (see box below) uses four questions to help the nurse (1) understand the context within which the ethical problem has occurred, (2) explore the significance of values central to the problem, (3) examine the meaning of the ethical problem to all parties involved, and (4) determine what should be done (Fry, 1994):

1. *What is the story behind the values conflicts?* By asking this question, the nurse begins to discover how the problem is defined by the parties experiencing the problem. The story needs to be told by each of the parties involved in terms of factual information (who did what), in terms of the values of the parties involved (why the situation is seen as an ethical question), and in terms of the conflicts of values perceived by the parties involved. It is important to allow the telling of the story in all its dimensions and through the eyes of all parties involved—the patient, the family members, the nurse, the physician, other health care workers,

---

Representative Framework for Case Study Analysis

1. What is the story behind the values conflicts?
2. What is the significance of the values involved?
3. What is the significance of the conflicts to the parties involved?
4. What should be done?

administrative officials, etc. When the full story of the problem is known, the context within which the problem arose will be made explicit, and the various interpretations of the problem and the values of the parties involved will become clear. In this way, the values conflicts will be clarified. Ethical questions *always* involve conflicts between values.

2. *What is the significance of the values involved?* In exploring the meaning of the values held by the parties involved, one gains insight into the nature of the values and their personal, religious, cultural, professional, and even political origins. Additional questions that might need to be asked include: What does it mean to "care" for this patient and what are my nursing responsibilities to this patient? Are there any legal questions that might need to be explored by a legal representative? How do I, as a professional nurse, maintain my ethical integrity in this situation? Exploring the significance of the values held by individuals in any situation is always very important. Ethical problems cannot be adequately resolved unless the value dimensions of the problem are known, respected, and considered in the decision-making process. This does not mean that all values will always be protected. In most conflict situations, the nurse assists the parties involved in examining their values and the values of others so that the parties can begin to negotiate. In other words, the parties to the conflict will need to decide which values are most important to preserve and protect in this instance and which values might be of lesser importance. The goal of the professional nurse is to help the parties involved respect each other's values and help individuals prioritize their values and preserve the most important ones in the process of decision making (Fry, 1989b). This can be done only when the significance of all values involved is known.

3. *What is the significance of the conflicts to the parties involved?* In answering this question, the nurse learns how the parties involved related their values to the present situation. Values are never static. They are dynamic in that they change over time and in relation to significant human events and relationships. Situations of value conflicts likewise do not occur in a vacuum. They have a history and a necessary social, economic, and political context that make them significant or nonsignificant to the parties involved. The conflicts of values might lead to a decision that affects the quality of a person's life, how long he or she might live, the amount of guilt that other parties to the conflict might experience, the emotional and psychological stress that individuals might experience following the resolution of the conflict, and the nurse's professional demeanor.

The acknowledgment of conflicts of values might also lead to the formation of policy that helps to resolve or prevent such value conflicts from occurring in the future. The nature of the value conflicts might have great significance for health professionals, who often must deal repeatedly with conflicts of values in the work environment.

4. *What should be done?* By asking this question, the nurse explores all the ways in which the values conflicts might be resolved. Seldom is there a single "ethically correct" solution to a situation. In most cases, ethical decisions are reached based

on the amount of information available at that time, the significance of the value dimensions, and the best judgment of the decision maker or the collective ethical stance of the group. Knowing a variety of possible ways in which the conflicts might be resolved gives the involved parties options to explore. These options should be explored in light of (1) the values held by the various parties, (2) outcomes that may occur, and (3) the moral rightness or wrongness of the various options. Some options might be ethically permissible (i.e., they do not conflict with the professional code of ethics) but may not support the values of the key decision maker, other parties to the situation, or the community group consensus. Some options might not be ethically permissible, although they might support important values. Some options (such as assisted suicide) might be ethically permissible for the patient, family members, or community group (i.e., consistent with their personal, cultural, and religious values) but not permissible for the nurse.

At some point, the key decision maker must choose a course of action based on his or her best judgment of what ought to be done. This decision is often very individual but is morally responsive in that it stems from a careful consideration of the context of the value conflicts, the values of all parties involved, the ethical relevance of these values, and the moral meaning of the situation to the individuals involved. It should also be a rational decision based on a careful process of ethical reflection and supported by the moral concepts of nursing and ethical principles.

Following the implementation of the choice or decision made, some assessment should be done about the outcome of the situation and the process that led to the decision. The nurse should always consider whether the process could have been improved and what implications, if any, the conflicts of values have for future patient care situations. To test your understanding of this framework for case study analysis, use the framework in deciding what the nurse should do in the following case study.

CASE STUDY: THE NURSE WHO THOUGHT THE ANA CODE FOR NURSES WAS WRONG*

Martha Long, a staff nurse, is caring for an 84-year-old man, Mr. Carson, who is being readmitted to the nursing home after a 6-week stay at the county medical center. Mr. Carson suffers from diabetes, chronic brain syndrome, frequent urinary tract infections, and heart disease. He is unaware of his surroundings but does move his extremities and moans loudly when the nursing staff try to talk to him or move him. He is also suffering from gangrene of the left foot, but his surrogate decision maker (his niece) has refused a surgical amputation. She refused on the basis that Mr. Carson would not have consented to the procedure if he were competent and able to state his wishes.

*Modified from Veatch, R.M., & Fry, S.T. (1987). *Case studies in nursing ethics.* Boston: Jones & Bartlett, pp. 38-39.

Mr. Carson was discharged from the medical center with a nasogastric tube in place to facilitate his feeding and nutritional intake. The nursing staff in the nursing home, however, note that he apparently does not like his tube feedings; he moans, turns his head, and waves his arms when the tube feedings are administered. The aides restrain his arms and hold his head while the tube feedings are given. Once given, the tube feedings are apparently tolerated well.

When his niece visits her uncle, she is visibly upset by the feeding tube. She asks that the tube be removed and calls the physician to remove it. The physician calls the nurse, Ms. Long, and asks her to remove the feeding tube. However, Ms. Long is not sure that she ought to remove the tube from Mr. Carson. She does not believe that Mr. Carson will be able to receive adequate nutrition without the tube and that removing the tube will contribute to a deterioration of his condition. She does not want to participate in what, in her opinion, might contribute to Mr. Carson's death despite his reactions to the tube feedings. Her reasons stem, in part, from her religious tradition. She believes that there is wisdom in this tradition, which has consistently taught that all life should be preserved. She believes that she should do whatever she can to assure that the risk of death to patients is avoided, or is at least minimized.

The other nurses on the unit, however, cite the right of the patient to refuse treatment, as exercised by his legal guardian, and the obligation of the nurse not to prolong the dying process. When Ms. Long reads the ANA Code for Nurses, she discovers that the obligation of the nurse to "provide services with respect for human dignity and the uniqueness of the client . . ." had recently been interpreted by the profession in the following manner: "Nursing care is directed toward the prevention and relief of the suffering commonly associated with the dying process. The nurse may provide interventions to relieve symptoms in the dying client even when the interventions entail substantial risks of hastening death" (Statement 1.3). Ms. Long reasons that if "relieving symptoms" in the case of Mr. Carson means removing his nasogastric tube, then the ANA Code for Nurses statement must be wrong. What should Ms. Long do?

RESEARCH ON NURSING ETHICS

The earliest record of a nursing ethics research project was Vaughan's study (1935) of the diaries of 95 student and graduate nurses who recorded the ethical problems they encountered in nursing practice over a 3-month period. Vaughan's analysis identified a total of 2265 moral problems, 67 problems of etiquette, and 110 questions about ethical behavior. The ethical problem the nurses faced most often was the lack of cooperation between nurses and physicians, and between nurses in general. Vaughan concluded that the problem of lack of cooperation her subjects experienced signaled nurses' growing awareness of their responsibilities to society and the role they were playing in patient care.

Despite this early interest in descriptive ethics, nursing ethics research did not begin in earnest until the 1980s. Research efforts initially focused on ethical reasoning abilities, and ethical behaviors and judgments among practicing nurses (Crisham, 1981; Ketefian, 1981a, 1981b; Murphy, 1976). Related studies focused on the moral reasoning levels of nursing students and nursing faculty (Munhall, 1980), and on patient values in relation to treatment choices (Gortner, 1984). More recently, studies have compared nurses' perceptions of moral problems in clinical practice with the perceptions of physicians (Gamelspacher et al., 1986) and have analyzed nurses' beliefs about medical ethical decision making into objective and subjective value dimensions (Self, 1987).

These studies have focused on the ability of the nurse to make moral judgments, on the hypothetical moral behavior of the nurse, on nurses' perceptions of moral problems, or on the value dimensions of nurses' and patients' beliefs about ethical decision making (Fry, 1987b). The measurement tools and the procedures employed have been designed to evaluate the cognitive ability of nurses to perceive value dimensions or to make moral judgments. In most cases, study results have been interpreted according to theoretical structures outside the context of nursing. Kohlberg's stage theory of moral development has been the most frequently cited theoretical structure (Kohlberg, 1981), but bioethics theory (Beauchamp & Childress, 1994) and value theory (Self, 1979) have also been cited.

During the 1980s and early 1990s, the focus of nursing ethics research shifted from the study of nurses' ethical perceptions and behaviors and how nursing ethics is taught to the study of how nurses make ethical decisions and plan patient care when confronted with complex moral issues. The use of nursing care resources by "do not resuscitate" (DNR) patients in medical intensive care units and the impact of the DNR order on nursing interventions has been studied (Lewandowski et al., 1985). The identification of variables that are the best predictors of a DNR classification and the extent of nursing care required by the DNR patient have been the focus of another research study (Tittle, Moody, & Becker, 1991). Other researchers have studied the effects of a nurse-initiated advance directive information program on patients' reactions and interests concerning advance directives (Silverman, Fry, & Armistead, 1994; see box on p. 281).

Observations that can be made about the current "state of the art" in nursing ethics research are the following:

- Values, value changes, moral judgment, and levels of moral reasoning among nurses or nursing students have not been adequately correlated with formal educational ethics content in nursing curricula. It is also not evident that the formal teaching of ethics affects the development of moral judgment in practicing nurses or that the development of moral judgment and increased levels of moral reasoning among nurses have any effect on the performance of nursing functions or patient care outcomes. These are all areas for further study. We tend to think that ethics is an important subject to learn and that the abilities to recognize values, make moral decisions, and be accountable for decisions are important to the quality of nursing care. Yet we do not really know what type of ethics content is truly effective in the education of nurses. Neither do we know to what extent the effective teaching of ethics influences the ability of the nurse to give more competent patient care. Is the morally accountable nurse a more competent nurse?
- The use of theoretical frameworks to interpret study results should be carefully evaluated. Since nursing is largely practiced by women, theoretical structures

---

Clinical Nursing Ethics Research Study

This study was conducted to determine how nurses perceive their roles in the implementation of the Patient Self-Determination Act (PSDA) and how they were prepared to undertake this role. Nineteen of the 20 nurses interviewed expressed a favorable reaction to being involved in the implementation of the PSDA on their units, and one nurse was neutral about this role ("it is part of my job"). All nurses stated that they felt comfortable asking patients or their families about advance directives, and most felt qualified to be involved in the PSDA implementation program. A majority of the nurses (11 of 20), however, expressed the opinion that nurses should have more responsibility in the implementation of the PSDA. Specifically, they believed nurses should do more than just ask patients about advance directives and give them a brochure. They believed that nurses have a moral duty or obligation to provide patients with detailed information about advance directives and promote meaningful discussions about treatment options. This duty or obligation stems from the close nursing relationship with patients, and nursing preparation to handle the emotional and psychological features that may surface from a discussion concerning end-of-life treatment decisions. Nurses developed and used several strategies to make the patient-provider interaction on advance directives less threatening to the patient and to reduce patient anxieties.

Modified from Silverman, H.J., Fry, S.T., & Armistead, N. (1994). Nurses' perspectives on implementation of the Patient Self-Determination Act. *Journal of Clinical Ethics, 5*(1), 30-37.

should include the process of ethical decision making by women, as well as by men. Kohlberg's theory, derived from cognitive psychology and based on studies of male children, has been strongly challenged for its lack of relevance to the moral development and ethical reasoning of women (Gilligan, 1982; Noddings, 1984). Furthermore, researchers should use structures that can account for the nature and process of ethical decisions made by nurses in contrast to those of other health care workers, such as physicians (Fry, 1989d).

• The evaluation of nursing research on ethics needs to address the subject matters of ethics rather than typical subject matters of nursing. Units of analysis, such as nurse, patient, and the environment, reflect traditional paradigms of nursing inquiry, but they tell us nothing about the discipline of ethics or the state of ethical inquiry in nursing. Ethical inquiry in nursing should be reviewed and evaluated according to the subject matters of ethics: descriptive ethics, normative ethics, and metaethics. We should also be encouraging nurse researchers to pursue research on ethics within these classifications.

• The particular roles of nurses in ethical decisions that affect patients are not very clear. Nurses' abilities to recognize moral values, make ethical decisions, and support patients' or family members' decisions are believed to be very important to the quality of patient care. However, little is known about the type of ethical decisions made by nurses and how they affect patient outcomes. Nursing ethics research should attend to this lack of information.

Key Points

- The discipline of ethics has different subject matters or areas of inquiry and often uses various methods of argumentation in its investigations of morality. As part of this process, analysis of moral concepts and ethical principles related to the practice of nursing is recommended.

- The moral concepts of advocacy, accountability, cooperation, and caring have important moral dimensions and constitute part of the conceptual framework for nurses' ethical decision making.

- The ethical principles of beneficence, justice, autonomy, veracity, sanctity of human life, and fidelity are action guides to moral nurse actions but often conflict with one another or with other significant human values. Because of these conflicts, nurses may find that the use of an ethical decision-making framework is useful in patient care situations.

- Many ethical decision-making frameworks are available in the nursing literature, and all seem to provide a systematic approach to ethical analysis of values conflicts and questions of what should be done in the nursing role.

- A representative framework for case study analysis is recommended, since it addresses values conflicts and their complex interactions.

- As nurses use ethical decision-making frameworks and engage in ethical analysis, the need for additional research on nurses' decision-making patterns and choices will become evident.

- Descriptive ethics research is at a very early stage of development in nursing, and few good metaethical studies of nursing's moral concepts have been conducted. Normative ethics as a form of inquiry in nursing is also at a very early stage of development.

- All nurses should become familiar with the methods of ethics, the use of ethical decision-making frameworks, and the current state of nursing ethics research so that they can contribute effectively to the growth of ethical inquiry within nursing.

- If one of the goals of nursing education is to produce a morally accountable individual who can contribute to the quality of patient care, then ethics occupies an important role in nursing education, practice, and research.

Critical Thinking Exercises

1. To what extent should one's personal code of ethics, integrated with religious beliefs and cultural values, influence moral decision making in nursing practice?

2. If terminally ill patients under your care asked you to help them end their lives or assist them in dying, what would you do? Why?

3. Some ethicists have argued that there is nothing morally unique to nursing practice (i.e., the same moral issues and questions arise in all health professionals' practices). Would you agree or disagree with this statement? Why?

4. The term "applied ethics" means the application of ethical theory, principles, and reasoning to a realm of practice. How would you apply ethics to your own area of nursing practice?

5. Consider a patient care situation where ethical principles seem to conflict with one another. How would you decide the right action(s) to take in providing ethical nursing care to the patient?

References

American Association of Colleges of Nursing. (1986). *Summary report: Generic baccalaureate nursing-data project.* Washington, DC: The Association.

American Association of Colleges of Nursing. (1988). *RN baccalaureate nursing education: Special report.* Washington, DC: The Association.

American Medical Association, Judicial Council. (1986). *Current opinions of the Council on Ethical and Judicial Affairs of the American Medical Association—1986: Including the principles of medical ethics and rules of the Council on Ethical and Judicial Affairs.* Chicago: American Medical Association.

American Nurses' Association. (1985). *Code for nurses with interpretive statements.* Kansas City, MO: The Association.

Aroskar, M.A. (1980). Anatomy of an ethical dilemma: The theory. *American Journal of Nursing, 80,* 658-660.

Beauchamp, T.L., & Childress, J.F. (1994). *Principles of biomedical ethics* (4th ed.). New York: Oxford University Press.

Benjamin, M., & Curtis, J. (1986). *Ethics in nursing* (2nd ed.). New York: Oxford University Press.

Benner, P., & Wrubel, J. (1989). *The primacy of caring.* Menlo Park, CA: Addison-Wesley.

Bergman, R. (1973). Ethics-concepts and practice. *International Nursing Review, 20,* 140-141.

Burnard, P., & Chapman, C.M. (1988). *Professional and ethical issues in nursing.* New York: John Wiley & Sons.

Callahan, D. (1983). On feeding the dying. *Hastings Center Report, 13*(5), 22.

Childress, J.F. (1982). *Paternalism in health care.* New York: Oxford University Press.

In re Conroy, No. A-108 (N.J. Sup. Ct. Jan. 17, 1985).

Crisham, P. (1981). Measuring moral judgment in nursing dilemmas. *Nursing Research, 30,* 104-110.

Cruzan v. Director, Missouri Department of Health, 110 S. Ct. 2841 (1990).

Curtin, L.A. (1978). A proposed model for critical ethical analysis. *Nursing Forum, 17,* 12-17.

Fleming, D., Scanlon, D., & D'Agostino, N.S. (1987). A study of the comfort needs of patients with advanced cancer. *Cancer Nursing 10*(5), 237-243.

Forrest, D. (1989). The experience of caring. *Journal of Advanced Nursing, 14*(10), 815-823.

Frankena, W. (1973). *Ethics* (2nd ed.). Englewood Cliffs, NJ: Prentice Hall.

Fry, S.T. (1986). Ethical inquiry in nursing: The definition and methods of biomedical ethics. *Perioperative Nursing Quarterly, 2,* 1-8.

Fry, S.T. (1987a). Autonomy, advocacy, and accountability: Ethics at the bedside. In M.D. Fowler & J. Levine-Ariff (Eds.), *Ethics at the bedside* (pp. 39-49). Philadelphia: J.B. Lippincott.

Fry, S.T. (1987b). Research on ethics in nursing: The state of the art. *Nursing Outlook, 35*(5), 246.

Fry, S.T. (1988). New ANA Guidelines on withdrawing or withholding food and fluid from patients. *Nursing Outlook, 36*(3), 122-123, 148-150.

Fry, S.T. (1989a). Ethical decision making: 1. Selecting a framework. *Nursing Outlook, 37*(5), 248.

Fry, S.T. (1989b). The ethics of compromise. *Nursing Outlook, 37*(3), 56.

Fry, S.T. (1989c). Measurement of moral answerability in nursing practice. In C.F. Waltz & O.L. Strickland (Eds.), *Measurement of clinical and educational nursing outcomes* (Vol. 3, pp. 169-180).

Fry, S.T. (1989d). Toward a theory of nursing ethics. *Advances in Nursing Science, 11,* 9-22.

Fry, S.T. (1994). *Ethics in nursing practice: A guide to ethical decision making.* Geneva, Switzerland: International Council of Nurses.

Gamelspacher, G.P., et al. (1986). Perceptions of ethical problems by nurses and doctors. *Archives of Internal Medicine, 146,* 577-578.

Gilligan, C. (1982). *In a different voice: Psychological theory and women's development.* Cambridge, MA: Harvard University Press.

Gortner, S.R., et al. (1984). Appraisal of values in the choice of treatment. *Nursing Research, 33,* 319-324.

In re Hier, 464 N.E. 2d Series 959, Mass. App. 1984.

Jameton, A. (1984). *Nursing practice: The ethical issues.* Englewood Cliffs, NJ: Prentice Hall.

Ketefian, S. (1981a). Critical thinking, educational preparation, and development of moral judgment among selected groups of practicing nurses. *Nursing Research, 30,* 104-110.

Ketefian, S. (1981b). Moral reasoning and moral behavior among selected groups of practicing nurses. *Nursing Research, 30,* 171-176.

Kohlberg, L. (1981). *The philosophy of moral development: Essays on moral development* (Vol. 1). New York: Harper & Row.

Larson, P.J. (1986). Cancer nurses' perceptions of caring. *Cancer Nursing, 9*(2), 86-91.

Leininger, M.M. (1984). Care, the essence of nursing and health. In *Care: The essence of nursing and health* (pp. 3-15). Detroit: Wayne State University Press.

Lewandowski, W., Daly, B., McClish, D.K., Juknialis, B.W., & Youngner, S.J. (1985). Treatment and care of "do not resuscitate" patients in a medical intensive care unit. *Heart and Lung, 14*(2), 175-181.

Lynn, J., & Childress, J.F. (1983). Must patients always be given food and water? *The Hastings Center Report, 13*(5), 17-21.

Mayer, D.K. (1987). Oncology nurses' versus cancer patients' perceptions of nurse caring behaviors: A replication study. *Oncology Nursing Forum, 14*(3), 48-52.

Mezey, M., Evans, L.K., Golub, Z.D., Murphy, E., & White, G.B. (1994). The Patient Self-Determination Act: Sources of concern for nurses. *Nursing Outlook, 42*(1), 30-38.

Munhall, P. (1980). Moral reasoning levels of nursing students and faculty in a baccalaureate nursing program. *Image: Journal of Nursing Scholarship, 12,* 57-61.

Murphy, C.P. (1976). *Levels of moral reasoning in selected groups of nursing practitioners.* Unpublished doctoral dissertation, Teachers College, Columbia University, New York.

Murphy, M.A. & Murphy, J. (1976). Making ethical decisions systematically. *Nursing 76, 6*(5), CG 13-14.

Noddings, N. (1984). *Caring: A feminine approach to ethics and moral education.* Berkeley, CA: University of California Press.

Nutting, A., & Dock, L.L. (1907). *A history of nursing* (Vol. 2). New York: G.P. Putnam's Sons.

Omery, A. (1989). Values, moral reasoning, and ethics. *Nursing Clinics of North America, 24*(2), 488-508.

Paris, J.J., & Fletcher, A.B. (1983). Infant Doe regulations and the absolute requirement to use nourishment and fluids for the dying infant. *Law, Medicine, and Health Care, 11*(5), 210-213.

Pellegrino, E. (1985). The caring ethic: The relation of physician to patient. In A.H. Bishop & J.R. Scudder (Eds.), *Caring, curing, coping: Nurse, physician, patient relationships* (pp. 8-30). Birmingham, AL: University of Alabama Press.

Prescott, P.A., Dennis, K.E., & Jacox, A.K. (1987). Clinical decision making of staff nurses. *Image: Journal of Nursing Scholarship, 19,* 56-62.

Robb, I.H. (1921). *Nursing ethics: For hospital and private use.* Cleveland: E.C. Loeckert.

Rokeach, M. (1968). *Beliefs, attitudes, and values.* San Francisco: Jossey-Bass.

Ross, W.D. (1939). *The right and the good.* London: Oxford University Press.

Self, D.J. (1979). Philosophical foundations of various approaches to medical ethical decision making. *Journal of Medicine & Philosophy, 4,* 20-31.

Self, D.J. (1987). A study of the foundations of ethical decision making of nurses. *Theoretical Medicine, 8,* 86-95.

Shelly, J.A. (1980). *Dilemma: A nurse's guide for making ethical decisions.* Downer's Grove, IL: Intervarsity Press.

Silverman, H.J., Fry, S.T., & Armistead, N. (1994). Nurses' perspectives on implementation of the Patient Self-Determination Act. *Journal of Clinical Ethics, 5*(1), 30-37.

Stanley, Sr. T. (1980). Ethics as a component of the curriculum. *Nursing and Health Care, 1,* 63-72.

Tittle, M.B., Moody, L., & Becker, M.P. (1991). Preliminary development of two predictive models for DNR patients in intensive care. *Image: Journal of Nursing Scholarship, 23*(3), 140-144.

Vaughan, R.H. (1935). *The actual incidence of moral problems in nursing: A preliminary study in empirical ethics.* Unpublished dissertation, Catholic University of America, Washington, D.C.

Veatch, R.M. (1978). Truth-telling attitudes. In W.T. Reich (Ed.), *Encyclopedia of bioethics* (Vol. 4, pp. 1677-1682). New York: The Free Press.

Veatch, R.M., & Fry, S.T. (1987). *Case studies in nursing ethics.* Philadelphia: J.B. Lippincott.

Social and Cultural Dimensions of Health and Health Care

13

Kathryn Hopkins Kavanagh

 Objectives

At the completion of this chapter, the reader will be able to:

- Understand ways in which cultural and lifestyle differences between nurses and clients affect nursing care.

- Describe influences of cultural values and social norms on health, health care, and nursing.

- Discuss how a balance of sensitivity, knowledge, and skills allows nurses to manage diversity effectively.

- Identify strategies for culturally acceptable nursing assessment, communication, and intervention.

Profile in Practice

Sandra Tyler, MS, MAA, RN
Part-Time Instructor,
School of Nursing, University of Maryland,
Baltimore, Maryland

I first became interested in learning about cultural differences and how they affect patient care when I was working with an oncologist in Washington, D.C., and we had patients from all over the world and from many different cultures in the United States. I could see that people reacted very differently to their diagnoses, treatment alternatives, and side effects of the chemotherapy. There were, however, patterns to their different reactions that reflected their cultural differences, and I became interested in finding out what those differences were all about. I started out by just sitting down with patients and getting them to talk. I became further involved by spending time in South America, India, and New Zealand. I also went back to school for a second masters degree in applied an-

---

thropology to learn more about how people in different cultures respond to health and illness.

One of the biggest problems that I have observed in terms of patients from different cultures is that often the health care system expects them to come for care bringing their own interpreter. Often, the interpreter ends up being a school-age child in the family who has the best English skills. This frequently means that the child misses school. Of even more concern is that this is a very great responsibility for the child, who is asked to correctly interpret very intimate problems or very serious problems for an adult family member.

One of the greatest challenges I have found in trying to teach students how to be more sensitive about cultural differences is that they frequently become overwhelmed. They think that they must know all the nuances of each culture or have a degree in anthropology as I do. I try to tell them to just relax and use their strong nursing skills of listening and observation. If they think that for some reason they are not communicating with the person, they should just sit down and discuss it. Most people are pleased that someone in the health care system is interested in learning about them, and they are pleased when you don't make assumptions. They are happy to tell you about themselves.

Nurses are increasingly being challenged to provide care to individuals and groups of people with diverse backgrounds, values, and expectations. This requires great flexibility on the part of the nurse because there is no single way to provide such care. Expectations vary widely with the many standards people have for what constitutes "care" and "caring," how those are perceived and recognized, and how quality of care is evaluated. Nurses must be innovative to provide care that is recognized for its quality and is acceptable to members of diverse groups. This chapter is devoted to facilitating development of the sensitivity, knowledge, and skills that are essential to providing high-quality nursing care in a diverse and multicultural society.

VISITING: A CASE STUDY

When Ellen began her clinical rotation on a large Indian reservation, her thinking revolved around what she could teach the community workers there. She spent days traveling many miles with various community health representatives (CHRs). These were Indian men and women who had about 1 month's training (sometimes in addition to other training and student experiences). They then assumed roles as providers, visiting homes of other Indians, doing routine and basic care, and acting as liaisons between the Indian population and the biomedical system. Slowly Ellen realized how Lakota culture shaped the Indians' perceptions of health, illness, and their expectations for treatment and care. As the weeks went on and Ellen learned to be open to new ways of knowing and doing things, her interpretations changed, as her journal entries indicate:

Week 1. "The CHRs don't really do anything. They just go and drink coffee and sit down and visit."

Week 2. "I think they just visit because they don't know what else to do. They even talk about themselves there. And they are all quiet a lot. Sometimes they hardly talk about the patient's problem."

Week 3. "You know, something happens when the CHRs visit, but I don't know what it is. I don't see how their visiting works, but I see that the people appreciate it."

Week 4. "The patients do what the CHRs want them to do. Something goes on, but I don't get it—they never actually tell the patients what to do."

Week 5. "I still don't see how the visiting works when the CHRs don't do much instruction. They do other things—wash the quadriplegic man's long hair, dress decubiti, weigh babies, but mostly they visit. Somehow it works."

Week 6. "I've got it. Visiting is what the CHRs do. It is what is important and how they intervene. It is because of the visiting that the patients respond, not because of what the CHRs do when they visit."

As Ellen became more observant and sensitive to Lakota culture, and more knowledgeable about it, she began to understand how members of that society perceived the situation. When she no longer tried to fit what they did and valued into her non-Indian frame of reference, she became open to knowing that visiting was the expected intervention, as well as the socially acceptable medium for more active intervention. As with many other groups, being together was not the means to an end, as visiting usually is in the Euro-American biomedical culture, but an end in itself. Ellen's new knowledge allowed her to build on Lakota ways to provide culturally appropriate nursing care.

DIVERSITY AND HEALTH

Health and health care are influenced by *culture,* with its shared values and beliefs, and *society,* with its behavioral expectations referred to as social norms. The theme of this chapter is diversity and its impact on nursing. *Diversity* is not defined here as ethnicity, with which it is commonly associated. Rather, it is defined as differences that may be rooted in age, culture, health status, experience, gender, sexual orientation, racial or ethnic identity, or other aspects of sociocultural description and socioeconomic position (Kavanagh & Kennedy, 1992).

Effective interventions are founded in informed decisions, not chance happenings. In the management of diversity, *manage* is defined, not as manipulation to get compliance, but as affirmation and encouragement focused on development of full potential (Thomas, 1990). In assisting people with personal concerns and losses, nurses encounter patterns of similarities and differences that shape client care needs. Providing culturally appropriate care involves learning to balance sensitivity, knowledge, and skills to respectfully accommodate social and cultural, as well as biological, psychological, and spiritual needs.

Why should nurses be concerned about diversity? Because groups and individuals interpret the world in ways that reflect how they view the world (i.e., from their perspectives and in the context of their own experience). What is considered normal or abnormal, caring or noncaring, appropriate or a waste of time, or even offensive, depends on context. Health and illness are perceived in diverse ways, and there are many different expectations for appropriate care and treatment. Cultural values and social norms are major influences, and these often come from groups other than the Euro-American one most prevalent in nursing and health care in the United States.

The model of transcultural nursing (Fig. 13-1) relates the commonalities and differences among cultural worldviews that reflect various aspects of society to the diverse health systems (Leininger, 1991). This depiction of the many interrelated dimensions of culture and care is helpful for exploring important meanings and patterns of care. When working with clients who have cultural orientations that are different, in minor or major ways, from those of the nurse, these considerations are particularly significant.

VALUES THAT SHAPE NURSING AND AMERICAN CULTURE

Nursing as a discipline reflects the generalized values of society, which in the United States is predominantly Eurocentric, middle class, Christian, and androcentric in view. Over time, American culture has generated social expectations that tend to minimize recognition of differences in both opportunity and experience. The American culture values personal freedom, independence, and individual achievement over the common good. The notion that everyone should be treated exactly the same is idealized. These themes fit well with the American values of action, productivity, materialism and consumerism, competition, and time as money (DeVita & Armstrong, 1993; Stewart & Bennett, 1991). In combination, these predilections lead to routinizing health care for efficiency, resulting in a "one size fits all" model of treatment and care. Americans typically assume that problems can be fixed and should (and can) be done so economically and quickly.

Presumptions inherent in the American culture typically flow from this set of values. For example, it is presumed that each individual should be in control of his or her own destiny. Another presumption is that one's efforts should be rewarded, and if they are not rewarded, the efforts must not have been good enough. A further presumption is that people have the right and ability to control as much of nature as possible (in contrast to living in harmony with it and/or being controlled by it in a fatalistic manner). Progress is defined in terms of technology and the future. Regarding health care, the presumption is that health care providers know more about clients' needs than clients do, although we are learning to listen to clients' desires and goals, and to recognize their beliefs, practices, and worldviews as resources. Because these ideals drive American society, they strongly influence its medical and health care systems. Yet values are merely abstract preferences, beliefs, and ideals that are inherently neither good nor bad. However, they should not be left unexamined or taken for granted because they strongly influence everyday life.

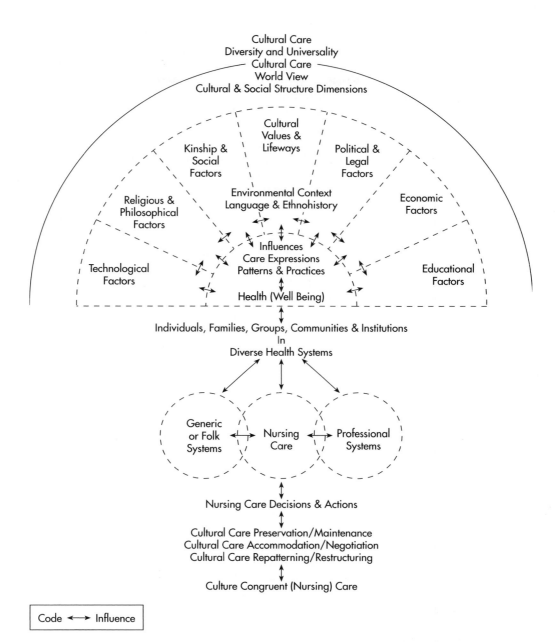

Fig. 13-1　Leininger's model of transcultural nursing. (Redrawn from Leininger M. [1991]. *Culture care diversity and universality: A theory of nursing.* New York: National League for Nursing.)

Critical Examination of Values

With nursing education comes an often unarticulated set of values and norms that must be made explicit and examined if nurses are to become competent managers of diversity. Values require serious critique, not only because they strongly and subtly influence how society operates, but also because they empower better and informed decisions about what aspects of society to accept, reject, ignore, or work to change. Some choices are in order. Nurses are in a situation in which a relatively firm and historically successful (at least from some points of view) set of values is reflected throughout health care and in nursing. However, both humanity and the interactive rules are changing, and some of the values that predominate in society today do not fit well with the high-quality care that nurses strive to provide.

Much of the public is willing to accept the rules and directives of health care providers and facilities. The medicalization of American society reflects its commitment to, and investment in, a nearly singular model of medical care. Even when consumers are told that they have rights and are expected to be involved in decision making about their own treatment and care (goals that are influenced by the values of individualism and independence), professional providers often continue to control the situation. However, today's consumer population is far more demographically and attitudinally diverse than it was in the past. Health care and nursing, reflecting society at large, are pressed to accommodate diverse values and beliefs. At present, health care is an aggregate of institutions built on a value system too inflexible to reflect its consumers' diverse needs.

VALUES THAT SHAPE WORLDVIEWS IN GENERAL

Despite the vast variability found among humans and within and between groups, we are all more alike than we are different. Every group and every individual must manage the same basic requirements of living to survive and to thrive. It is often helpful to visualize the basic, universal categories of values on a continuum. Ask yourself where you would place yourself along the continua of cultural values (Fig. 13-2) and how others' worldviews might differ from yours. Categories of values include orientations toward nature (including the supernatural), time, activity, relationships with other people, and the nature of humankind (Kluckhohn, 1971). Because worldviews and value orientations are often taken for granted, they may be difficult to discern. The more you get to know yourself, your colleagues, and your clients, the more effective you will be at accurately recognizing your own and others' perspectives and their influence on relationships.

Health care professionals are increasingly aware of a need to consider their clients' views of the world. However, they may not be aware of the ways in which values influence the discipline of nursing, the expectations that common nursing practices communicate to others, or the influence of values in the formation of goals and priorities. The following example illustrates how values can influence clinical practice.

ORIENTATIONS TOWARD PERSON/NATURE RELATIONSHIPS

| External forces control life (fate) | Living in harmony with nature | Mastery over nature |

PREDOMINANT ORIENTATIONS TOWARD TIME

| Past | Present and immediate issues and concerns | Future |

PREDOMINANT ORIENTATIONS TOWARD ACTIVITY

| Being is enough | Individuals must develop themselves | Efforts to develop will be rewarded |

PREDOMINANT ORIENTATIONS TOWARD SOCIAL RELATIONS

| There are leaders, and there are followers | Ask others how to solve problems | All have equal rights and control |

| Dependence is okay | Interdependence is valued | Independence is best |

THE NATURE OF HUMANKIND

| People are basically good and can be trusted | | People are basically evil and can't be trusted |

Fig. 13-2 Continua of cultural values. Ask yourself: "Where is _____ on each continuum? Where am I?"

"YAVIS" and "QUOIDS"

Research going back to the 1960s indicates that even when the intent is to treat people fairly, implicit values may result in quite different outcomes. Members of some groups receive better care than others. Some people get less positive attention, have fewer choices and more pressure to conform to others' standards, or receive less vigorous treatment. Clients who exemplify the predominant values (reflected by the acronym "YAVIS") often get more and quicker attention and better treatment than those clients characterized by the acronym "QUOIDS" (Kavanagh & Kennedy, 1992; Pedersen, 1988). The YAVIS are *Y*oung, *A*ttractive, *V*erbal, *I*ntelligent, and *S*uccessful (or at least potentially successful)—all traits that are highly valued in European-American culture. In contrast, QUOIDS might be *Q*uiet, *U*gly, *O*ld, *I*ndigent (poor), *D*issimilar (in lifestyle, language, or culture), or suspected of being *S*tupid. None of these characteristics bodes well in a youth-oriented, affluent, highly educated, technologically dependent, industrialized, and information-oriented society. Although someone carefully observing interactions in health care settings might quickly discern preferential patterns involving YAVIS and QUOIDS characteristics, those who work there are often oblivious to the biases that result when strong cultural values are not critically examined.

Nursing's Challenge

Decades ago, nursing moved beyond an emphasis on physical care into consideration of psychological factors. This shift provided a more comprehensive picture of the complex social realities experienced by people but still limited the focus of attention to individuals. Meanwhile, the presumption that one type of care fits everyone's needs, linked with a conviction that professionals' views are more valuable than clients' views, ignored the multifaceted contexts of actual experience. Despite empathy for its client populations, nursing's progress toward diversity management has focused on increasing tolerance rather than on appreciation and utilization of diversity.

Contemporary American society is a composite of disparate populations. Nursing is in the position of providing care to diverse groups with diverse expectations, problems, and goals. Quite often, nursing's clients are people who are generally underserved. Today's nurses attend to both population-based and individual patterns and needs. In so doing, they realize that respectful encounter with topics such as race, ethnicity, religion, politics, and belief systems outside of biomedicine is essential to providing acceptable and effective care. Being blind to the impact that those aspects of life have on actual experience creates obstacles to effective health care. On the other hand, integrating them into nursing care can result in high-quality and acceptable care that is rewarding to clients and nurses alike.

Even as nurses embrace both individuals and populations (Butterfield, 1990) and engage in more sincerely holistic and negotiated models of care that include intuitive subjective aspects of clients' realities (Kenney, 1995), those transformations occur more slowly than changes in society. However, the major concern is not catching up with increasing diversification. Rather, it is that nurses become competent and confident managers of diversity.

Relatively few nurses are prepared in nursing school to manage diversity effectively. The risk is that stereotypes, which by definition are incomplete and inflexible, may be reinforced. Another barrier to confronting diversity in nursing practice is the failure to critically examine the distribution of power. The discipline of nursing is remarkably ambivalent in its response to hierarchy. Nursing and nurses must scrutinize their attitudes toward strategies that promote true collaboration and participation in education, research, and practice. Sooner or later, nurses must learn to manage diversity humanely and effectively. The alternative is to be forced to change on others' terms.

Whether nursing acts or reacts, the trends are clear. The U.S. society continues to diversify rapidly while the world becomes symbolically smaller. Increasingly, it is acknowledged that members of diverse groups have the right to their own lifestyles, values, and norms, including expectations for culture-specific care. In nursing, the ability to communicate and work interculturally and to understand culture-based care and caring practices is viewed as essential to providing high-quality, effective, and acceptable illness-alleviating and/or health-promoting care (Leininger, 1985, 1991).

Protecting Against Bias

There are more than 3000 cultural groups, each of which interprets the world, including health and illness, somewhat differently. Combined with innumerable individual interpretations and experiences, it is obvious that no one can know everything about diversity. There are no reliable "how-to" manuals for nursing in a diverse society. It takes flexibility, willingness to learn, and ability to explore and understand multiple perspectives for nurses to provide acceptable care across significant cultural differences. To manage diversity well, nurses must be sensitive to both differences and commonalities, knowledgeable about expectable patterns of belief and behavior, and skillful at integrating their sensitivity and knowledge into appropriate assessment, communication, and intervention modalities. However, information about expectable patterns of behavior and their interpretation must always be tested against an individual's perception of a specific situation.

It is natural to have *biases* (i.e., to prefer some ideas, things, or behaviors and to find others less appealing). It is important to identify our biases, or they can distort the interpretation of the world around us. *Objectivity* does not imply a lack of bias; rather, it is the ability to avoid distortion of facts by personal or other preferences. Natural biases become negative when they are allowed to misrepresent and distort facts. People tend to see what they expect to see, and stereotypes hamper interpretation by supplying built-in blind spots. Communication ideally facilitates open, nonprejudicial relationships that can maximize understanding of clients' views and resources. A flowchart illustrating the outcomes of open and closed information processing is presented in Fig. 13-3.

Society and Resources

American society does not always manage diversity well. Many people shy away from issues involving race, sex, or other aspects of life that, although important in everyday life, may be considered too personally or politically sensitive to discuss. Despite the United States' image as a land of opportunity where effort is correlated with accomplishment and many people "get ahead" (although not always equitably so), society is stratified. Resources are distributed through patterned social processes involving numerous interrelated factors. Among others, these factors include sex, education, in-

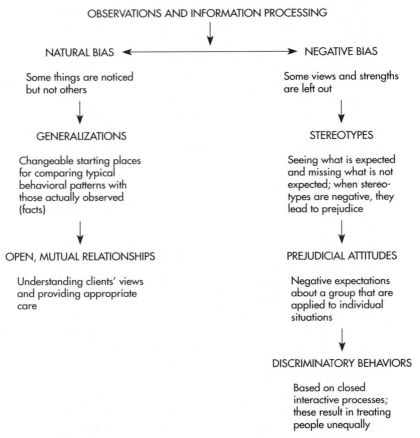

Fig. 13-3   Open versus closed information processing.

come, occupation, religion, material possessions, health status, appearance, race, ethnicity, family name, residence, family composition, and landedness. The extent of influence of a given factor differs with time and circumstance. Despite civil rights to protect against discrimination, different opportunities are likely to be experienced by certain individuals and groups. Some examples are a single-parent versus a two-parent family, a wheelchair-bound worker versus his or her able-bodied peer, and a taxpayer who rents a home versus another who lives with a mortgage but, by "owning" property, qualifies for a more favorable tax return.

Social categories exist because some social criteria are weighted as more valuable than others. Classifying social worth is so much a part of everyday social life that it is often taken for granted. However, the outcome of social stratification is social inequality, which implies unequal life chances and opportunities. The long-term result of unexamined social processes may be unequal opportunity to achieve the basic resources of status, power, and wealth. In contrast to a middle-class individual with adequate health insurance, for example, an economically disadvantaged or socially disenfranchised person may not receive attention for a health problem until it seriously impedes his or her ability to function productively in society.

In the United States, the only industrialized country except South Africa without a national health care system, there is limited societal pressure to provide equitable care for all. Significant variation in mortality and morbidity rates is one outcome of unequal distribution of health care. American infant mortality rates are higher than those of most other industrialized countries and are particularly high among poor and nonwhite groups (Boone, 1989). Similarly, rates of premature deaths among nonwhite males below age 65 greatly exceed mortality rates for white males. These statistics exemplify the costs of limited access to health care for large underserved populations.

The "ISMs"

Several interaction patterns that are grounded in bias, prejudicial in attitude, and discriminatory in their behavioral expression have acquired the label "ISM" because of their common word endings (see box on p. 296). Each *ISM* involves a tendency to judge others according to their match or lack of fit with a standard that is considered ideal or presumed to be "normal." Whatever the issue or level (personal or group), an *ISM* is centered on one's own judgment (Brislin, 1993). The three most powerful *ISMs* in America are racism, sexism, and classism.

Racial and ethnic diversity. When America was originally envisioned as a cultural "melting pot," nearly all of its immigrants came from northern Europe, and most had Protestant origins. When members of culturally and racially different groups began to arrive in sizable numbers, the merged population experienced some painful, unassimilated lumps. The melting pot idea worked well only for those groups that would and could assume the values of the predominant population.

People did not blend in if they resisted giving up cultural values and traditions (i.e., they chose to keep their ethnic identities) or if they were physically "different." Race in American society has perpetuated a system of stratification based on skin color, hair texture, and other biological differences presumed to be significant. Many ethnic groups moved, with time, toward acculturation and assimilation. A few, such as the Amish and Hutterites, steadfastly maintained their specific cultures. People of color, however, experienced systematic barriers to "melting in," even if motivated to do so.

Advances in the physical and social sciences long ago redefined race as a social, rather than a biological, phenomenon, which left racist themes of inherent superiority and inferiority untenable. If the earth's more than 5.5 billion inhabitants were mustered somehow into a single line, starting with the darkest skinned on one end and ending with the lightest skinned on the other, that vast multitude could not be sorted reliably into races. Some are light and some are dark, but the great majority are every shade of brown. Skin color does not occur in discrete categories and surely cannot be used to predict ability.

Although ethnicity is a more viable tool than race for examination of similarities and differences, the United States remains a society in which one's race influences ev-

The "ISMs"

Egocentrism The assumption that oneself is superior to others. This occurs when someone who has never been diagnosed as mentally ill (a staff member, for instance) thinks he or she is better than those who are diagnosed as ill.

Ethnocentrism The assumption that one's own cultural or ethnic group is superior to that of others. (*Ethnicity* refers to cultural differences rather than race.) Ethnocentrism occurs, for example, when everyone is expected to speak English and to know the rules, many of which are implicit, for living in this society.

Sociocentrism The assumption that one society's way of knowing or doing is superior to the ways of other societies. It may be assumed, for instance, that biomedicine is effective and folk medicines are not. Actually, there is strong evidence that this is not always the case. Many traditional societies have highly effective, community-oriented forms of treatment.

Racism The assumption that members of one race are superior to those of another. (Race refers to presumed biological differences.)

Sexism The assumption that members of one sex are superior to those of the other. For example, women have historically been viewed as being less rational and more emotional than men.

Heterosexism The assumption that everyone is, or should be, heterosexual and that heterosexuality is superior and expectable. It is relatively recent that homosexuality was redefined as a lifestyle rather than a disease.

Ageism The assumption that members of one age group are superior to those of others. Young patients and staff may not be taken as seriously as those who are older, whereas in other circumstances, older persons may be discredited in favor of those who are younger.

Adultism The assumption that adults are superior to youths and can or should control, direct, reprimand, and reward them or deprive them of respect. Children in American society are often interrupted or ignored by adults. They may not be given choices that allow them to feel they have some control over a situation.

Sizism The assumption that people of one body size are superior to or better than those of other shapes and sizes. Positions involving interaction with the public, for example, may be denied to individuals who are very heavy or who otherwise fail to meet the standards of ideal appearance.

Classism/elitism The assumption that certain people are superior because of their social and economic status or position in a group or organization. This often assumes that those with more money or education are superior. A poorly dressed high school dropout, for example, may not be given the same treatment options offered to a well-dressed college graduate.

Ableism The assumption that the able-bodied and sound of mind are physically or developmentally superior to those who are disabled, retarded, or otherwise different. An example of ableism is not offering a chronically ill patient choices because of the assumption that he or she does not want to, or cannot, make decisions.

eryday social experience. Nursing is strongly criticized for avoiding real confrontation with racism (Barbee, 1993; Jackson, 1993), and race is one of the major issues to be dealt with if nurses are to manage diversity effectively. As with other *ISMs,* failure to address the issue leaves important dimensions of health and health care unrecognized and potential resources unused.

Sex and gender diversity. Sexism is one of the most obvious *ISMs,* and one directly pertinent to nurses, whether male or female. As with other *ISMs,* problems involving sexism cannot be completely resolved within the context of the health care system alone, for they reflect processes that permeate all of society. However, it is important to be aware of gender differences in opportunities to acquire status, power, and wealth. Similarly, it is important to be aware of the influence of those differences on health, access to health care, and adequacy of care, as well as on opportunities for professional career development in nursing.

In the United States, women earn significantly less money than men do for the same work and with the same level of preparation for that work. Single parents are typically women, a fact that reflects differences in gender-based rights and responsibilities, and their presence on the welfare rolls has greatly expanded. As more women assume roles as heads of households, bias toward the worth of women and their work is increasingly becoming apparent in undervalued, largely female occupations, such as nursing.

Manipulation of women's roles in society has not left men unaffected. As industrialization moved the locus of economic earning away from homes and farms and into factories and offices, men were removed from traditional familial involvement. While women, like children, were viewed as needing control and protection, Western men were deprived of equitable companionship and forced to assume stereotypically paternalistic roles. Characteristically stressed by expectations of achievement in the marketplace and estranged from emotional involvement at home, male roles only now are returning comfortably to the family. Society remains a long way from androgynous interchangeability of roles, however, as is illustrated by the relatively small proportion of men in nursing, although nurses comprise an otherwise educationally, ethnically, and experientially heterogeneous group. It should be kept in mind that sexism and gender issues are not limited to heterosexual populations. Advocacy of gay and lesbian providers and clients also requires sensitivity to, and knowledge of, social processes that are often overlooked by those unaware of their impact.

Classism. *Class* is defined as the ability to muster economic resources. It does not imply specific preferences, behaviors, or lifeways. Elitist attitudes often lead to assumptions that certain people are superior or inferior because of their social or economic status. The client who is poorly dressed, uses poor grammar, or otherwise "looks low class" may not be given the same treatment options offered to others whose appearance or behavior gives the impression of greater fiscal assets.

Class is related to health and health care in several ways. Universally, the greatest threat to positive health status is poverty. In the United States, although specific ethnic and racial groups are often stereotyped as having more or fewer health problems, it is really differences in socioeconomic status that are directly associated with health status (Centers for Disease Control, 1993). Race and ethnicity became confounded with class because of long-term inequality in the distribution of educational and occupational opportunities. Today there are significant class differences within racial and ethnic categories, and there is definite ethnic and racial variation within each socioeconomic class. The important points are to avoid stereotypic associations across categories and to recognize the impact that poverty has on access to, and eligibility for, care, priorities and coping patterns, relationships with health care providers, and overall health status. For example, people who live "hand to mouth" must be oriented toward present concerns and may not prioritize health practices that tend to pay off only in the future—such as immunizations, dietary restrictions, or even disease prevention strategies such as those associated with reducing risk for HIV infection.

Costs of Inequality

The desire to avoid confronting difficult issues often results in "colorblindness," "genderblindness," and similar phenomena. By pretending that everything is the same for everyone, societal patterns of differential treatment based on race or gender go unrecognized and are perpetuated. They are nonproductive because they deny variations in life experience that are both real and meaningful. It is painful to not have important characteristics recognized and acknowledged.

Overlooking or ignoring differences implies that specific experiences of individuals and groups are not important and that change is not necessary. Since many aspects of racism, sexism, and other systems of unequal opportunity (all those other *ISMs*) are institutionalized in the social system, failure to recognize and change them perpetuates, as well as condones, them. Effective and acceptable health care involves critical thinking and problem solving on all levels. Understanding social processes that underlie the perpetuation of social inequality empowers change by providers, as well as consumers, of health care.

EVER-CHANGING, DIVERSIFYING SOCIETY

The challenge of providing appropriate care becomes more manageable as we learn more about it and more demanding as society continues to change. According to Census Bureau projections, before the middle of the next century the average U.S. resident will neither trace his or her heritage to Europe nor be what is commonly referred to as "white" (Henry, 1990). However, societal and cultural change does not occur readily or easily. It is predicted that the nation's crisis of values and ethics will deepen and racial and cultural tension will mount in response to pressures of intensified diversity. Creating and maintaining a sense of community will become more challenging (Hechenberger, 1994). While some people find these projections threatening and others find them hopeful, nursing at times seems to be stuck between fight and flight in dealing with such change.

Every nurse has encountered clients who seemed steadfastly resistant to every professional ministration. Some health care providers, in their belief that they know what is best for clients, label a client's failure to respond as "noncompliance." This biased label deserves a closer look. In the beginning of this century, pressure to move toward the dominant value system was the norm; indeed, it was how one became "Americanized." Authority was granted to those in charge to control the attitudes and behaviors, as much as possible, of those who chose or were forced to use the institution's services. Other perspectives, including the client's, were rendered marginal, trivialized, or even overtly discredited. Times have changed. As the century closes, it is no longer acceptable to demand conformity to a single set of values and norms. Great social variation persists despite a homogenized culture that permeates nearly every household with standardized versions of fast foods, media event analysis, and consumer expectations. There is no longer a clear distinction between members of a provider group who set the goals and rules, and clients who must deny their own preferences to comply with the controlling group's expectations. As a society, we are moving toward a truer participatory democracy. In client care, democratic participation goes beyond a patient's bill of rights posted on the wall and soon forgotten.

Ways of Understanding: Explanatory Models

Since health, illness, and death are part of life, all people have conscious health-related needs. Knowledge about health and health care is not limited to professionals or professional ways of knowing. Every cultural group has at least one system of beliefs, diagnosis, treatment, and care to maximize control over distressing and life-threatening phenomena. How illness is defined, ideas about what caused it, and what is to be done about symptoms (when and by whom) are important concerns in every cultural system.

Explanatory models are the sets of explanations used to put ideas about the meaning, cause, process, and treatment of illness into familiar, workable frameworks (Kleinman, 1988). These models are used to understand health, health care, and illness within the context of complex cultural phenomena, including religion, economic situation, education, language, family and social organization, interaction patterns, ethnic orientation, and general perceptions of the world and self.

Biomedicine tends to view health problems as the consequence of trouble within the client or as resulting from interaction between the client and the natural world with its pathogens, environmental risks, and stressors. Members of social and cultural groups that do not use science as the basic explanation for everything often base their explanatory models within society (e.g., illness resulting from disharmonious social relations) or in supernatural belief systems (e.g., viewing disease as a punishment for sin or breaking a taboo).

Westernized definitions of health and illness are vague. There are numerous definitions of health, whereas illness is the culturally influenced individual experience of sickness. Biomedical science, in contrast, defines disease in objective terms of deviance from clinical norms or as the result of environmental insult. Mental health and mental illnesses are more difficult to delineate than physical status because of a lack of readily observable, discrete, and organic evidence. The result is reliance on assessment of behaviors rather than on definitive symptomatology. Diagnoses involve extent of social competence, which, to be valid, must be assessed against culture-specific criteria.

To members of many societies, concepts such as mental health have little or no meaning. One is either ill or not, and that distinction is based on somatic criteria that either allow or impede the ability to perform one's normal roles in society. A diagnosis and prognosis based on unobservable phenomena (as opposed to that obtained from laboratory or diagnostic tests) may seem absurd, and only impaired function motivates health care attention. Despite the predominance of biomedicine in the United States, popular (over-the-counter) and folk systems also proliferate and are widely used. *Popular systems* of health-related knowledge and resources are available through drug and health stores, in all forms of the media, and through information passed among personal acquaintances and networks. *Folk* or *ethnomedical systems* of beliefs and practices originate in traditional cultures and include healing rituals, herbal medicines, and systems of knowledge that reflect diverse cultural values and social norms. Within American society, professional biomedical systems, popular medicine (over-the-counter and nonprescription alternatives), and a variety of folk medical systems provide more varied services to consumers than many nurses imagine. Often more than one system is used at a time. Nurses can have powerful intermediary roles in negotiating the varied options.

Individual Versus Group Identity

One assumption often taken for granted in nursing is that nurses care for individuals. It is important to realize that members of many societies do not perceive themselves first as individuals but as members of groups (typically, extended families). As an Asian nursing student explained it, she (an individual in Western eyes) is in her view a "small *i*"; her family is the "large *I*." Decisions are made by groups or by heads of groups for the good of the group. Individuals are first part of the whole family, and only secondly are they autonomous and separate persons. Therefore, although care may be appropriately individualized for each client, nurses must become more comfortable with perceiving clients in collective terms. Orientation to common units that are more than aggregates of individuals is traditional in some cultures.

It is similarly risky to assume that love is the idealized primary emotion in a relationship. Many cultural groups place far more value on respect and honor. Nor should nurses assume that biological relationships or formal ties such as marriage are the most significant ones. The individual who culturally is expected to make decisions is often a dominant male, regardless of who in the group is considered the focus of care or treatment. For example, community health nurses who try to encourage mothers to have their children immunized may have little impact unless the heads of households or community leaders are convinced of the value of inoculations.

Care Barriers and Resources

There are numerous cultural and social phenomena that pose potential barriers in health care but also can serve as potential resources. Language, both verbal and nonverbal, is an obvious obstacle to, as well as a vehicle for, communication. Strong identities, such as with racial, ethnic, or gender groups, are reflected in attitudes, expectations, and practices related to health and care. Likewise, differences in ideas about relationships may encourage or discourage resource utilization (e.g., expectations of hierarchy or mutuality, independence or dependence, others who are perceived as different). Expectations of self-care or personal involvement in decision making may be perceived as an inappropriate imposition in some cultures. Many people view health professionals as experts who are expected to provide advice and direction. Furthermore, cultural expectations may be that illness results in a sick role that is characterized by dependence on others.

PROVIDING ACCEPTABLE AND CONGRUENT CARE

Given the diversity within society, its patterns of social interaction, and sundry cultural understandings of health and illness, it is not surprising that there is great variation in expectations for appropriate treatment and care. Overly simplified explanations of culture and health care can cause more problems than they solve. Nursing, like other health care disciplines, is learning to manage this diversity, which requires some substantive changes in care delivery systems.

To enhance health care, diversity must be understood in terms of the plasticity and flexibility of culture. This means avoiding stereotypes about people, being open to their many ways of understanding and adapting to the world, and allowing for a multidirectional flow of ideas. As barriers between health care professions are broken down, ideas also can flow creatively across disciplinary boundaries. Barriers between clients and care providers must also be broken down so that the sensitivity, knowledge, resources, and skills that *both* have can be incorporated into client care. In this multicultural view, boundaries are artificial and social identities are continuously renegotiated. Where cultures come together, there is creative ground (Kessler-Harris, 1992; Wali, 1992). Providers and clients can learn about and from each other and can negotiate appropriate goals, care strategies, and outcomes. The essential element is that respect be maintained by all involved so that mutual communication can be open to multiple perceptions.

Nursing's Unique Position

Nurses function as gatekeepers between clients and the health care system, and at times between clients' cultural backgrounds and American culture as it is reflected in health care. Nurses must therefore become comfortable with care meanings, patterns, and processes that allow flexibility in practice. Nursing has a unique opportunity to help other health care disciplines to negotiate their way in an ever-changing environment without a loss of collective identity and with a sense of the diversity that is inherently American. It takes a sense of the whole to appreciate the individual. Nursing's value of holism encourages awareness that each individual is like some others, like all others, and like no others. To be acceptable and appropriate, that individual's health care must follow the same pattern.

Culturally Congruent Care

Care is the central, dominant, and unifying feature of nursing (Leininger, 1991). Providing care that is comprehensive must take into account culture-based factors related to systems of values and norms, technology, religion and philosophy, kinship and social relations, politics and law, economy, and education (Leininger, 1991). Language and environmental contexts are threads throughout those systems and further influence care patterns and expressions of individuals, families, groups, and societies. Nurses providing culturally congruent and culture-specific nursing care can intervene by preserving, accommodating, or repatterning (Leininger, 1988).

There are many strengths associated with traditional and popular (i.e., nonprofessional) systems of knowledge, care, and treatment. They are familiar and understandable to the client. Moreover, they are usually readily accessible, inexpensive, and noninvasive. Many clients find traditional healing systems more humanistic than scientific medicine and more sensitive to, and compatible with, their quality of life. Many health practices are harmless, some are useless, and others are harmful. Providing culturally congruent care involves being open to exploring the client's beliefs and practices, recognizing and reinforcing those that are positive and promoting change only in those that are known to be harmful. *Cultural care preservation* serves to maintain a state of health, aid recovery from illness, or assist with the dying process through reinforcement of traditional cultural values and lifeways that provide familiar, available, and nonthreatening resources.

Culture care accommodation involves negotiation between professional and folk, biomedical, or nonscientific healing approaches. Rather than assuming that professional ways are better, interventions that are acceptable and relevant to clients can be negotiated using both the prescribed treatments of the biomedical system and the views and practices of the client's personal reference group. It is in this realm that most culturally acceptable nursing care takes place. For example, the nurse who wants to teach a special diet to a client can effectively do so by negotiating that diet within the client's normal framework of food practices, resources, and preferences.

Many cultural groups believe that all of life should be balanced: hot foods balanced with cold, hot illnesses treated with cold remedies, and so forth. This "hot-cold theory" does not relate to temperature but to meanings that are culturally ascribed to things and events. Dietary and treatment regimens can be "balanced" to fit the client's expectations, as well as the professional's. The only requirement is that the nurse inquire about the client's beliefs and practices, treat the information with respect, and take the time to negotiate mutually acceptable plans and goals.

Cultural care restructuring or repatterning is the category in which most nursing care traditionally occurs. As change agents, nurses often act as culture-bearers, frequently discrediting alternative ways of doing things without understanding them. Occasionally it is essential to repattern behavior, as in cases of abuse or neglect. However, clients are generally more likely to value and follow nursing care that fits their ways of thinking.

Communication

Communication is the core of much of nursing care. Clients always have a relationship with the problem as they see it, which may or may not be similar to professional assessment of the situation (Pedersen, 1988). Effective intervention requires the ability to understand the problem from both the insider's (client's) and the outsider's (nurse's) point of view. One must learn what the client views as the problem, who the client sees as being responsible for the problem, what the problem means to the client, and who the client thinks has control over the problem. It should be kept in mind that the influence of the nurse is less than the influence of the problem, unless the nurse's influence can be combined with that of the client to form a coalition. It is when the client and provider work together that they can problem solve (Pedersen, 1988; Pedersen et al., 1981).

As nurses move away from dependency on Eurocentric assumptions and references and become more sensitive to other ways of viewing the world, they become more comfortable learning about other explanatory models. Understanding various ways of thinking is important. Clients' beliefs about what causes problems are often directly related to what they view as solutions. A client who believes his illness resulted from a failure to pray or to go to church, for example, is likely to have little faith in medication as the resolution. Nurses interact well with clients and potential clients, so they are in an ideal position to explore over-the-counter and folk remedies that people use. When nurses work with a specific cultural group, it is useful to learn as much as possible about the folk illnesses and folk practices common to that group. While there is a large body of medical anthropological literature on such topics, the easiest way to access the information is to respectfully ask people about their beliefs and practices. When a sincere interest and nonjudgmental attitude accompany such questions, clients often openly share their perspectives. Recommended approaches for culturally appropriate care are presented in the box on p. 304.

Cultural Assessment Strategies

Cultural assessment in nursing involves systematic appraisal of values, beliefs, and practices to learn the context of client needs and to determine appropriate nursing interventions (Tripp-Reimer & Afifi, 1989). Such assessments are useful to identify general lifestyles and patterns that assist or interfere with nursing intervention or treatment regimens (Brink, 1984; Tripp-Reimer, Brink, & Saunders, 1984). There are several available assessment guides (e.g. Bloch, 1983), as well as guides for interviewing (Leininger, 1984; Kavanagh & Kennedy, 1992). Categories for a basic cultural assessment are presented in the box on p. 305.

All comprehensive assessment plans attend to value orientations, personal and family health histories, and social and cultural backgrounds. One cannot assume what beliefs, practices, or supports do or do not exist. Expected patterns must always be contrasted with actual, individual situations. It is often useful to explore local groups for information about an ethnic population in the area, and to solicit the assistance of the group leaders for problem solving and information about acceptable interventions when it does not involve disclosure of individual clients' circumstances.

In addition to cultural assessment, with its inclusive sociological and psychological dimensions, there must be consideration of biological and physiological norms for different groups. These include racial anatomical characteristics; growth and development patterns; variations in body systems; physiology of skin, hair, and mucous membranes; and diseases and illnesses common to the group.

•   •   •

Approaches Recommended for All Cultural Groups

- Provide a feeling of acceptance.
- Establish open communication.
- Present yourself with confidence. Introduce yourself. Shake hands if it is appropriate.
- Strive to gain your client's trust, but don't resent it if you don't get it.
- Understand what members of the cultural or subcultural group consider to be "caring," both attitudinally and behaviorally.
- Understand the relationship between your client and authority.
- Understand your client's desire to please you and his or her motivations to comply or not to comply.
- Anticipate diversity. Avoid stereotypes by sex, age, ethnicity, socioeconomic status, etc.
- Don't make assumptions about where people come from. Let them tell you.
- Understand the client's goals and expectations.
- Make your goals realistic.
- Emphasize positive points and strengths of health beliefs and practices.
- Show respect, especially for men, even if it is women or children you are interested in. Men are often decision makers about follow-up.
- Be prepared for the fact that children go everywhere with some cultural groups, as well as with poorer families, who may have few options. Include them.
- Know the traditional, health-related practices common to the group you are working with. Don't discredit them unless you *know* they are harmful.
- Know the folk illnesses and remedies common to the group you are working with.
- Try to make the clinic setting comfortable. Consider colors, music, atmosphere, scheduling expectations, pace, tone, seating arrangements, and so on.
- Whenever possible and appropriate, involve the leaders of the local group. Confidentiality is important, but the leaders know the problems and often can suggest acceptable interventions.
- Respect values, beliefs, rights, and practices. Some may conflict with your own or with your determination to make changes. But every group and individual wants respect above all else.
- Learn to appreciate the richness of diversity as an asset, rather than a hindrance, in your work.

Diversity is here to stay. Both clients and health care professionals, reflecting the mosaic of society, continue to become more diverse. Failure to recognize diversity can be painful when what people value is not respectfully acknowledged and they are forced to comply with values and norms that are not their own. Every client has a right to culturally congruent care. Nursing is in a unique position to use its assessment, communication, and intervention skills to help delineate care appropriate and acceptable to specific clients. Competent management of diversity empowers all involved to work toward development of full potential.

Categories for a Basic Cultural Assessment

- Ethnic origin, identity, affiliation, and values (ideas about health and illness, human nature, relationships between humankind and nature, time, activity, and interpersonal relationships); also relevant rites of passage, customs, art and symbols, and history
- Racial identity (Ask, do not assume.)
- Place of birth; relocation and migration history
- Habits, customs, and beliefs associated with health, disease, illness, health maintenance, illness prevention, and health promotion; explanatory models; connections between health and religion
- Cultural sanctions and restrictions (what behaviors are encouraged or discouraged)
- Language and communication processes (verbal and nonverbal patterns; eye contact; touching; use of, and toleration for, silence; tempo; styles of questioning and persuasion; styles of decision making)
- Gender rules
- Healing beliefs and practices (relationships with folk, popular, and professional health systems; symbolism related to health and illness; what behaviors are considered normal or abnormal; care associated with unusual or abnormal behavior; care associated with body fluids, body excretions, and body temperature; activities included in tending to one's body; substances and practices used in rituals; myths about health and taboos [substances and events to be avoided]; ideas and practices related to death, dying, and grief)
- Nutritional factors; food preferences, preparation, and consumption patterns (kinds of foods and amounts, schedules and rituals, eating environments, utensils and implements, taboos, changes with illness)
- Sleep routines, bedtime rituals, and environment (kinds of covering, sleepwear, comforting materials used, rules for sleeping and for awakening)
- Environmental resources and strains (the "fit" within the community)
- Economic status, resources, and living situation
- Educational history and background
- Occupational history and background
- Social network (types and amount of support available from family, other individuals and group resources; who and where kin and significant others are; what is expected and expectable of them; social interaction patterns)
- Self-identity/concept and sense of well-being
- Religious history, background, and beliefs
- Other spiritual beliefs and practices
- Usual response to stress and discomfort
- Meaning of care and caring (expectations, beliefs, and practices related to care; fit between nurse as provider and client as cultural seeker of health care, and between client and health system)

Key Points

- Cultural and social views of individuals and groups influence perceptions of health and health care.

- Diversity management uses affirmation and encouragement to move toward development of the client's full potential.

- Universal categories of values include orientation toward nature, time, activity, relationships with other people, and the nature of humankind.

- Open information processing can facilitate nurse-client relationships that maximize understanding of clients' views and resources.

- Nurses can protect against bias by recognizing and building on strengths found in diverse perspectives and experiences.

- Society has numerous built-in *ISMs* that result in social inequities.

- The three most powerful *ISMs* in America are racism, sexism, and classism.

- Explanatory models are used to understand health, health care, and illness within the context of complex cultural views and perceptions.

- Culturally congruent care must take into account culture-based factors related to systems of values and norms, technology, religion and philosophy, kinship and social relations, politics and law, economy, and education.

- Cultural assessment in nursing involves systematic appraisal of values, beliefs, and practices of the client.

- Nurses will either learn to manage diversity or be managed by it.

Critical Thinking Exercises

1. What benefits are derived from understanding how cultural and lifestyle differences between nurses and clients affect nursing care?

2. Formulate strategies that nurses can use to effectively manage the influences of cultural values and social norms on health, health care, and nursing.

3. How could a nurse develop a balance of sensitivity, knowledge, and skills necessary to manage diversity effectively?

4. Discuss the effect on the client and the nurse when the *nurse's* perspective dominates the setting of goals and priorities, planning and intervention strategies, and assessment and evaluation criteria.

5. Discuss the effect on the client and the nurse when the *client's* perspective is used as the basis for setting goals and priorities, planning and intervention strategies, and assessment and evaluation criteria.

6. Describe an example of an *ISM* that you have observed in your professional experience. What measures were taken to reduce the effects of this bias on the individuals or groups involved? What measures could have been taken that were not?

7. In your experience, what strategies work well for the practice of culturally acceptable nursing assessment, communication, and intervention?

References

Barbee, E.L. (1993). Racism in U.S. nursing. *Medical Anthropology Quarterly 7*(4), 346-362.

Bloch, B. (1983). Bloch's ethnic-cultural assessment guide. In M.S. Orque, B. Bloch, & L.S.A. Monrroy (Eds.), *Ethnic nursing care: A multicultural approach* (pp. 49-75), St. Louis: Mosby; reprinted in part in B. Kozier & G. Erb. (1988). *Concepts and issues in nursing practice* (pp. 376-379). Menlo Park, CA: Addison-Wesley.

Boone, M.S. (1989). *Capital crime: Black infant mortality in America.* Newbury Park, CA: Sage Publications.

Brink, P.J. (1984). Value orientations as an assessment tool in cultural diversity. *Nursing Research, 33*(4), 198-203.

Brislin, R. (1993). *Understanding culture's influence on behavior.* Fort Worth: Harcourt Brace College.

Butterfield, P.G. (1990). Thinking upstream: Nurturing a conceptual understanding of the societal context of health behavior. *Advances in Nursing Science, 12*(2), 1-8.

Centers for Disease Control. (1993). Use of race and ethnicity in public health surveillance. *Morbidity and Mortality Weekly Report, 42*(RR-10), 1-17.

DeVita, P.R., & Armstrong, J.D. (1993). *Distant mirrors: America as a foreign culture.* Belmont, CA: Wadsworth.

Hechenberger, N. (1994). Higher education: Organizational changes in structure and roles of faculty and administrators. *Strategies for graduate faculty: Internal demands vs. external realities.* Atlanta, GA: Southern Council on Collegiate Education for Nursing in Affiliation with the Southern Regional Education Board.

Henry, W.A. (1990, April 9). Beyond the melting pot. *Time,* pp. 28-31.

Jackson, E.M. (1993). Whiting-out difference: Why U.S. nursing research fails black families. *Medical Anthropology Quarterly, 7*(4), 363-385.

Kavanagh, K.H., & Kennedy, P.H. (1992). *Promoting cultural diversity: Strategies for health care professionals.* Beverly Hills, CA: Sage Publications.

Kenney, J.W. (1995). Relevance of theoretical approaches in nursing practice. In P.J. Christensen & J.W. Kenney (Eds.), *Nursing process: Applications of conceptual models* (4th ed., pp. 3-23). St. Louis: Mosby.

Kessler-Harris, A. (1992, October 21). Multiculturalism can strengthen, not undermine, a common culture. *Chronicle of Higher Education,* pp. B3, B7.

Kleinman, A. (1988). *Rethinking psychiatry: From cultural category to personal experience.* New York: Free Press.

Kluckhohn, F.R. (1971). Dominant and variant value orientations. In C. Kluckhohn & J.A. Murray (Eds.), *Personality in nature, society, and culture* (pp. 342-357). New York: Alfred A. Knopf.

Leininger, M. (1984). Transcultural interviewing and health assessment. In P. Pedersen, N. Sartorius, & A.J. Marsella (Eds.), *Mental health services: The cross-cultural context* (pp. 109-133). Beverly Hills, CA: Sage Publications.

Leininger, M. (1985). Transcultural caring: A different way to help people. In P. Pedersen (Ed.), *Handbook of cross-cultural counseling and therapy* (pp. 107-115). Westport, CT: Greenwood Press.

Leininger, M. (1988). Leininger's theory of nursing: Cultural care diversity and universality. *Nursing Science Quarterly, 1*(4), 152-160.

Leininger, M.M. (1991). The theory of culture care diversity and universality. In M.M. Leininger (Ed.), *Culture care diversity and universality: A theory of nursing* (NLN Publication No. 15-2402, pp. 5-68). New York: National League for Nursing.

Pedersen, P. (Ed.). (1988). The three stages of multicultural development: Awareness, knowledge, and skill. In *A handbook for developing multicultural awareness* (pp. 3-18). Alexandria, VA: American Association for Counseling and Development.

Pedersen, P.B., Draguns, J.G., Lonner, W.J., & Trimble, J.E. (Eds.). (1981). *Counseling across cultures.* Honolulu: University of Hawaii Press.

Stewart, E.C., & Bennett, M.J. (1991). *American cultural patterns: A cross-cultural perspective.* Yarmouth, ME: Intercultural Press.

Thomas, R.R. (1990, March-April). From affirmative action to affirming diversity. *Harvard Business Review,* pp. 107-117.

Tripp-Reimer, T., & Afifi, L.A. (1989). Cross-cultural perspectives on patient teaching. *Nursing Clinics of North America, 24*(3), 613-619.

Tripp-Reimer, T., Brink, P.J., & Saunders, J.M. (1984). Cultural assessment: Content and process. *Nursing Outlook, 32*(2), 78-82.

Wali, A. (1992). Multiculturalism: An anthropological perspective. *Report from the Institute for Philosophy and Public Policy* (University of Maryland at College Park), *12*(1), 6-8.

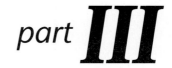

part **III**

THEMES IN PROFESSIONAL NURSING PRACTICE

Concepts common across all areas of professional nursing practice are referred to as themes. Of interest to nurses in a variety of practice settings, these themes serve as unifying threads for nursing practice. For example, regardless of the population being served or the setting, caring is an integral part of nursing. Health promotion and wellness are major thrusts in today's health care, and the effect of the environment on individual and community health is of paramount concern at local and national levels. Nurses may use interpersonal communication techniques in any nurse-client interaction, and teaching is a fundamental nursing responsibility, whether the client is young or old, ill or well. Presented as new chapters to the second edition, critical thinking and change challenge today's nurse to be flexible and creative to meet the ever-changing health care environment. Nursing research will continue to direct our patient care activities and promote improved treatment and care modalities. Finally, the impact of information technology on the planning and delivery of nursing care is a current theme that will become increasingly important in the future. These themes are discussed in this section.

Caring

14

Janet B. Younger

Objectives

At the completion of this chapter, the reader will be able to:

- Understand the essential nature of care.
- Distinguish between human care and professional care.
- Understand care as a context for nursing intervention.
- Understand care as an intervention in itself.

Profile in Practice

Robyn Rice, MSN, RN
Clinical Associate Professor,
Barnes College of Nursing–The University of Missouri at St. Louis,
St. Louis, Missouri;
Home Health Clinical Nurse Specialist,
Saint Anthony's Health Center,
Alton, Illinois

I suspect nurses are nurses because they are *born to care*. For me, caring is that inner force that we nurses draw on in order to make life and death better for our patients and their families. It represents science and a sensitivity in practice and a political platform for support within our profession.

In describing the concept of caring, many images come to mind. I think of the intensive care nurse who stays by his or her patient's bed all night long, keeping a close watch so that the patient wakes up to better days. I think of the oncology nurse educator hugging his or her patient while trying to explain treatment options for cancer. I think of school nurses giving immunizations and lots of smiles to tearful children. I think of home health nurses fostering self-care management in patients and, at times, caring for the patient's caregiver. I think of hospice and parish nurses who offer spiritual comfort. I think of nurse educators and managers who teach, lead, write, and speak out in order to make things better for our profession.

From working in health care for over 20 years, I can recall more images of caring than I have ink in my pen or printer. I think of all of us out in the public who, when the call sounds, resolutely come forward to offer our assistance . . . our caring . . . ourselves. Such actions are not driven by money or profit; we do it because *we care* to do it. Because it is the quintessence of giving and elemental to our personhood as nurses.

Care is a basic and necessary condition of life. Most animal species care for their young, and without this care the young would not survive. For example, some species of birds keep the same mate and same nest for life. They care for their eggs, they feed and protect their young, and the mates feed each other while nesting. These birds may fly away for thousands of miles to obtain food and then return to the same nest to care for the mate and the young. Most of this care is not only growth promoting, but also is necessary for life.

In human beings maternal care normally begins before birth with the care a mother takes of herself during pregnancy and the care the father takes to provide for the addition to the family. Soon after birth parental care takes the form of feeding, clothing, nurturing, socializing, and loving the child. Caring parents engage their infants in a watchful gaze that has been termed *en face* (Ainsworth et al., 1978). This means that the parent's attentiveness is manifested by canting her face in the same plane as the infant's and imitating the infant's expressions. Parental care is a great deal more than just satisfying the physical and material needs of the infant. In fact, a startling scientific discovery of this century was that infants in orphanages who had every physical and material need met, but who did not have the consistent presence of parental care, developed anaclitic depression and failed to thrive. *Anaclitic depression* is a term that means severe loss of vitality of anaclitic origin, literally meaning "without care" (Spitz, 1946). If the absence of parental care is nearly absolute, even if physical needs are met, most children die.

As a child grows, care is the most fundamental ingredient in the secure base provided by families that enables the child to develop. The certain knowledge of care enables exploration, experimenting, venturing out, developing and deploying talents, and developing a high level of self-reliance (Bowlby, 1969, 1979). Also of fundamental importance is the fact that the care a growing person receives is a critical ingredient in that person's later ability to care for others and to form affectional bonds (Bowlby, 1979). Noddings (1984) grounds caring in the universal memory of being cared for. She traced one root of human caring to the longing to maintain, recapture, or enhance our most caring and tender moments. Noddings further claims that caring is the universal basis of morality.

The ability to care is further developed throughout life. Erikson's (1982) theory of psychosocial development includes a stage of adult life that he calls generativity versus self-absorption. In this stage, care is the human strength that emerges from the struggle of the stage. Also, the principal mode of expressing generativity involves caring for future generations through family, work, community involvement, and similar pursuits. Erikson (1982) defines care as "the broadening concern for what has been generated by love, necessity, or accident—a concern that must consistently overcome the ambivalence adhering to irreversible obligation and the narrowness of self-concern" (p. 10). The stages in Erikson's theory are hierarchically related in a way that requires previous stages to be largely successful in their completion before success is likely at a later stage. This then implies that a person who is developmentally capable of generative care would have previously acquired the developmental strengths of trust, autonomy, initiative, industry, identity, and intimacy and have these skills available to use in caring. Thus care as Erikson describes it is not likely to occur in individuals who are immature in their own development.

It is no accident that health professionals refer to what they do in their practices as care. We as a nation are concerned about the availability of health CARE. We want insurance for dental CARE and for medical CARE. Hospitals are places where people go to obtain nursing CARE. Other kinds of efforts are not typically referred to as care but as services. We obtain legal services and postal services. But, suppose you see two advertisements and assume both to be true. One says they provide car services, and the other says they provide car care. What would you assume to be the difference? Of central importance to us, then, is to understand what distinguishes care from services and professional care from human care.

WHAT IS THE ESSENCE OF CARING?

Earlier Definitions

The word *care* comes from the Old English and Gothic word *kara,* which meant grief, lament, sorrow, or bed of sickness (Gaut, 1983). The *American Heritage Dictionary of the English Language* (third edition) defines care as "a state of mind; a responsibility; mental suffering; an object of worry, attention, or solicitude; a caution in avoiding harm or danger; close attention; painstaking application; maintenance; watchful oversight; attentive assistance or treatment; to be concerned or interested; to have an attachment; the function of watching or guarding or overseeing; an organization, CARE (Cooperative for American Relief Everywhere); and feeling and exhibiting concern and empathy for others."

Marcel, an early existentialist philosopher, characterized a *caring attitude* in terms of "disposability, the readiness to bestow and spend oneself and make oneself available, and its contrary, indisposability." Those who are disposable recognize that they have a self to invest, to give. They do not identify themselves by their objects and possessions. They are present to the one who is cared for. Those who are indisposable, on the other hand, come across, even though physically present, as being absent, as being elsewhere. Marcel said, "When I am with someone who is indisposable, I am conscious of being with someone for whom I do not exist; I am thrown back on myself" (Blackham, 1959, p. 80).

Present Definition

Caring is a function of the whole person in which concern for the growth and well-being of another is expressed in an integrated application of the mind, body, and spirit of the one who is caring toward maximizing positive outcomes in the one who is cared for. The expressions of caring, therefore, are quite broad and include, but are not limited to, the following: a feeling of compassion; an attitude of concern; a philosophy of commitment; a moral disposition in the situation; acts of doing for another; conscious attention to the monitoring, surveillance, and protection of well-being; the nurturance of growth; the courage of venturing into the experience of another and being fully present; and advocacy on behalf of another. Caring denotes a primary mode of being in the world and thus is fundamental to our understanding of human nature (Benner & Wrubel, 1989; Griffin, 1983). It may be expressed in a wide variety of activities, such as providing information, doing things, listening, helping, showing respect, and communicating (Warren, 1988). Leininger identified 27 caring activities, which included helping, touching, nurturing, protecting, and supporting (Gaut, 1983). Leininger believed caring to be a universal phenomenon, although she noted that expressions, processes, and patterns varied among cultures (Leininger, 1988). Much of present writing in nursing theory suggests that caring is an essential component of nursing (Boykin & Schoenhofer, 1990; Watson, 1985). Swanson (1993), for example, describes nursing as "informed caring for the well-being of others" (p. 352).

A more abstract form of care is existential care, which is compassion and care as a result of awareness of the common bonds of humanity, common fates, common experiences, and common feelings (Younger, 1995). Care may occur as a product of an individual relationship that has grown into a rapport, but it does not always. Existential care does not necessitate rapport with another, at least at first, but simply the acknowledgment of a shared human experience. This awareness enables us to care for another, not as a stranger, but as another "I." Thus, as the philosopher Heidegger (1962) said, care is "a priori and primordial" no mere generalization, but a real structure that appears in all (pp. 243-244).

Care as an Ideal

As a philosophical concept, Care is an ideal, like Truth, Justice, or Beauty. Both the word *ideal* and the use of capitalization denote that Care can never be perfect or fully attained in human expression. Human beings are not capable of perfect Care any more than we are capable of perfect Truth, Justice, or Beauty. However, in striving for the ideal, we occasionally come close and by so doing achieve something quite wonderful. A danger is in viewing such ideals concretely and expecting that they "should" be achievable and that they should be measured, and that those who fall short should be ashamed. A nurse who expected to Care would likely feel guilty about moments of feeling selfish or about being unable to Care for a particular patient. Another danger is to be too discouraged about the impossibility of perfection and fail to strive for that part of the ideal that might be achievable.

Professional Care

Professional caring adds the additional defining characteristic of applying the knowledge of the discipline, including its art, science, theory, and practice, to the situation of concern. This is what distinguishes professional caring from basic human caring. Human caring therefore is necessary for professional caring, but it is far from sufficient. It is also necessary to know what to care about and to be competent in the professional activities that operationalize care. Professional caring, like human caring, is an activity of the whole person. Activities and techniques alone do not constitute care, just as provision for basic needs of the infant is insufficient. Also, compassion alone, without knowledge and competence, is insufficient. The involvement of the whole person is a necessary condition for caring, and in the case of professional caring, involvement of the whole of the art and science of the discipline is needed.

Different Meanings of the Word *Care*

Not everyone who uses the word *care* or *caring* means the same thing. Some interpret it to mean only an emotional state and resent its use as devaluing the scientific and instrumental activities of nursing. Some others may use the expression "provide nursing care" to mean only performing technical skills. Again, this may be resented as denying the intellectual, humanistic, and existential component of nursing. Another use is to say "care" with an automaticity that lacks specific meaning, such as the phrase "nursing care plan." Still others see caring as a human trait and consider nurses' claim to caring as egocentric. This is particularly true of other health professionals. To be sure, any of the above interpretations fall far short of the meaning that is conveyed here. Given the possible confusion, it is usually a good idea to define the term before using it and assuming the same interpretation.

Caring in Nursing

The expression of caring in nursing is well directed by Henderson's (1966) definition of nursing, which is "to do those things the patient would do unaided for himself if he had the necessary strength, will or knowledge; and to do this in such a way as to help him gain independence as rapidly as possible" (p. 15). The American Nurses' Association (ANA) definition of nursing, which is "the diagnosis and treatment of human responses to health and illness," further guides the area of concern in nursing (ANA, 1980). Both of these definitions help us know what to care about. Thus, while there are aspects of caring in nursing that are specific to the purposes of nursing, the foundation of caring is common to human professions, to human beings, and, indeed, to most living beings.

CARING AS A CONTEXT FOR INTERVENTION

Benner and Wrubel (1989) assert that caring is primary. Caring means being connected and having that connection matter. It is the force that fuses thought, feeling, and action. It sets up what matters to a person; it also sets up what counts as stressful and what options are available for coping. Caring creates possibility and gives meaning. This is the first way in which caring is primary (Benner & Wrubel, 1989).

When patients feel cared for, it sets up the perception of a safe environment. The safety is like what the child experiences in an environment of parental care. It is predicated on the sense that someone more knowledgeable is monitoring the situation and will invariably act for well-being. This state is then accompanied by a lowering of vigilance, a sense of comfort, a willingness to explore, and a willingness to reveal more of the vulnerable self. It is helpful to contrast the sense one has when the environment is experienced as indifferent or dangerous. Nursing research has pursued the question of this contrast (Brown, 1986; Riemen, 1986; Swanson-Kauffman, 1986). Findings suggest that most people under those circumstances assume a guarded, defensive posture, and their stress level is much higher.

Caring and Illness

The experience of illness is very personal and, at the same time, universal. The personal experience is that illness always has a story. It is the story of a life interrupted. The nature of the interruption is very specifically related to the life itself. What plans have been changed? What meanings were assigned to whatever has been lost? What is the personal meaning of the reminder that life is vulnerable and time limited? To acknowledge the reality of pain and suffering means saying to oneself: "I may lose at any moment, through the play of circumstances over which I have no control, anything whatsoever that I possess, including those things which are so intimately mine that I consider them as being myself" (Weil, 1969, p. 287). This is true even when the illness is minor, but it is especially true when the illness produces a long-term or permanent change. Consider the trivial example of a person who has a flat tire en route to somewhere. Although the flat tire is trivial, the story of that journey to somewhere is epic. These stories are very personal, but in every illness there simultaneously exists an encounter with the universal. Caring involves learning the universal patterns of human fate. It is a voluntary involvement in the universality of pain, suffering, aloneness, fear, and a looming death. Caring also means involvement in the universal characteristic of constructing a life and restructuring meaning. Even a new mother is, in a day's time, interrupted from her old life and finds herself constructing a new life with a new person. This ceaseless activity of inventing, restructuring, and reinterpreting is universal, even though the outcomes are personal. For the nurse, it also means responding to a universal appeal that is made by one who suffers—that is, to care, the potential for which is in all.

Another type of activity that is not usually associated with the affective component of caring is careful monitoring. For example, a nurse in an intensive care unit spends much of the day monitoring information provided by machines. Is that caring? Certainly, the activity of very careful watching, like that the mother does with her infant or the bird does with its nest, is a component of the living prototypes of care. The fact that the patient may not talk is immaterial in answering the question. The full integration of the monitoring information is a necessary element in order to call this professional care. The only issue that remains in answering the question is whether the nurse integrates this information with other kinds of information obtained from monitoring this patient as a whole person, and whether this nurse acts as a whole person on behalf of the patient's well-being.

Caring is the force that takes the nurse into the patient's life while monitoring the patient's condition and selecting actions in an integrated goal-corrected movement toward well-being. Caring is the integrative force that organizes and binds together all of the resources of the nurse. Since nursing actions are really functional only when integrated, it is the context for nursing intervention.

CARING AS AN INTERVENTION

The most demanding and deeply human aspect of caring is the expressive art of being fully present to another person (Davis, 1981). In the deepest sense, caring for the other is extending a human and humane presence to a fellow being—an action that reinforces caring. It transcends role obligations and acknowledges the vulnerable humanness of us all. To be present means to unconceal, to be aware of tone of voice, eye contact, affect, and body language—to be in tune with the patient's messages. The effect of this interaction is the reinforcement of one's self-esteem, the strengthening of one's spirit, and the healing and nurturing of the self. This is the ability to "convey by presence that my own fears and ego needs have been laid aside and I am yours." An act of human contact and concern provides the alienated with a human self-extension and, in itself, partially recreates the connection. Being present and available so that the patient's needs are responded to appropriately, so that "one's existence is acknowledged by another who cares" is confirmation (Drew, 1986, p. 40). The one who is caring sees the best self in the one who is cared for and works with this person to actualize that self (Noddings, 1984).

The suffering of another illuminates essential humanity under threat and is thus a profound call for the attention of the giver of care; a protector of humanity (Griffin, 1983). Since the nature of suffering is to call forth deep questioning of the truth of one's being and its meaning, care becomes a midwife of rebirth of a reconstructed life (Younger, 1995). Caring acknowledgment of patients' suffering legitimizes their experiences and gives them a feeling of personal integrity, wholeness, and value (Suchman & Matthews, 1988).

It is a frequent mistake to believe that people who do not speak of their caring in fact do not care. This may be inaccurate and a misjudgment of the true situation. In our society this misjudgment happens to men more often than to women, to physicians more often than to nurses, and to quiet nurses more often than to talkative ones. It is well to remember that caring may or may not be related to claims of caring. Furthermore, it may be demoralizing to one who cares to be accused of not caring. It has the effect of making the person feel misunderstood and alienated. Those conditions may then actually interfere with that person's ability to care or to receive support for caring and thereby result in less care. Consider the situation of a nurse who believes that a mother who does not come often to see her hospitalized child does not care. If the nurse subsequently communicates that to the mother, is the mother more likely or less likely to feel supported in caring for the child?

Not all emotional involvement with another person constitutes caring as herein defined. If the mother of a young child is overprotective and because of her own fearfulness prohibits the child from engaging in normal play activities, which the child needs for development, that is not maternal care. Although the mother may feel much concern for the child, her actions do not promote the growth and well-being of the child and therefore fall short of caring. Sometimes a nurse becomes personally involved with a patient, and the relationship becomes a friendship. When that occurs and the relationship itself becomes of highest importance or the nurse loses the ability to use professional knowledge fully for the well-being of that patient, then the nurse's involvement is no longer professional care.

Sometimes the patient has something wrong that the nurse has also experienced. That experience can become a source of knowledge and skill, or it can be a personal experience that the nurse cannot get beyond. In such instances the nurse is actually absorbed in the continued care of himself or herself.

There are also times when the nurse is unable to bear the pain or suffering of the patient without giving up the ability to care in one of two ways. First the nurse may become quite detached and cease to engage the patient with the same watchful gaze, studied concern, or available presence. The patient may become the object of some technical intervention that regardless of how skillfully it is done, is not a product of the whole person of the nurse. In the second case, the nurse may give alcohol to an alcoholic or morphine to an addict, or tell patients that things will be fine when they will not. In these instances the nurse is so wrapped up in the patient's suffering that the focus on well-being is lost.

In all of these cases the nurse has much feeling but is not engaged in professional care. It is a common, human mistake. It does not mean the nurse is never capable of caring, but in these instances the actions are short of that.

Care Versus Cure

Medicine is primarily concerned with the prevention, diagnosis, and treatment of disease. As such, it has sometimes been associated with cure in contrast to nursing, which has primarily been associated with care. Proposing that medicine is concerned with cure and nursing with care therefore may highlight some of the primary distinctions of the two disciplines. Would it be valid, though, to think that care is the province of nursing and that cure belongs to medicine? Consider these questions. When a nurse debrides an ulcer, is that caring or curing? When a physician orders pain medication, what is that? Pain is a response to disease or trauma. Treatment of pain rarely cures the underlying problem. When a nurse practitioner orders aspirin for fever, is that medicine or nursing? Fever is a response to disease and not the disease itself. Treating it does not cure the disease. Is a surgical procedure necessarily done for the purpose of cure? Each of these questions illustrates the ambiguity in trying to distinguish medicine and nursing by their caring or curing activities.

Given the definition of caring presented in this chapter, caring would encompass curing if that possibility were present (Jecker & Self, 1991). Similarly, curing often involves altering the relationships among the disease process and the patient's natural defenses. Placing the patient in the best possible position to fight the disease or injury often involves acts of caring. Therefore, to believe that caring is confined to nursing and that curing is confined to medicine is unduly simplistic and unrealistically confining. Although the concepts of care and cure may be distinguished, in practice they are often well blended.

DEVELOPING MORE CARING ABILITY

There may be several things beginning nurses could do to develop their caring abilities. These involve strengthening capacities in each of the areas of mind, body, and spirit, as well as increasing the ability to integrate these. Everything nurses can discover or learn about the science of illness or its manifestations and about nursing interventions improves the ability to assess problems and understand what helps. Every technical skill that is perfected, whether it is the ability to give an injection with skill or to move a patient painlessly contributes to care. The task of eliciting from the patient what is being experienced is tremendously complex. How do you get a patient to tell you how much pain, how much worry, how much knowledge he or she is experiencing? This is an artful combination of the questions asked and how they are asked, and there is never enough practice.

There is a type of knowledge of what it is like to be ill or to suffer or to be in pain that is not entirely intellectual and not entirely personal. Nurses may learn about this from listening to the experiences of their patients if they can listen without too much defensive avoidance. A lower level of exposure to that learning may be through artistic depictions of those experiences in literary works, artwork, and movies (Younger, 1990). Writers often draw on the very material that nurses encounter daily, and literary themes are often the same as the human themes that nurses need to recognize: endurance in the face of suffering, the quest for meaning, and acceptance of loss. The depictions of suffering and illness are closer in their expression to the way patients describe their experiences than are descriptions found in textbooks. The human condition is expressed sensitively and articulately in literature, and the esthetic appeal of these often calls forth compassion that is crucial to nursing. These literary works convey something complex in a more simple metaphorical form that can be grasped as a whole and understood. This is because they convey not only the facts, but also the context and meaning of the experience. The inexperienced nurse can risk entering into the vicarious experience of a story that would be beyond the professional level of experience. Also, performance is not required, so personal defenses may be relaxed, enabling the nurse to grow in knowledge, understanding, and compassion. Thus literary works offer a way for nurses to gain maturity, understanding of human responses, and depth of compassion for others (Younger, 1990).

Another means of increasing one's ability to care is to use as professional models those nurses who demonstrate caring and avoid those who do not care. Nurses who are not very knowledgeable and highly skilled or who have become so detached as to not know what their patients are experiencing may model behaviors that seem attractive because they are easier, but these behaviors will not result in professional care. However, an experienced nurse who is able to care may help by allowing a less experienced nurse to watch or to hear the stories of important experiences. Even more helpful is for the more experienced nurse to hear the problems of the novice and help with approaches and with encouragement. Much of caring requires some courage, so those individuals who encourage are very valuable colleagues.

Finally, nurses who wish to increase their ability to care for others must care for their own spirits (Lane, 1987). Lane tells us that we all desire to push back the horizons of our present life, aspiring to be something more, and that life is a journey on the road to somewhere. We are restless to know more, to love more, to create more, and to express a generosity within us that desires to give to the other, to make life better. Lane advises us to engage in inward turning to get in touch with the "wounded self" (Nouwen, 1972), which eventually helps us to be at home with ourselves, to be who we are, to accept the limitations life has imposed on us, and to go on.

EXAMPLES OF CARING

Each of the following clinical examples depicts certain aspects of caring. The situations differ, as does the form that caring takes.

EXAMPLE 1: THE NEUROINTENSIVE CARE UNIT

Ms. A is a nurse on the unit, and her patient is a young man who is an illegal immigrant. He has been in a car accident and has a serious head injury. He has no family in this country. The patient has been unconscious since his accident. Ms. A is quite concerned about the well-being of her patient. She thinks about his possible recovery and wants to assist him in regaining his health and function. She does not condone his illegal activity, but that is not her concern in this situation. He is in need of help. She is very knowledgeable about neuroanatomy and physiology and realizes that she must monitor every change in the patient's condition. She watches carefully all of the equipment that helps her assess the condition of his brain. She also uses all of her physical assessment skills to detect any complication that may arise. She assesses his level of consciousness at least every hour and talks to him in an attempt to penetrate his coma with some sense of life. He, however, cannot talk to her, nor is he at this moment aware of her care. Nonetheless, this is care. It is a product of her whole person on behalf of the patient's well-being.

EXAMPLE 2: THE ONCOLOGY UNIT

Mr. B, a nurse on the oncology unit, has been the primary nurse for his patient, a 53-year-old grandmother who has advanced cancer. She has been in pain and is aware that her prognosis is quite poor. While Mr. B is adjusting her IV, she says to him, "Are you a religious man, Mr. B?" Actually, Mr. B does not consider himself a particularly religious man, and, fur-

thermore, he has much to do this morning. A part of him sighs at being called on to enter into this patient's suffering. This morning, at least, he would rather attend to other things. He is human and is not capable of perfect Care. However, he is also an expert clinician in oncology, and he recognizes that is it not his religion that is at issue here; rather, the patient is seeking a human connection. He recognizes the pattern of the question and the way she asks it. He sits down on her bed, but not because he plans to stay a long time. This will not take very long. He wants to signal his intention to be fully present to her and to enter into her experience. Beginning truthfully, he says, "My own religion has its ups and downs—does yours provide you some comfort now?" The question is gentle and not very demanding. The patient may choose to say a few more things about her religion and remain silent about other concerns. However, she may also choose to accept his gentle acknowledgement that there is really something here that is in need of comfort, and she may share this with him. In fact, she says, "I know that I have not much longer to live. I long to watch my grandchild grow a bit longer and offer more support to his parents. My comfort is in knowing that the Lord does things in His own good time and that He will provide for my children." He takes her hand for a moment and says, "Your faith that the Lord will provide for your children seems a comfort to you now indeed." His answer is brief and tacitly accepting of everything she has said. He waits to see where she needs to go with this next. She pats his hand and says, "Well, you have others to take care of. Thank you so much."

EXAMPLE 3: THE NURSING STUDENT

Ms. C is a junior nursing student who is assigned to a 16-year-old girl who, because of a chronic illness that has worsened, is now in multisystem failure, including renal and hepatic shutdown. The patient wants to live, and the student perhaps identifies with this patient and recognizes that in a 16-year-old there is much living that can be lost. The student assesses the patient very carefully and spends nearly the whole night before her clinical experience researching what should be done for this patient. She arrives the next morning and presents her instructor with an excellent and exhaustive nursing care plan. The instructor looks at the care plan and then at the patient. From her experience she recognizes in this patient the unmistakable signs of impending death, and in this student she recognizes the lack of awareness of that reality. In the morning the student cares for the patient exhaustively. In the afternoon the patient dies. The instructor finds the student alone in an out-of-the-way corner of the unit. The student is maintaining a stiff upper lip and is nearly mute. The instructor talks to the student for a while, and the student says, "I should have done more." The instructor replies, "There was too much wrong. She couldn't be saved." The instructor begins to talk about the overwhelming problems of this patient and the unmistakable signs of impending death. The instructor then begins to take out a tissue to wipe the tears from her own eyes. The student says, "Nurses don't cry like this." The instructor replies, "Maybe not while things are happening and people need your help immediately, but after it is over we sometimes need a good cry." The student is then able to let go of her stiff upper lip and, in the safety of her instructor's acceptance, give way to her feelings.

In this situation the student is showing deep human care and excellent beginning professional care. The instructor also shows human care and mature professional care.

She also, as a professional, is creating more potential for care in this developing student. As she helps her develop professionally and learn to fuse her knowledge, humanness, and professionalism, she helps create a nurse more capable of care.

EXAMPLE 4: THE WELL-CHILD CLINIC

Mr. D is a nurse practitioner in a well-child clinic based in a neighborhood with much social and economic deprivation. His patient this morning is an 18-month-old and his mother. Mr. D is aware that this mother has had cultural experiences quite different from his own and that English is her second language and his only language. He thinks about that for a moment before entering the patient's room. He will do his best to understand, but this understanding can never be perfect. He is quite committed to fostering the health and growth of young people in this community. His knowledge of the normal growth and development of the child is excellent. Using that knowledge, he carefully assesses this child. The child, who was premature, is underweight; speech is nonexistent; the hematocrit is below normal; the immunizations are markedly behind; but most troublesome to him is the pattern of bruises with uneven levels of healing. He sits down and asks the mother, "How do you manage?" She says in broken English, "Life is very hard—three children, no money, no man—this boy bad." He asks a clinic helper who speaks her language fluently to help him talk to the mother. The mother denies abusing the child and indicates only normal punishment for misbehavior. Mr. D carefully considers the legal and ethical requirements of his situation. He must be an advocate for the child. He calls protective services. While waiting for them to come, he and the clinic helper talk at length to the mother about normal behavior of children that age and their needs. Although momentarily he feels like shaking the mother, he listens to her and feels compassion for her while at the same time he is providing protection for the child.

Each of these vignettes is an example of caring. All demonstrate a primary human quality finely honed by professional training and expressed humanly rather than perfectly. Each demonstrates some defining characteristic(s) of care. They depict nurses engaged with the whole of their professional knowledge, as well as their human spirits.

Key Points

- Caring is a function of the whole person in which concern for the growth and well-being of another is expressed in an integrated application of the mind, body, and spirit of the one who is caring toward maximizing positive outcomes in the one who is cared for.

- Professional caring adds the defining characteristic of applying the knowledge of the discipline, including its art, science, theory, and practice, to the situation of concern. This is what distinguishes professional caring from basic human caring. Human caring, therefore, is necessary for professional caring, but it is far from sufficient.

- Definitions of nursing direct us in what to care about in professional practice.

- Caring as a context provides for the integration of activities of the mind, body, and spirit of the nurse on behalf of the well-being of the patient.

- Caring as an intervention is effective in giving patients a sense of personal integrity, wholeness, and value. In the suffering patient it helps to bear the burden.

- Caring as an activity integrates the information gained from monitoring the patient and activities on the patient's behalf into a constantly readjusted, goal-corrected intervention for the patient's well-being.

Critical Thinking Exercises

1. Consider situations in which you have felt cared for. Analyze the situation. How did you know you were cared for? What was the effect of that care?

2. Consider situations in which you have been unable to care. Analyze the situation. What were barriers? What aspects of you as a whole person were affected?

3. What do you have to do to care for an individual who lives a life so adverse to your values as to create a conflict in you?

4. What is the difference between caring for someone you love, like your own child, and caring for someone you do not love, like a stranger?

5. Consider the example of a nurse who comes to work at 3:00 PM. The assigned patient's chart reveals that a dressing, which is ordered once a shift, was done at 2:30 PM. It is now 3:30; the nurse has time to do the dressing and considers doing it now. What does it mean in terms of caring to do it now?

6. Consider your development as a professional. What is missing from your full ability to provide professional care?

References

Ainsworth, M.D.S., Blehar, M.C., Waters, E., & Wall, S. (1978). *Patterns of attachment.* Hillsdale, NJ: Lawrence Erlbaum Associates.

American Nurses' Association. (1980). *Nursing: A social policy statement* (ANA Publication No. NP-63). Kansas City, MO.

Benner, P., & Wrubel, J. (1989). *The primacy of caring.* Menlo Park: Addison-Wesley.

Blackham, H. (1959). *Six existentialist thinkers.* New York: Harper & Row.

Bowlby, J. (1969). *Attachment and loss: Vol. 1. Attachment.* New York: Basic Books.

Bowlby, J. (1979). *The making and breaking of affectional bonds.* London: Tavistock Publications.

Boykin, A. & Schoenhofer, S. (1990). Caring in nursing: Analysis of extant theory. *Nursing Science Quarterly, 4,* 149-155.

Brown, L. (1986). The experience of care: patient perspectives. *Topics in Clinical Nursing, 8*(2), 56-62.

Davis, M. (1981). Compassion, suffering, morality: Ethical dilemmas in caring. *Nursing Law and Ethics, 2,* 1-2, 6.

Drew, N. (1986). Exclusion and confirmation: A phenomenology of patients' experiences with caregivers. *Image: Journal of Nursing Scholarship, 18*(2), 39-43.

Erikson, E. (1978). Life cycle. In J. Gardner (Ed), *Readings in developmental psychology* (pp. 3-12). Boston: Little, Brown.

Erikson, E. (1982). *The life cycle completed.* New York: W.W. Norton.

Gaut, D. (1983). Development of a theoretically adequate description of caring. *Western Journal of Nursing Research, 5*(4), 311-324.

Griffin, A.P. (1983). A philosophical analysis of caring in nursing. *Journal of Advanced Nursing, 8,* 289-295.

Heidegger, M. (1962). *Being and time.* New York: Harper & Row.

Henderson, V. (1966). *The nature of nursing.* New York: Macmillan.

Jecker, N., & Self, D. (1991). Separating care and cure: An analysis of historical and contemporary images of nursing and medicine. *The Journal of Medicine and Philosophy, 16,* 285-306.

Lane, J. (1987). The care of the human spirit. *Journal of Professional Nursing,* 332-337.

Leininger, M. (1988). The phenomenon of caring: Importance, research questions and theoretical considerations. In M. Leininger (Ed.), *Caring: An essential human need.* Thorofare, NJ: Slack.

Noddings, N. (1984). *Caring: A feminine approach to ethics and moral education.* Los Angeles: University of California Press.

Nouwen, H. (1972). *The wounded healer.* New York: Doubleday.

Riemen, D. (1986). Noncaring and caring in the clinical setting: patients' descriptions. *Topics in Clinical Nursing, 8*(2), 30-36.

Spitz, R.A. (1946). Anaclitic depression. *Psychoanalytic Study of the Child, 2,* 313-342.

Suchman, A., Matthews, D. (1988). What makes the patient-doctor relationship therapeutic? Exploring the connexional dimension of medical care. *Annals of Internal Medicine, 108,* 125-130.

Swanson, K. (1993). Nursing as informed caring for the well-being of others. *Image: Journal of Nursing Scholarship, 25*(4) 352-357.

Swanson-Kauffman, K. (1986). Caring in the instance of unexpected early pregnancy loss. *Topics in Clinical Nursing, 8*(2), 37-46.

Vaillot, M. (1966). Existentialism: A philosophy of commitment. *American Journal of Nursing, 66,* 500-505.

Warren, L. (1988). Review and synthesis of nine nursing studies on care and caring. *Journal of the New York State Nurses' Association, 19*(4), 17-21.

Watson, J. (1985). *Nursing: Human science and human care.* Norwalk, CT: Appleton-Century-Crofts.

Weil, S. (1969). Personality as affliction. In M. Lipman (Ed.), *Discovering philosophy.* Englewood Cliffs, NJ: Prentice Hall.

Younger, J. (1990). Literary works as a mode of knowing. *Image: Journal of Nursing Scholarship, 22*(1), 39-43.

Younger, J. (1995). Alienation of the sufferer. *Advances in Nursing Science, 17*(3), 53-72.

Health and Health Promotion

15

Patty J. Hale

Objectives

At the completion of this chapter, the reader will be able to:

- Compare and contrast several definitions of health.

- Describe Smith's (1983) four models of health.

- Compare and contrast several models of health behavior.

- Apply the health belief model to a selected health behavior (i.e., smoking cessation).

- Apply the theory of planned behavior to the use of condoms.

- Describe the use of the health risk appraisal.

- Describe societal influences on health and health promotion.

- Describe the goals and four major activities of *Healthy People 2000.*

- Describe a community-level health promotion program.

Profile in Practice

Janet S. Wyatt, PhD, RN, NP
Chief, Community Health Nursing–Preventive Medicine Service,
U.S. Army Health Clinic, SHAPE,
Brussels, Belgium;
Adjunct Assistant Professor,
Graduate School of Nursing,
Uniformed Services University of the Health Sciences,
Bethesda, Maryland

With advances in technology, pregnant patients in our OB clinic are quickly supplied information about their due date, fetal growth, and even the probable gender of the fetus. Yet none of these technological advances contributes to promoting and protecting the health and well-being of the mother and baby. Simple and straightforward health promotion activities remain a primary focus for each patient's prenatal plan of care.

As good detectives, nurse practitioners construct a detailed summary of each patient's health history, emphasizing investigation of lifestyle behaviors that may promote and protect or destroy and undermine health. Health-damaging lifestyles that include tobacco use, excessive alcohol intake, and utilization of potentially harmful medications alert the nurse to the need for immediate patient care interventions to minimize these threats and promote and protect health. Through examination of lifestyles, areas of positive health behavior are also revealed. Reinforcement and enhancement of these health behaviors, such as nutrition and exercise, help to increase levels of well-being and self-esteem among patients.

Recognition of both positive and negative health lifestyles represents only the assessment phase of health promotion. Implementation of strategies to change and enhance health behaviors remains a daunting task. In all health promotion interventions we attempt to incorporate principles of teaching and learning, building on previous learning, and offering social support to enhance adoption of behaviors, including strategies to motivate clients to change. While we maintain a multidimensional approach to implementing our health promotion activities, we have learned what helps and what hurts as patients work to enhance personal health and wellness. Advice has rarely been therapeutic. We try to avoid directive statements and cringe when we find ourselves preaching, "You should . . ." to our patients. Successful health promotion and personal behavior change has never occurred when we haven't demonstrated caring. Recognition and praise for the work invested in each patient's personal growth is essential to ensuring continued health promotion progress.

At a recent physical examination, Jane Smith, a 45-year-old woman, was told that she must modify her behaviors to reduce her risk for cardiac disease. She is overweight, smokes one pack of cigarettes per day, and has a sedentary lifestyle. Her father died at age 53 from a cerebrovascular accident. Pam Jones, RN, a home health nurse, will visit Mrs. Smith and work with her to improve her health by promoting healthy behavior changes.

Many people are advised to change their behavior to promote health, but it remains a formidable challenge to actually make these changes. Thus the concepts of health and health promotion have received great attention in nursing research and practice. This attention is warranted because a primary goal of nursing has been preventing disease and restoring health. Nurses use aspects of health promotion with individuals, families, and groups in virtually every practice role in the profession.

There is good reason to emphasize health and the prevention of disease over cure of illness. As early as 1979, it was recognized that 50% of the mortality from the 10 leading causes of death could be traced to lifestyles (U.S. Public Health Service [U.S. PHS],

1979). Adoption of healthy behaviors, such as refraining from smoking, reducing fat and caloric intake, exercising, and reducing alcohol consumption, improves the health of individuals. Thus, through choices that individuals make about their behavior, they can influence their health status.

There is evidence that individuals are increasingly engaged in health-promoting habits. For example, the number of deaths due to motor vehicle accidents has declined sharply and is partly a result of the greater use of seat belts. The number of people who monitor their fat intake and amount of exercise has also increased, resulting in a decline in deaths from cardiac disease since the 1960s (U.S. PHS, 1990).

In addition to the achievement of a higher quality of life for individuals, a primary motivating factor in preventing disease is the enormous economic cost incurred by treating illnesses after their onset. Diseases often require expensive diagnostic and treatment procedures. Waiting to first intervene with clients after the onset of symptomatic disease is not cost-effective, and it is increasingly recognized that society can no longer afford unlimited use of such technology. For example, acquired immunodeficiency syndrome (AIDS), a preventable disease, costs an average of $119,274 per person for illness care (Hellinger, 1993). This awareness has focused new attention on prevention of HIV infection.

This chapter begins by exploring definitions of health and health promotion. The importance of lifestyle and environment are considered for their impact on personal health behavior. Selected theories of health behavior are described, and interventions to change health behaviors targeted toward individuals and communities are discussed.

DEFINITIONS OF HEALTH

The concept of health has been the source of much contemplation and writing by nursing and other disciplines. Consequently, many definitions of health have evolved, as have ways of thinking about how to intervene to improve health. It is vital to understand these meanings because of their implications for how nurses incorporate the concept of health into their practices.

Some of the earliest work on health was that of Dunn (1959, 1971). His health continuum illustrates the dynamic interaction of health and environment as individuals move toward high-level wellness. Health is depicted as being dynamic, requiring continuous health-promoting activity in order to be maintained and improved (Fig. 15-1).

The World Health Organization (WHO) has defined health as a state of complete physical, mental, and social well-being and not merely the absence of disease and infirmity (WHO, 1958). A criticism of this definition is that it is too idealistic to be achievable. However, its strength is that it emphasizes the social components of health (e.g., environment, social support) and thus challenges health care providers to think of health more broadly than as simply the absence of illness.

A particularly useful way to understand the various meanings of health is based on Smith's (1983) four models of health depicted in Table 15-1. Smith analyzed definitions of health and categorized them into four models. There may be some overlap in these models, but they generally build from a narrow to a broader perspective of health.

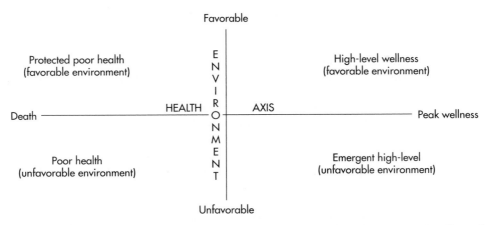

Fig. 15-1   Continuum of high-level wellness. (From Dunn, H.L. [1959]. High level wellness for man and society. *American Journal of Public Health, 49,* 88.)

Table 15-1   **Models of Health**

Model	Conception of Health
Clinical	Elimination of disease as identified through medical science
Role performance	Ability to perform social, occupational, and other roles
Adaptive	Ability to engage in effective interaction with physical and social environment
Eudaimonistic	Self-actualization of individual; optimal well-being

Data from Smith, J. (1983). *The idea of health: Implications for the nursing profession.* New York: Teachers College Press.

The first and most narrowly defined of Smith's models is the *clinical model,* which refers to health as the absence of disease. The clinical model is the definition of health adopted by modern medicine. It places emphasis on ridding individuals of symptomatic illness. The second model, *role-performance,* defines health from the perspective of capability of meeting role obligations related to work, family, and other positions. Moving to a multidimensional conception of health, the *adaptive model* refers to individuals' ability to purposefully interact with their physical and social environment. Here the emphasis is on adaptation to changes in the environment, such that social, as well as physical, health is addressed. Finally, the *eudaimonistic model* views health as all-encompassing and focuses on well-being and self-actualizing. This model aspires to complete development of the person and represents a holistic view of individuals.

Smith's models represent various perspectives that can be used as a basis for evaluating health status. Smith advises that nurses focus on the adaptation and eudaimonistic models, where quality of life is of interest. Thus nurses would move beyond care based only on the clinical model of health to care that addresses social, environmental, educational, and other factors related to well-being. In this context, defining health more broadly has implications for the types of nursing roles and interventions provided to clients.

HEALTH PROMOTION AND DISEASE PREVENTION

Health promotion is defined by Pender (1987) as increasing the level of well-being and self-actualization of a given individual or group. It includes behaviors such as weight control, balanced nutrition, stress management, and exercise.

Health promotion and *disease prevention* have sometimes been used interchangeably to refer to the same activities. Nurses who have explored these phenomena stress the importance of differentiating health promotion from disease prevention in order to recognize the distinct contribution each makes to nursing practice (Brubaker, 1983; Pender, 1987). Specifically, *health promotion* aims to achieve a healthier state; it takes on a positive view of moving toward greater health. In contrast, *disease prevention* focuses on maintaining health through avoiding behavior that may result in disease. For example, maintaining a low-fat diet is a health-promoting activity because it promotes overall health status. On the other hand, if an individual eats a low-fat diet because of a high cholesterol level and a family history of heart disease, this would be interpreted as disease prevention.

Leavell and Clark's (1965) classic work on levels of disease prevention views prevention based on the stage of disease progression. These authors proposed three levels of disease prevention—primary, secondary, and tertiary—to identify and differentiate the activities and goals of prevention for each specific phase of an illness. *Primary prevention* is protection from a disease while still in a healthy state. Thus it includes aspects of health promotion and disease prevention. Examples of primary prevention include preventing diseases through immunization or condom use and practicing positive health habits, such as good nutrition and exercise. *Secondary prevention* involves early detection and treatment of disease. This includes all types of screening programs, such as mammography and cholesterol screening. The goal of *tertiary prevention* is to prevent complications and to maintain health once the disease process has occurred. Tertiary prevention includes activities such as performing range-of-motion exercises to prevent contractures following a stroke. Table 15-2 illustrates application of primary, secondary, and tertiary prevention to AIDS.

HEALTH BEHAVIOR

Analysis of the leading causes of death can provide a basis for identifying health behaviors that are important to modify. The ten major causes of death are heart disease, cancer, cerebrovascular disease, accidents, chronic obstructive pulmonary disease, pneumonia and influenza, diabetes, suicide, chronic liver disease, and HIV (Centers for Disease Control and Prevention [CDC], 1994).

Table 15-2   **Primary, Secondary and Tertiary Prevention Activities Applied to AIDS**

Levels of Prevention	Prevention Activities
Primary prevention	Assess risks and teach clients how to change risky behaviors (e.g., condom use)
Secondary prevention	Test for antibody to human immunodeficiency virus (HIV); provide treatment if test is positive
Tertiary prevention	Manage physical symptoms of AIDS and provide psychosocial support

However, it is imperative to distinguish between the actual causes of death and the reported causes of death. Although these are reported to be the primary causes of death, they are often just the pathophysiologic manifestations of health behaviors (or the lack thereof). McGinnis and Foege (1993) identify the true causes that underlie these reported causes as tobacco use, unhealthful diet and activity patterns, alcohol misuse, microbial agents, toxic agents, unsafe sexual behavior, unsafe practices with motor vehicles and firearms, illicit use of drugs, and other factors, such as poverty and lack of access to primary care. These are lifestyle factors that strongly influence health but have very little to do with where most of the resources for health care are placed—in the hands of the health care system and professionals who provide care.

OVERVIEW OF SELECTED HEALTH BEHAVIOR THEORIES

Mr. Lee is a 36-year-old man with a 20-year history of smoking 1 to 1½ packs of cigarettes a day. He has a strong desire to quit smoking. He has tried to stop in the past and has not been successful. This time, he is serious. He has a chronic cough on waking in the morning, believes that his voice has changed because of smoking, feels smoking wastes time, and finds the habit expensive. In addition, all of his co-workers frown on smoking, he is a health care professional, and he smokes only in his personal life. After attempting to stop in the past, he has found that after a few days, when he is in a situation where he usually smokes a cigarette, he craves one so strongly that he ends up smoking again. Usually his intention is to have just one, but he finds himself smoking a complete pack again within a few days. So why can't he quit?

The above case study illustrates the difficulty with changing behaviors and the importance of personal responsibility and motivation in influencing individual health status. Although some factors, such as heredity, are not modifiable, health behavior is a way that individuals can improve health and prevent disease. Because health behavior has a great impact on health status, research has focused on explaining the determinants of health behavior. As a result of this research, several models have been developed to explain why people engage in health-promoting behaviors. These models are extremely important because they can direct how nurses work with clients to facilitate behavior change. Selected models are presented here.

Health Belief Model

The first research on health behavior was done in the 1950s by a group of social psychologists who were attempting to explain the public's low response to free or low-cost screening programs (Hochbaum, 1958). The health belief model (HBM) evolved from this work. Since this early work, the HBM has been used to predict safer sex behavior, seat belt use, and breast self-examination, among others (Champion, 1994; Gerhart, 1992; Lux & Petosa, 1994).

As depicted in Fig. 15-2, the HBM consists of five main dimensions: perceived susceptibility, perceived severity, perceived benefits, perceived barriers, and cues to action. According to this model, an individual's readiness to take action is influenced by the

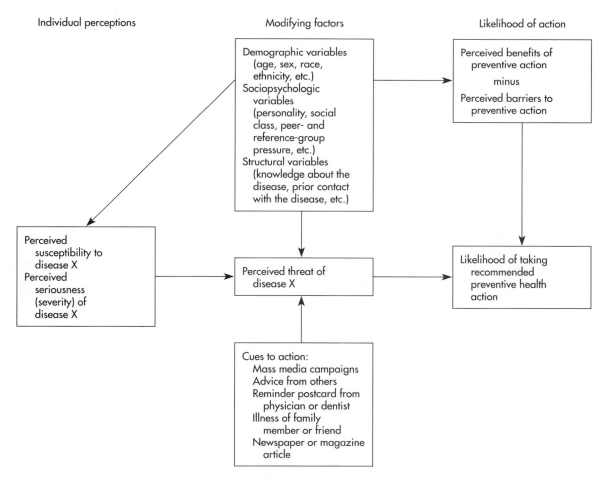

Fig. 15-2   Health belief model. (Redrawn from Becker, M.H., et al. [1977]. Selected psychosocial models and correlates of individual health-related behaviors. *Medical Care 15*[5], 27-46.)

perceived susceptibility and perceived seriousness of contracting illness. Subsequently, the model depicts that perceived benefits and barriers influence the likelihood and direction of the action that is taken. To illustrate how the HBM can assist in facilitating behavior change, specific strategies can be developed to facilitate behavior change. Table 15-3 illustrates the HBM applied to smoking cessation.

Health Promotion Model

Pender's (1987) health promotion model (HPM) is organized similarly to the HBM and represents the factors that may influence whether an individual engages in health-promoting behaviors (Fig. 15-3). The major areas within the model that are thought to influence the likelihood of engaging in health-promoting behaviors include factors that affect individual perception of health and health behavior, and factors that modify these perceptions.

According to the HPM, participation in health-promoting behaviors is determined by how important health is to the individual; perceived control of health, or whether an individual attributes changes in health to personal efforts or to external factors; perceived self-efficacy, defined as individuals' perceptions of their ability to perform a health behavior; definition of health; perceived health status; and perceived benefits and perceived barriers to engaging in the behavior. The second groups of factors, modifying factors, are those that modify the cognitive-perceptual factors identified above. These include demographic variables (age, gender, education, socioeconomic status), biological factors (e.g., body weight), interpersonal influences (e.g., support from others for engaging in behavior), situational factors (e.g., availability of healthy food), and

Table 15-3   **Example of Application of Health Belief Model Factors and Related Interventions With Smoking Cessation**

Factors	Interventions
Perceived susceptibility	Teach about disease process and risk factors, such as gender and age (morbidity and mortality statistics of smokers versus nonsmokers).
Perceived severity	Illustrate what happens to lungs and other organ systems when smoking; show pictures of diseased lungs.
Perceived barriers	Counsel client to avoid situations that are associated with smoking, such as spending time with smokers. Identify other barriers unique to individual and assist in overcoming.
Perceived benefits	Identify benefits, such as money saved from not smoking, morning cough reduced, improved health (as if person were nonsmoker 10 years after quitting)
Cues to action	Identify cues and substitute with another behavior other than smoking (e.g., when talking on the telephone and usually have a cigarette, drink water instead).

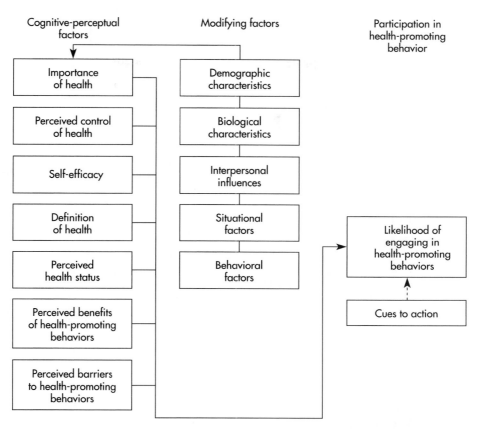

Fig. 15-3 Health promotion model. (Redrawn from Pender, N.J. [1987]. *Health promotion in nursing practice* [2nd ed.]. Norwalk, CT: Appleton & Lange.)

behavioral factors (e.g., previous experience with exercise program or healthy cooking). Cues to initiate action are anything in the environment that stimulate individuals to seek health care or practice healthy behavior. Cues might include information given from a friend or mass media programs.

Theory of Planned Behavior

Like the HBM, the theory of planned behavior (TPB) is a theory that emphasizes the influence of persons' beliefs on their intention to perform a behavior, and thus their actual behavior (Ajzen, 1988). This theory identifies three factors that influence intention to perform a behavior: attitude, subjective norms, and perceived control (Fig. 15-4). *Attitude* refers to the positive or negative feelings that one attaches to performing the behavior. Citing condom use in preventing sexually transmitted disease as an

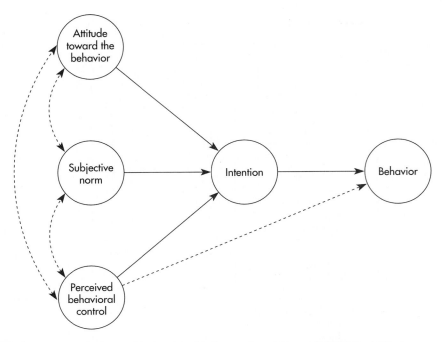

Fig. 15-4   Theory of planned behavior. (Redrawn from Ajzen, I. [1988]. *Attitudes, personality, and behavior.* Chicago: Dorsey Press.)

example, a nurse would want to determine a client's positive or negative feelings about condom use.

The second factor, *subjective norms,* is defined as the perceived social pressures to perform the behavior. These beliefs are those based on interpretations of what significant others believe should be done, as well as the individual's motivation to respond to this pressure.

A third element, *perceived control,* adds an important dimension for recognizing behaviors that are not solely under the individual's control. Perceived control refers to the individual's perception of whether he or she can perform the behavior and accounts for the influence of emotions, whether or not opportunities are available to actually perform the behavior, and dependence on others. For example, perceived control is significant in understanding women and safer sex, because some women may not have control over whether a male condom is used.

Interaction Model of Client Health Behavior

The interaction model of client health behavior (IMCHB) is a theory that incorporates some elements of the previous theories but in addition recognizes the influence of the nurse-client interaction on behaviors (Cox, 1982, 1986). The model is depicted in Fig. 15-5. The three major domains of the IMCHB are client singularity, client-professional interaction, and client health outcomes. The client singularity element contains variables that reflect the uniqueness that each individual brings to a situation. The client-professional interaction segment includes four factors reflecting nursing interventions and competencies: professional capabilities of the nurse, affective support, health information, and decisional control. An example of enactment of this part of the model is that nurses can choose to provide information or emotional support in any given situation. The health outcomes portion of the IMCHB includes utilization of health care services, clinical health indicators, severity of health problems, adherence to health behaviors, and satisfaction with health care.

• • •

This discussion of health behavior models has provided an overview of the variables contained within each model. These models have provided a basis for several research studies that can influence clinical practice. An example of how the determinants of health behavior can be applied to behavior change is depicted in the box on p. 337, which displays a newspaper article illustrating how this information can be useful for the lay public. It also provides an example of how nurses can use such models to help clients make a health behavior change.

MODIFYING INDIVIDUAL HEALTH BEHAVIOR

An assessment of factors that influence the client's health should take place before specific recommendation about changes can be made. Information about an individual's family history and about lifestyle factors will provide guidance about how behavior should be modified. Nurses must first know which behaviors need to be changed to prevent specific diseases. For example, it is commonly accepted that smoking, alcohol misuse, lack of exercise, and unhealthy diets are risk factors for disease.

Health Risk Appraisals

A *health risk appraisal* (HRA) is a tool that can be used for the purpose of determining how clients could benefit from purposeful behavior changes. It is a survey that is completed by the client about behavior, environmental conditions, emotional support, lifestyle choices, stress, and family history. Based on individuals' unique circumstances, recommendations are made for behavior change.

Some health risk appraisals assess broad areas, including the environment, education, health behavior, and stress. Others are more limited in their scope and focus only on a specific area, such as the Coronary Risk Profile (Wellsource, 1989). An example of a health risk appraisal that covers a broad view of health, the Healthier People Health Risk Appraisal, is shown in Fig. 15-6.

Depending on the type of HRA used, the results may be obtained through either self-scoring or computerized scoring. The Healthier People HRA assesses risks based on the 10 most common causes of death for the age and gender of the individual com-

Text continued on p. 342.

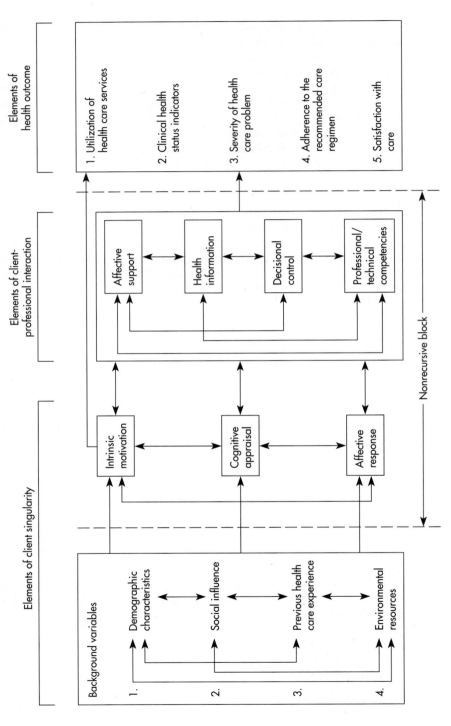

Fig. 15-5   Interaction model of client health behavior. (Redrawn from Cox, C.L. [1986]. The interaction model of client behavior: Application to the study of community-based elders. *Advances in Nursing Science, 9*[1], 40-57.)

Unhealthy Habits Can Be Changed

Most of the major causes of death in the United States result from our lifestyle. If we simply made changes in our behavior, odds are that we would live longer and lead a higher-quality life. Among the unhealthy habits that contribute to the leading causes of death are a sedentary activity level, smoking and alcohol abuse, and inappropriate diet, including excessive fat, refined sugar, and calories.

It seems that changing behavior would be easy—simply a matter of making up your mind to change and then doing it. To the contrary, those who have tried to quit smoking, eat lighter, or maintain an exercise program know that it can be extremely challenging to make behavior changes last. In fact, research has shown that it takes repeated efforts to be successful in changing.

Given this challenge, what factors are associated with success in adopting healthy habits? Research has revealed that there are many. The first is having the knowledge you need to take care of yourself, and the skills and resources to follow through on it. Information about specific health problems can be obtained from voluntary organizations. For example, the American Lung Association and American Cancer Society provide information about how to stop smoking, and the American Heart Association has material on low-fat eating. Health care professionals can also provide information.

Believing that you are susceptible to a disease may motivate you to take action to improve your health. For example, if you feel that it is possible for you to become ill from heart disease, you are more likely to exercise regularly and eat a low-fat diet. Learning about the risk factors for a specific disease can help you identify how susceptible you are to a disease. Examples of risk factors for some diseases are smoking, having a family history of the disease, and being overweight.

Another factor is a strong desire to change. This provides the necessary motivation to make a change in behavior and is extremely important to overcome urges to go back to unhealthy behaviors such as not exercising, smoking, or eating high-calorie foods.

Rewards can serve as motivation to change behavior. For example, saving money can be a positive motivator for quitting smoking. Weight loss can be a motivator for exercise. You can supply your own rewards for achieving success.

Support from other people also improves success. It is vitally important to spend time with people whose behaviors reinforce your own healthy behavior. Encouragement from others will also enhance your success. Having a buddy to exercise with can motivate you by making a commitment to the friend and the activity.

Finally, feeling confident and capable about performing the behavior is likely to make you more successful. You can increase your confidence that you will succeed in several ways—one way is to imagine yourself performing the behavior over and over again. This mental rehearsal makes behaviors like exercise easier. You might also try giving yourself encouragement and praise for your effort and success through positive self-talk. A technique that has been successful for some people is to envision yourself in front of a crowd applauding your success!

Although behavior change is difficult, it is possible. If you find you fall back into unhealthy behavior patterns, don't be self-critical, simply try again. Being unforgiving of yourself may actually depress your energy and the optimism needed to continue with your goals.

In summary, there are many strategies to help with behavior change, including understanding why you want to change, setting realistic goals for yourself, having a strong desire to change, obtaining support from other people, believing that you can make the change, and rewarding yourself. You are in control of your behavior and can choose whether to practice a positive, healthy lifestyle.

From Unhealthy habits can be changed. (1995, March 26). *Daily Progress.*

Healthier People
Health Risk Appraisal
The Carter Center of Emory University

No. _____

_____

Health risk appraisal is an educational tool. It shows you choices you can make to keep good health and avoid the most common causes of death for a person your age and sex. This health risk appraisal is not a substitute for a checkup or physical exam that you get from a doctor or nurse. It only gives you some ideas for lowering your risk of getting sick or injured in the future. It is NOT designed for people who already have HEART DISEASE, CANCER, KIDNEY DISEASE, OR MOST OTHER SERIOUS CONDITIONS. If you have any of these problems and you want a health risk appraisal anyway, ask your doctor or nurse to read the report with you.

DIRECTIONS: Your answers will be treated as confidential. Please keep the coupon with your participant number on it. You will need it to claim your computer report. To get the most accurate results, answer as many questions as you can and as best you can. If you do not know the answer leave it blank. Questions with a ★ (star symbol) are important to your health, but are not used by the computer to calculate your risks. However, your answers may be helpful in planning your health and fitness program.

Please put your answers in the empty boxes. (Examples: ☒ or ☐125)	
1. SEX	1 ☐ Male 2 ☐ Female
2. AGE	☐ Years
3. HEIGHT (Without shoes) (No fractions)	☐ Feet ☐ Inches
4. WEIGHT (Without shoes) (No fractions)	☐ Pounds
5. Body frame size	1 ☐ Small 2 ☐ Medium
6. Have you ever been told that you have diabetes (or sugar diabetes)?	1 ☐ Yes 2 ☐ No
7. Are you now taking medicine for high blood pressure?	1 ☐ Yes 2 ☐ No
8. What is your blood pressure now?	☐ / ☐ Systolic (High number)/Diastolic (Low number)
9. If you *do not* know the numbers, check the box that describes your blood pressure.	1 ☐ High 2 ☐ Normal or low 3 ☐ Don't know
10. What is your total cholesterol level (based on a blood test)?	☐ mg/dl
11. What is your HDL cholesterol (based on a blood test)?	☐ mg/dl
12. How many cigars do you usually smoke per day?	☐ cigars per day
13. How many pipes of tobacco do you usually smoke per day?	☐ pipes per day
14. How many times per day do you usually use smokeless tobacco? (Chewing tobacco, snuff, pouches, etc.)	☐ times per day

Fig. 15-6   Healthier People Health Risk Appraisal. (© Computer Outfitters, Tucson, Arizona. Used with permission.)

15. CIGARETTE SMOKING
How would you describe your cigarette smoking habits?

1 ☐ Never smoked   ☛ Go to 18
2 ☐ Used to smoke   ☛ Go to 17
                      ☛ Go to 16

16. STILL SMOKE
How many cigarettes a day do you smoke?
      ☛ GO TO QUESTION 18

[_____] cigarettes per day   ☛ Go to 18

17. USED TO SMOKE
a. How many years has it been since you smoked cigarettes fairly regularly?

[_____] years

b. What was the average number of cigarettes per day that you smoked in the 2 years before you quit?

[_____] cigarettes per day

18. In the next 12 months how many thousands of miles will you probably travel by each of the following?
(NOTE: U.S. average = 10,000 miles) a. Car, truck, or van:

[_____] ,000 miles

b. Motorcycle:

[_____] ,000 miles

19. On a typical day how do you USUALLY travel?
(Check one only)

1 ☐ Walk
2 ☐ Bicycle
3 ☐ Motorcycle
4 ☐ Subcompact or compact car
5 ☐ Mid-size or full-size car
6 ☐ Truck or van
7 ☐ Bus, subway, or train

20. What percent of the time do you usually buckle your safety belt when driving or riding?

[_____] %

21. On the average, how close to the speed limit do you usually drive?

1 ☐ Within 5 mph of limit
2 ☐ 6-10 mph over limit
3 ☐ 11-15 mph over limit
4 ☐ More than 15 mph over limit

22. How many times in the last month did you drive or ride when the driver had perhaps too much alcohol to drink?

[_____] times last month

23. How many drinks of alcoholic beverage do you have in a typical week?

☛ *(MEN GO TO QUESTION 33)*

(Write number of each type of drink)

[_____] Bottles or cans of beer
[_____] Glasses of wine
[_____] Wine coolers
[_____] Mixed drinks or shots of liquor

WOMEN

24. At what age did you have your first menstrual period?

[_____] years old

25. How old were you when your first child was born?

[_____] years old
(If no children write 0)

26. How long has it been since your last breast x-ray (mammogram)?

1 ☐ Less than 1 year ago
2 ☐ 1 year ago
3 ☐ 2 years ago
4 ☐ 3 or more years ago
5 ☐ Never

Fig. 15-6, cont'd   For legend see opposite page.   *Continued*

27. How many women in your natural family (mother and sisters only) have had breast cancer?	[_____] women

28. Have you had a hysterectomy operation?	1 ☐ Yes 2 ☐ No 3 ☐ Not sure

29. How long has it been since you had a pap smear?	1 ☐ Less than 1 year ago 2 ☐ 1 year ago 3 ☐ 2 years ago 4 ☐ 3 or more years ago 5 ☐ Never

★ 30. How often do you examine your breasts for lumps?	1 ☐ Monthly 2 ☐ Once every few months 3 ☐ Rarely or never

★ 31. About how long has it been since you had your breasts examined by a physician or nurse?	1 ☐ Less than 1 year ago 2 ☐ 1 year ago 3 ☐ 2 years ago 4 ☐ 3 or more years ago 5 ☐ Never

★ 32. About how long has it been since you had a rectal exam? ☛ *(WOMEN GO TO QUESTION 34)*	1 ☐ Less than 1 year ago 2 ☐ 1 year ago 3 ☐ 2 years ago 4 ☐ 3 or more years ago 5 ☐ Never

MEN ★ 33. About how long has it been since you had a rectal or prostate exam?	1 ☐ Less than 1 year ago 2 ☐ 1 year ago 3 ☐ 2 years ago 4 ☐ 3 or more years ago 5 ☐ Never

★ 34. How many times in the last year did you witness or become involved in a violent fight or attack where there was a good chance of a serious injury to someone?	1 ☐ 4 or more times 2 ☐ 2 or 3 times 3 ☐ 1 time or never

★ 35. Considering your age, how would you describe your overall physical health?	1 ☐ Excellent 2 ☐ Good 3 ☐ Fair 4 ☐ Poor

★ 36. In an average week, how many times do you engage in physical activity (exercise or work which lasts at least 20 minutes without stopping and which is hard enough to make you breathe heavier and your heart beat faster)?	1 ☐ Less than 1 time per week 2 ☐ 1 or 2 times per week 3 ☐ At least 3 times per week

★ 37. If you ride a motorcycle or all-terrain vehicle (ATV), what percent of the time do you wear a helmet?	1 ☐ 75% to 100% 2 ☐ 25% to 74% 3 ☐ Less than 25% 4 ☐ Does not apply to me

★ 38. Do you eat some food every day that is high in fiber, such as whole-grain bread, cereal, fresh fruits, or vegetables?	1 ☐ Yes 2 ☐ No

★ 39. Do you eat foods every day that are high in cholesterol or fat, such as fatty meat, cheese, fried foods, or eggs?	1 ☐ Yes 2 ☐ No

Fig. 15-6, cont'd   For legend see p. 338.

★ 40. In general, how satisfied are you with your life?	1 ☐ Mostly satisfied 2 ☐ Partly satisfied 3 ☐ Not satisfied
★ 41. Have you suffered a personal loss or misfortune in the past year that had a serious impact on your life? (For example, a job loss, separation, jail term, or the death of someone close to you.)	1 ☐ Yes, 1 serious loss or misfortune 2 ☐ Yes, 2 or more 3 ☐ No
★42a. Race	1 ☐ Aleutian, Alaska Native, Eskimo, or American Indian 2 ☐ Asian 3 ☐ Black 4 ☐ Pacific Islander 5 ☐ White 6 ☐ Other 7 ☐ Don't know
★42b. Are you of Hispanic origin, such as Mexican-American, Puerto Rican, or Cuban?	1 ☐ Yes 2 ☐ No
★ 43. What is the highest grade you completed in school?	1 ☐ Grade school or less 2 ☐ Some high school 3 ☐ High school graduate 4 ☐ Some college 5 ☐ College graduate 6 ☐ Postgraduate or professional degree
★ I.	A ☐ B ☐ C ☐ D ☐ E ☐ F ☐ G ☐ H ☐ I ☐ J ☐ K ☐ L ☐
★ II.	A ☐ B ☐ C ☐ D ☐ E ☐ F ☐ G ☐ H ☐ I ☐ J ☐ K ☐ L ☐

Last Name   First Name   M.I.

Address   City   State   Zip

Fig. 15-6, cont'd   For legend see p. 338.

pleting the HRA. The HRA gives an appraised age of each individual that is an estimate of that person's age based on lifestyle and risk. An achievable age is also provided and is based on what is possible if the person modifies his or her behavior and makes it healthier. The results provide specific information about how to improve health through changes in health behavior.

An HRA is best used in conjunction with laboratory findings, such as cholesterol and triglyceride levels, to provide clients with more information about their health status and the need to make changes. Although giving individuals feedback does not ensure that they will necessarily make behavior changes, the HRA does provide information that clients are able to understand about their risk and possible ways to reduce it.

Contracting may also be used with the HRA to formalize the agreed-on commitment between the client and the nurse. The contract may be verbal or written. This gives individuals specific goals and activities to work toward and underscores the importance of improving behavior.

Clinical Preventive Services

Another strategy for improving disease prevention is to educate health care providers about the need for such services. Griffith (1993) has noted that nurses and other primary care providers do not provide screening tests, immunizations, and counseling for improving health as often as they could. Possible reasons are that such services are not reimbursed and that providers are uncertain about who should get these services.

A prevention program developed by the U.S. Public Health Service Office of Disease Prevention and Health Promotion called "Put Prevention Into Practice" (PPIP) includes specific materials for nurses to use in facilitating disease prevention and health promotion. A handbook entitled *Guide to Clinical Preventive Services* provides an overview of specific interventions to prevent 60 diseases (Griffith & Rahman, 1994). A separate manual for health care providers, *The Clinician's Handbook of Clinical Preventive Services*, offers guidance on how to provide clinical preventive services. Another component is a booklet that is given to each client to serve as a reminder of when to seek services, as an educational tool on specific topics, and as a record of findings of the various laboratory and other diagnostic procedures. Separate booklets are available for adults (the *Personal Health Guide*) and for children (the *Child's Health Guide*). The box on p. 343 lists information contained in the *Child's Health Guide*.

SOCIETAL INFLUENCES ON HEALTH

The focus of the preceding section is on models of health behavior that emphasize individual factors such as health beliefs, attitudes, and knowledge. Butterfield (1990) contends that nurses must look beyond individual perceptions and capabilities if we are to be successful in helping clients to become healthier. Continuing to focus solely on the individual in one-to-one nurse-client interactions will not rectify many of the problems that influence health. Such additional interventions have long been used by

> ## Contents of *Child's Health Guide*
>
> Check-up visits (visit schedule)
> Immunization record
> Tests and exams
>   Growth
>   Blood pressure
>   Anemia
>   Lead
>   Vision and hearing
> Preventive care time line
> Health guidance
>   Development
>   Nutrition
>   Dental/oral health
>   Physical activity
>   Smoking
>   Safety
>   Message about sudden infant death syndrome
>   Child abuse
>   As your child grows up (alcohol, AIDS, birth control, etc.)
> Visit and illness record

From U.S. Public Health Service, Office of Disease Prevention and Health Promotion. (1993). *Child's health guide*. Washington, DC: U.S. Department of Health and Human Services.

public health nurses and include advocating for general economic and environmental improvement, for access to health care, and for quality of health care services to the populations served.

Healthy People 2000 Objectives

Healthy People 2000—National Health Promotion and Disease Prevention Objectives is a document that is widely used as a guide for actions to improve health (U.S. PHS, 1990). It focuses on both individual and societal influences on health. It recognizes not only that individual responsibility is necessary in order to achieve health, but also that environmental and socioeconomic factors that impact health are sometimes outside the control of individuals. For example, a client with few financial resources who is burdened by caring for an aging mother and a teenage daughter who has recently delivered a baby is more vulnerable to illness if she cannot seek health services when she needs them.

Healthy People 2000 is a guide to focusing efforts on three main goals. The first is to increase the span of healthy life for Americans rather than simply to prolong life in an unhealthy state. The second is to reduce health disparities among Americans. Because poverty strongly correlates with health, specifically focusing services on these groups is important. The third goal is to improve access to preventive services for all Americans, which emphasizes teaching people how to take better care of their health and to seek health care before disease has developed in order to prevent major illnesses.

To meet these goals, four major activities are emphasized:

1. Health promotion strategies, defined as those activities influenced by individual lifestyle
2. Health protection strategies, involving those related to regulatory measures that provide protection for large groups within a population, such as workers
3. Preventive services, including screening, counseling, and chemoprophylactic interventions for individuals
4. Continuing surveillance of the above three areas to note progress toward meeting the objectives

The box on p. 345 lists the specific content areas of *Healthy People 2000* that are addressed within the three main areas: health promotion, health protection, and prevention services.

Healthy Community Interventions

Recognition that health behavior change in individuals is likely to be more successful with support from the larger community has resulted in interventions that focus on the entire community. Community-wide norms that define healthy behaviors as acceptable and expected may influence individuals within the community.

One type of community intervention has focused on improving the cardiovascular health status of entire communities. Among these programs have been the Stanford Five City Project, the Pawtucket Heart Health Program, and Minnesota Heart Health Program (National Heart, Lung, and Blood Institute, 1990). These programs attempt to reduce risk factors such as obesity, high blood pressure, smoking, sedentary lifestyles, and serum cholesterol. Interventions include involvement of community members in providing community education on the prevention of cardiovascular disease using media campaigns. Partnership between the community and health care professionals is fostered and includes using community resources to develop health programs. Distinct programs are set up for different groups within the community, and the programs must be marketed so that community members are aware of them. Points of contact with the community include supermarkets, work sites, schools, churches, and other locations.

Preliminary results of the programs using a community health promotion strategy are encouraging but have varied. Noted benefits of these community programs have been reduced tobacco use, less weight gain, lowered blood pressure, reduced blood cholesterol levels, and lower coronary heart disease risks in general (Mittelmark et al., 1993; Salonen et al., 1989). In the Minnesota Heart Health Program, there were no differences in cholesterol levels, blood pressure, smoking activity, and exercise between communities that received health promotion interventions and communities that did not. All communities generally had trends toward improved cardiac health. Improvements in health promotion behavior have occurred generally across most communities, which has made the impact, if any, of these programs unclear (Luepker et al.,

---

Contents of *Healthy People 2000*

Health Promotion

Physical activity and fitness
Nutrition
Tobacco
Alcohol and other drugs
Family planning
Mental health and mental disorders
Violent and abusive behavior
Educational and community-based
    programs

Health Protection

Unintentional injuries
Occupational safety and health
Environmental health
Food and drug safety
Oral health

Preventive Services

Maternal and infant health
Heart disease and stroke
Cancer
Diabetes and chronic disabling conditions
HIV infection
Sexually transmitted diseases
Immunization and infectious diseases
Clinical preventive services

From U.S. Public Health Service. (1990). *Healthy People 2000.* Washington, DC: U.S. Department of Health and Human Services.

1994). Further research will continue into the effectiveness of community interventions and will become available in the future.

A second type of community program that has developed is the healthy cities initiatives. The model for these programs was first developed in Canada and Europe. The first site in the United States, the Indiana Healthy Community Project, was developed by a nurse (Flynn, Rider, & Bailey, 1992). Rather than focus on a predetermined health problem such as cardiovascular risk, the healthy cities initiatives focus on a broad range of health concerns that are identified by community members. The process is designed to build coalitions of community groups to develop programs to improve health. The California Healthy Cities Project (1994) has initiated programs focused on environmental protection, healthy behavior, and economic development. Issues such as gang violence, smoking cessation, and job creation are examples of these projects. The bases of such programs are community leadership, collaboration, and innovation to ultimately improve individuals' health status. These programs have provided a forum for community members to take action to address problems specific to their community.

Both the Healthy Cities initiatives and community-wide health promotion programs are examples of focusing interventions on entire communities. These projects recognize the importance of communication and support among people for healthy behavior change.

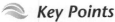 *Key Points*

- Health may be defined as simply the absence of disease, or it may be defined so that it reflects social and environmental dimensions of health.

- Smith's four models of health are the clinical, role performance, adaptive, and eudaimonistic models. Nurses will be more effective in promoting health if they function from the adaptive and eudaimonistic models.

- The three levels of disease prevention are primary, secondary, and tertiary prevention. Primary prevention is protection from a disease while still in a healthy state; secondary prevention is early detection and treatment of a disease; and tertiary prevention is prevention of complications and maintenance of health.

- Health promotion and disease prevention are differentiated in that health promotion activities aim to achieve a healthier state and disease prevention activities are specific to one disease.

- The major causes of death are related to lifestyle and individual choices in behavior.

- Determinants of why people engage in healthy or unhealthy behaviors are depicted in various health behaviors models. Four that are described in this chapter are the health belief model, the theory of planned behavior, the health promotion model, and the interaction model of client health behavior.

- Tools used to modify individual health behavior include health risk appraisals. Efforts to educate health professionals about preventive services will ultimately influence individuals to whom they provide care.

- Community norms and standards influence individuals' health behaviors. Health promotion programs, such as the healthy cities projects, have been developed to target entire communities.

 Critical Thinking Exercises

1. Assess your behavior by reviewing your exercise, diet, sleep, and recreation patterns. Select one behavior that you wish to change. Using the behavior theories in this chapter as a foundation, describe possible reasons why you engage in the behavior. Develop a plan to help you achieve a change in your behavior.

2. Interview three persons for their definition of health. Write their definition and determine under which of Smith's four models their definition could be categorized.

3. Select one of the four health behavior models described in this chapter. Considering behaviors that reduce cardiac risk, identify nursing interventions derived from this model to assist clients in making a behavior change.

References

Ajzen, I. (1988). *Attitudes, personality, and behavior.* Chicago: Dorsey Press.

Becker, M.H., Haefner, D.P., Kasl, S.V., Kirscht, J.P., Maiman, L.A., & Rosenstock, J.P. (1977). Selected psychosocial models and correlates of individual health-related behaviors. *Medical Care, 15*(5), 27-46.

Brubaker, B.H. (1983). Health promotion: A linguistic analysis. *Advances in Nursing Science, 5*(3), 1-14.

Butterfield, P. (1990). Thinking upstream: Nurturing a conceptual understanding of the societal context of health behavior. *Advances in Nursing Science, 12*(2), 1-8.

California Healthy Cities Project. (1994). *Connections, 6*(2), 1-5.

Centers for Disease Control and Prevention. (1994). Advance report of final mortality statistics, 1992. *Monthly Vital Statistics Report, 43,* 6.

Champion, V.L. (1994). Strategies to increase mammography utilization. *Medical Care, 32,* 119-129.

Cox, C.L. (1982). Motivation in health behavior: Measurement, antecedents, and correlates. *Advances in Nursing Science, 9*(4), 1-15.

Cox, C.L. (1986). The interaction model of client health behavior: Application to the study of community-based elders. *Advances in Nursing Science, 9*(1), 40-57.

Dunn, H.L. (1959). High level wellness for man and society. *American Journal of Public Health, 49,* 88.

Dunn, H.L. (1971). *High level wellness.* Arlington, VA: Beatty.

Flynn, B.C., Rider, M.S., & Bailey, W.W. (1992). Developing community leadership in healthy cities: The Indiana model. *Nursing Outlook, 49*(3), 121-126.

Gerhart, S.L. (1992). *The use of child car safety restraints: A test of the health belief model.* Unpublished doctoral dissertation, Indianapolis, Indiana University.

Griffith, H.M. (1993). Needed—A strong nursing position on preventive service. *Image: Journal of Nursing Scholarship, 25*(4), 272.

Griffith, H.M., & Rahman, M.I. (1994). Implementing the Put Prevention Into Practice Program. *Nurse Practitioner, 19*(10), 12-19.

Hellinger, F. (1993). The lifetime costs of treating a person with HIV. *JAMA, 270,* 474-478.

Hochbaum, G.M. (1958). *Public participation in medical screening programs: A sociopsychological study* (U.S. PHS Publication No. 572). Washington, DC: Department of Health and Human Services.

Leavell, H.R., & Clark, D.W. (1965). *Preventive medicine for the doctor in his community.* New York: McGraw-Hill.

Luepker, R.V., Murray, D.M., Jacobs, D.R., Mittelmark, M.B., Bracht, N., Carlaw, R., Crow, R., Elmer, P., Finnegan, J., Folsom, A.R., Grimm, R., Hannan, P.J., Jeffrey, R., Lando, H., McGovern, P., Mullis, R., Perry, C.L., Pechacek, T., Pirie, P., Sprafka, J.M., Weisbrod, R., & Blackburn, H. (1994). Community education for cardiovascular disease prevention: Risk factor changes in the Minnesota Heart Health Program. *American Journal of Public Health, 84*(9), 1383-1393.

Lux, K.M., & Petosa, R. (1994). Using the health belief model to predict safer sex intentions of incarcerated youth. *Health Education Quarterly, 21,* 487-497.

McGinnis, J.M., & Foege, W.H. (1993). Actual causes of death in the United States. *Journal of the American Medical Association, 270,* 18.

Mittelmark, M.B., Hunt, M.K., Heath, G.W., & Schmid, T.L. (1993). Realistic outcomes: Lessons from community-based research and demonstration programs for the prevention of cardiovascular diseases. *Journal of Public Health Policy, 14*(4), 437-461.

National Heart, Lung, and Blood Institute. (1990). Three community programs change heart health across the nation. *[Special edition]. Infomemo.*

Pender, N.J. (1987). *Health promotion in nursing practice.* Norwalk, CT: Appleton & Lange.

Risk Assessment Systems. (1991). *Healthier people health risk appraisal.* Memphis, TN: Risk Assessment Systems, Inc.

Salonen, J.T., Tuomilehto, J., Nissinen, A., Kaplan, G.A., & Puska, P. (1989). Contribution of risk factor changes to the decline in coronary incidence during the North Karelia project: A within community analysis. *International Journal of Epidemiology, 18,* 595-601.

Smith, J. (1983). *The idea of health: Implications for the nursing profession.* New York: Teachers College Press.

U.S. Public Health Service. (1979). *Healthy people: Surgeon General's report on health promotion and disease prevention.* Washington, DC: U.S. Department of Health and Human Services.

U.S. Public Health Service. (1990). *Healthy people 2000.* Washington, DC: U.S. Department of Health and Human Services.

Wellsource. (1989). *Coronary risk appraisal.* Clackamas, OR: Wellsource.

World Health Organization. (1958). *The first ten years of the World Health Organization.* New York: The Organization.

Challenges in Teaching and Learning

16

Joan Garity

Objectives

At the completion of this chapter, the reader will be able to:

- Discuss the principles and practices of an effective teaching-learning experience.
- Compare and contrast major teaching-learning theories.
- Distinguish between child-centered and adult-centered teaching and learning.
- Design teaching-learning experiences for individuals and groups.

Profile in Practice

Janet S. Wyatt, PhD, RN, NP
Chief, Community Health Nursing–Preventive Medicine Service,
U.S. Army Health Clinic, SHAPE,
Brussels, Belgium;
Adjunct Assistant Professor,
Graduate School of Nursing,
Uniformed Services University of the Health Sciences,
Bethesda, Maryland

While beliefs, attitudes, motivation, culture, and many other variables influence how, what, and why we learn, knowledge and information remain the foundation for many patient education encounters. One of our most important responsibilities as nurses is to remain current regarding our knowledge of disease, treatment, and health promotion.

The many questions generated by patients in our TB clinic have required that all of our community health nurses become TB experts. Recent changes in methods for TB skin testing and interpretation have made many clients suspicious and confused. Clients think that technology has moved backward when they learn that the simple four-pronged tine skin test, with its self-read card, is now scientifically inaccurate. When TB skin test results are positive, clients immediately flood the nurse with questions; "Am I contagious?" "Does this mean I will get sick with TB?" "Should my family members get tested?" "Since I've always been negative before, why is my skin test positive now?" We are challenged to offer clear and simple, scientifically sound explanations to help reasonable people make reasonable decisions regarding their health care.

Initially our patient education had to focus on helping individuals unlearn and discard information that has for many years been trusted. Explanations of why old testing methods are no longer valid have been immediately followed with information about the accuracy of new methods and a clear decision pathway regarding recommendations for laboratory tests and drug treatment. Fears of disease and concern about infecting others have been eased as new information about the epidemiology, transmission, and progression of TB infection is presented.

Despite our desire to package our teaching in appropriate amounts to foster progressive and sequential learning, many patients want to know everything about their treatment immediately. As we have tried to meet patients' immediate needs for knowledge and reassurance, we have varied our teaching strategies to enhance learning. Colorful posters have provided a visual display of information about skin-testing methods and results. Written one-page handouts summarize each component of verbal teaching. Since compliance with any health treatment has often been linked to attitude, we have spent time at the end of each visit discussing how test results, treatment plans, and medication have personally affected each individual. As we get smart about TB, our clients get smart, and make us even smarter with information about their health experiences during treatment. This teaching-learning partnership recognizes and values the unique contribution of professionals and patients to the process of health education. The importance of this partnership in our TB clinic has continually been reinforced. Our current clients remain one of our best referral sources.

The nurse's role with patients and families encourages, promotes, and frequently demands planned teaching-learning experiences. Most readers have probably encountered patient-teaching situations similar to the following:

- *The mother of a 2-year-old newly diagnosed with juvenile diabetes needs to learn how to monitor her child's blood sugar and give his insulin injections.*
- *A 54-year-old African-American male security guard has just been diagnosed with hypertension. He will need follow-up care in the ambulatory clinic of the local medical center for continued teaching about the signs and symptoms of the disease, the side effects of his medications, and the importance of diet and exercise in relation to this health problem.*
- *A hospice nurse visits a new patient, who has terminal cancer, at her daughter's home. The daughter, who is 32, married, and the mother of two young children (3 and 6), is also blind. She very much wishes to be her mother's primary caregiver and needs to learn how to change her mother's colostomy bag.*

- *An 18-year-old girl who comes to the family-planning clinic for birth control pills has little knowledge about safe sex. She is dating a man with a history of intravenous drug use.**

Few nurses have had formal preparation or coursework in teaching and learning (DeYoung, 1990; Heinrich & Scherr, 1994). While nursing textbooks emphasize the teaching role of the nurse, most provide little information about the process of teaching and learning. Even within nursing education, there is a dearth of articles and studies addressing teaching-learning skills and the evaluation of learning outcomes (Tanner, 1994). Redman (1993a), a prominent nurse author on the topic of patient education, reported the following observations in a 25-year review:

- Only 37 reviews or metaanalyses exist on the accumulated research in patient education.
- Development of patient education has occurred by field of specialization, notably in diabetes, prenatal/parenting, cardiovascular problems, medicine compliance, AIDS, cancer, and mental health. Surprisingly, given the ever-increasing age of the population, there has been almost no development in the field of geriatrics.
- Systematic review of master's programs in nursing shows courses in patient education to be quite rare.
- A preliminary review of 31 nursing textbooks showed that about 45% had substantial content on teaching. Maternity textbooks displayed the most developed model of patient education.
- Considerable focus exists on readability of patient education materials, but there is little or no focus on whom they are effective in teaching.
- Nursing diagnosis categories for expressing learning needs are incomplete. There is heavy reliance on the extremely limited category of "knowledge deficit."
- The increasing population with chronic disease will require practitioners skilled in addressing teaching and learning about functional loss, pain, and anxiety.

This chapter presents the principles and practices of effective teaching-learning experiences, reviews some of the major teaching-learning theories, distinguishes between andragogy and pedagogy, presents research on teaching-learning styles, provides tips for designing successful teaching-learning experiences, and reviews evaluation methods.

TEACHING AND LEARNING

Teaching is a set of planned, purposeful activities that assist the learner in acquiring new skills, knowledge, attitudes, or values. Since the late 1950s most teaching and training efforts have stressed a similar model with five parts: analysis, design, development, implementation, and evaluation/revision (Thompson, 1991). This model has led to an overemphasis on the process of teaching (i.e., writing instructor objectives and lesson plans) and a deemphasis on learning (i.e., learner outcomes and performance).

*The teaching plan for this client is presented at the end of the chapter.

Learning is defined as "the way in which individuals or groups acquire, interpret, organize, change, or assimilate a related cluster of information, skills, and feelings and construct meaning in their personal and shared family/work lives" (Marsick & Watkins, 1990, p. 4). According to these authors, 83% of all learning is informal and incidental. *Informal learning* may result from interactions with others through networking, coaching, and mentoring. Self-directed learning of a predominantly experiential and noninstitutional nature may also be termed informal learning. *Incidental learning,* on the other hand, consists of learning from mistakes, assumptions, beliefs, attributions, and internalized meanings and is a by-product of another activity. Perhaps this is one reason why the most successful client learning often takes place in groups such as weight loss groups, grief support groups, and parenting groups, where clients help one another.

Transfer of Learning

The key to successful application of learning is the perception of how important new learning is to the learner's ability to function effectively in his or her own milieu (Kemerer, 1991). Transfer of learning is linked to the extent to which the learning environment resembles the actual environment where the learning will be applied (Gagne, 1977; Knowles, 1980). Strategies to increase learning transfer include focusing on behavior rather than knowledge, setting realistic expectations, and establishing rewards. Factors that inhibit transfer of learning include unclear expectations, poor timing, no ownership by the learner, isolated teaching, and little opportunity for reinforcement (Kemerer, 1991).

Learner Responsibility for Learning

In today's permissive society, it has become all too common to hear, "If the learner doesn't learn, the teacher didn't teach." It is important that both the teacher and the learner understand teaching-learning theories and research in order to nurture learner growth and cultivate a responsibility for learning (Davis & Murrell, 1993; Pace, 1984). For example, a study of learner withdrawal patterns demonstrated the importance of social integration (belonging) to learner retention (Tinto, 1987). Another study found that learning and development are directly affected by the learner's interaction with teachers and peers plus the learner's quality of effort (Pascarella, 1985). Finally, Astin (1985) presented a theory relating learner involvement to the level of learner development. The findings of these studies provide valuable insights about the teaching-learning experience.

Mutuality and Trust

It is important to remember that the most successful teaching-learning experiences involve a process in which an interpersonal relationship of shared mutuality and trust is established between the teacher and the learner. In such a relationship, the nurse is viewed as the knowledge and information expert on health, and the client is seen as the expert on the need for information, support, and related health behaviors within the particular context of his life. The accent is on the learner actively engaging, discovering, and taking responsibility for new ways of acting and problem solving. For example, a client in a short-term rehabilitation center who relearns activities of daily living following a stroke is actively engaged in the learning process.

Characteristics of Effective Teachers

Most of us teach the way we were taught, imitating the behaviors of the best teachers we have known and minimizing the worst behaviors of those teachers we did not like. To be an effective teacher, however, requires that we develop a sound educational theory and research base, learn the specifics of the teacher-learner roles, find new ways of interrelating, and continually explore new teaching methods. In addition, we must possess the ability to critique our own performance and possess the willingness to be critiqued by others (DeYoung, 1990).

Five characteristics are consistently attributed to excellent teachers in the college setting: (1) enthusiasm, (2) clarity, (3) preparation/organization of material, (4) ability to stimulate the learner, and (5) love of knowledge (Sherman et al., 1987). Although there are few studies that define and evaluate teaching effectiveness in nursing, categories such as availability to the learner, knowledge of subject, interpersonal style, teaching methods, teaching style, and evaluation methods have emerged (Reeve, 1994). Surprisingly, no studies were found that identified effective teaching-learning characteristics with clients.

TEACHING-LEARNING THEORIES

There exists no shortage of theories relative to the teaching-learning process. Some theories focus on changes in the learner, whereas others describe the preferred teaching methods. Since no single approach to teaching and learning is effective for all clients, the nurse must draw from a variety of perspectives when designing teaching-learning experiences for the client. An overview of selected teaching-learning theories follows.

Theories of Learning

Theories of learning can be divided into three major classifications: behaviorist, cognitive, and humanistic.

Behaviorist theories. The *behaviorists* believe that changed behavior (new learning) results from a stimulus and a conditioned response that requires reinforcement (a reward). Behaviorist theories include modeling or repeated practice of a new behavior until it is internalized (Bandura, 1971), stimulus substitution (Wolpe & Lazarus, 1966), operant conditioning (Skinner, 1953), and stimulus response (Pavlov, 1927), all of which positively or negatively shape or condition the learner. Another behaviorist theory is connectionism or trial-and-error learning (Thorndike, 1913).

Teachers who subscribe to behaviorist theories will give learners feedback about their performance and reward movement toward the desired behavior. For example, "You've reached your long-term goal of a 20-pound weight loss this week. What tangible or intangible reward (other than food) are you going to give yourself? What is your plan for maintaining this weight over the next several months?" Table 16-1 summarizes the learning principles and teaching applications relative to behaviorist theory.

Cognitive theories. *Cognitive theory* is based on an internal change in the perception (information processing) of the individual. This change is neither obvious nor measurable and allows the individual to receive information from the environment in multiple ways. Cognitive theories include information processing or moving from simple to complex skill (Gagne, 1974), field theory in which the positive and negative forces for change are identified (Lewin, 1951), hierarchical structure or identification of lev-

---

Table 16-1   Learning Principles and Teaching Applications Relative to Behaviorist Theory

MAJOR THEORIES AND THEORISTS	
Connectionism	E. L. Thorndike
Stimulus-response	I. Pavlov
Operant conditioning	B. F. Skinner
Stimulus substitution	J. Wolpe and A. Lazarus
Modeling	A. Bandura
Learning Principle	**Teaching Application**
Humans learn through trial and error.	Provide opportunity for problem solving.
Learning develops over time.	Provide adequate practice time; plan retesting or repeat demonstrations both immediately and at later intervals.
Given a stimulus, the learner responds.	Plan teaching strategies to trigger desired response; avoid unnecessary information that may detract from desired response.
Positive and negative feedback influence learning; positive feedback is remembered longer.	Reward learner for all correct behavior; praising positive behavior is better than punishing mistakes.
Learning is strengthened each time a positive response is received or a negative consequence is avoided.	Continue praise and positive reinforcement throughout the teaching transaction.
Learning occurs through linking behavior with associated response.	Proceed from simple to complex; provide information to show that learning is occurring.
Learning remains until other learning interferes with original learned response.	Assess prior experience with subject; some "unlearning" may be needed before new learning can take place.

els of learning (Bloom, 1956), and discovery learning in which children progress through predictable stages of cognitive development (Piaget, 1954).

Teachers who use cognitive theories believe that when learners perceive a need to acquire new knowledge, skills, or attitudes, they will be motivated to learn. For example, alcoholics who become dedicated members of Alcoholics Anonymous following the loss of their job, family, and other social supports may have a high level of motivation to learn new behaviors. A summary of cognitive theory and applications is presented in Table 16-2.

Humanistic theories. In *humanistic theory,* learning is self-motivated, self-directed, and self-evaluated. The teacher provides information and support to help learners increase their cognitive and affective functioning. Humanistic theories include andragogy or adult-centered learning (Knowles, 1984), hierarchy of needs or motivation-based learning (Maslow, 1970), self-directed learning (Rogers, 1969), reality theory of self-awareness learning (Glasser, 1965), perceptual-existential theory or self-determined learning (Combs, 1965), and values clarification learning (Dewey, 1938).

Teachers who use humanistic theories will encourage learners to set their own goals and work toward them. For example, a nurse might ask a diabetic client, "When do you think you'll be ready to give your own insulin injection? What activities or steps would help you to get ready to do this?" Table 16-3 summarizes teaching applications and learning principles relative to humanistic theories.

Table 16-2   Learning Principles and Teaching Applications Relative to Cognitive Theory

MAJOR THEORIES AND THEORISTS	
Cognitive discovery	J. Piaget
Field theory	K. Lewin
Information processing theory	R. Gagne
Hierarchal structure	B. Bloom

Learning Principle	Teaching Application
Learning is based on a change in perception.	All learning cannot be readily observed; information must be internalized.
Perception is influenced by the senses.	Use multisensory teaching strategies; adjust environment to minimize distractions.
Perception is dependent on learning and is influenced by both internal and external variables.	Assess attitude toward learning, past experiences with similar situations, culture, maturity, developmental level, and physical ability before designing teaching plan.
Personal characteristics have an impact on how a cue is perceived.	Identify learning style and target it in the teaching process; develop a flexible approach.
Perceptions are selectively chosen to be focused on by the individual.	Focus learner on what is to be learned; provide support and guidance.

Table 16-3   **Learning Principles and Teaching Applications Relative to Humanistic Theory**

MAJOR THEORIES AND THEORISTS	
Self-directed learning	C. Rogers
Hierarchy of needs	A. Maslow
Perceptual-existential theory	A. Combs
Values clarification	J. Dewey
Reality theory	W. Glasser
Andragogy	M. Knowles
Learning Principle	**Teaching Application**
Learning is self-initiated.	Promote self-directed learning.
Learner is an active participant in teaching-learning transaction.	Serve as a facilitator, mentor, and resource for learner to encourage active learning.
Learning should promote development of insight, judgment, values, and self-concept.	Avoid imposing own values and views on learner; support development of learner's self-concept.
Learning proceeds best if it is relevant to learner.	Expose learner to new, necessary information; pose relevant questions to encourage learner to seek answers.

Patterns of Knowing

Before the 1950s the apprenticeship model of education in nursing often produced graduate nurses who determined what was right and wrong in nursing practice by observing more experienced nurses, memorizing rules and facts about specific tasks, and seldom asking questions (Ashley, 1976; Reverby, 1987). In contrast, today's graduates face an increasingly complex and specialized practice that requires a rich theory base, critical thinking skills, and a value system for making ethical decisions (Oermann, 1994). Jenks (1993) suggested that nurses could narrow the education-practice gap by developing teaching methodologies based on the patterns of knowing. Several patterns of knowing have been identified in the nursing literature and include the following: (1) ethics, the moral knowledge in nursing; (2) esthetics, the art of nursing; (3) personal knowledge in nursing; and (4) empirics, the science of nursing (Carper, 1978). *Ethical knowledge* seeks credibility for providing care and focuses on matters of obligation or what ought to be done. *Esthetic knowledge* is used to creatively structure, design, and implement nursing care. *Empiric* or *scientific knowledge* is based on objective evidence obtained by the senses, validated and verified by others, and used to describe or predict nursing actions and outcomes. *Personal knowledge* is a synthesis of knowing based on past experiences that is integrated into current situations. Chinn and Kramer (1995) built on Carper's work by developing the conceptualizations described in Table 16-4.

Andragogy and Pedagogy

Knowles (1980) described *andragogy* as the art and science of helping adults learn. The adult learner has a multitude of life experiences on which to build and is moti-

Table 16-4 **Patterns of Knowing**

Ethics	Esthetics	Empirics	Personal
Valuing	Engaging	Describing	Opening
Clarifying	Intuiting	Explaining	Centering
Advocating	Envisioning	Predicting	Realizing

Modified from Chinn, P.L., & Kramer, M.K. (1995). *Theory and nursing.* (4th ed.). St. Louis: Mosby.

vated by the desire for self-growth and self-direction. Characteristics of adult learners have implications for teaching methodology as illustrated in Table 16-5 (Knowles, 1970).

Pedagogy is the art and science of teaching children. In contrast to andragogy, pedagogy is primarily initiated, planned, and facilitated by the teacher. The nurse's understanding of growth and development and age-appropriate expectations ensures a successful teaching-learning experience with children. For example, nonverbal communication, use of touch, and a soothing tone of voice can be effective teaching strategies with infants and very young children who have not yet developed language skills. The use of play, exploration, and observation with puppets have all proved to be useful teaching strategies with toddlers and preschoolers. Since school-age children have a larger vocabulary and greater repertoire of problem-solving skills and abilities, they can learn better through formal teaching interactions, such as coloring, creating, handling objects, and asking questions. Finally, adolescents, who are struggling for their identity and are strongly influenced by their peers, challenge the teacher to respect their growing intelligence by designing more creative teaching-learning experiences. For example, the hazards of substance abuse can be effectively communicated to adolescents by posters displayed outside cafeterias or other popular gathering places.

Pedagogy requires different assumptions than does andragogy. While the life experiences of adults serve as a rich resource for learning, the life experiences of children are minimal. In addition, the child's orientation to learning is usually subject centered, whereas the adult's is problem centered. Table 16-6 presents a comparison of the assumptions underlying pedagogy and andragogy.

The design of teaching-learning experiences necessarily differs for children and adults. For example, the climate for pedagogy is more formal and authority oriented, whereas the climate for andragogy is more collaborative and informal. Learning objectives are usually formulated by the teacher in pedagogy while being mutually negotiated in andragogy. A comparison of pedagogy and andragogy design elements is shown in Table 16-7.

Learning Styles and Preferences

Few would argue that each of us learns in different ways. For example, some individuals prefer a lecture, others a group discussion, and still others problem solving a

Table 16-5   **Characteristics of Adult Learners and Implications for Teaching**

Characteristics	Implications
Adults want to learn but do not always respond to traditional methods of teaching.	Diverse ways of learning, such as small project groups, teams, independent study, etc., need to be offered.
Life experiences influence how adults learn.	Learning can be enhanced by sharing these life experiences through use of discussion, role-playing, and case method.
Adults learn best if they can actively participate in learning.	If adults help to plan and conduct their own learning experiences, they will learn more than if they are passive recipients.
Identifying usefulness of the learning to the individual can enhance overall motivation of adult learner.	Learner must be involved in a mutual process of formulating learning objectives in which needs of learner, subject, institution, and society are taken into account.
Adults can be anxious about their ability to succeed.	Learning environment needs to be characterized by physical comfort, mutual trust, respect and helpfulness, freedom of expression, and acceptance of differences.
Adults enter learning experiences with different levels of learner readiness.	Learning will be more effective when programs are sequenced to allow for different levels of learner readiness.
Adults like to apply learning to more immediate life problems or situations.	Learning experiences organized around life problems will be more relevant than those organized around subject topics.

Table 16-6   **Comparison of the Assumptions of Pedagogy and Andragogy**

	Pedagogy	Andragogy
Self-concept	Dependence	Increasing self-directiveness
Experience	Needs to be built on	Learners are a rich resource for learning
Readiness	Biological development Social pressure	Developmental tasks of life roles
Time perspective	Postponed application	Immediate application
Orientation to learning	Subject centered	Problem centered

Modified from Knowles, M. (1980). *The modern practice of adult education: From pedagogy to andragogy* (Rev. ed.). Chicago: Follett.

Table 16-7   Comparison of the Design Elements of Pedagogy and Andragogy

	Pedagogy	Andragogy
Climate	Authority oriented Formal Competitive	Mutual Collaborative/informal Respectful
Planning	By teacher	Mechanism for mutual planning
Diagnosis of needs	By teacher	Mutual self-diagnosis
Formulation of objectives	By teacher	Mutual negotiation
Design	Logic of the subject matter Content units	Sequenced in terms of readiness Problem units
Activities	Transmittal techniques	Experiential techniques (inquiry)
Evaluation	By teacher	Mutual rediagnosis of needs Mutual measurement of program

Modified from Knowles, M. (1980). *The modern practice of adult education: From pedagogy to andragogy* (Rev. ed.). Chicago: Follett.

case study. A rich literature and research base exists on these individual differences in preferences and learning styles (Kolb, 1984; Witkin et al., 1977). Kogan (1971) defines *learning styles* as "individual variations in modes of perceiving, remembering, and thinking, or distinctive ways of apprehending, storing, transforming and utilizing information" (p. 244).

There are more than 11 learning style models (Partridge, 1983). Two of the most frequently used are Witkin's field dependence-independence model and Kolb's experiential learning theory model.

According to Witkin's model, the *field-dependent* individual perceives the whole, but not the parts, of a learning situation, whereas the *field-independent* person separates the background information from the whole. These differences are reflected in both the interpersonal characteristics and the learning behaviors of these individuals (Witkin, 1977a). For example, field-dependent individuals learn in a global fashion, have a short attention span, view the teacher as a facilitator, and prefer the discussion method. Field-independent individuals, on the other hand, are analytical in their learning, focus on ideas and concepts, have long attention spans, view the teacher as an information giver, and prefer the lecture method.

Differences in learning styles also influence how teachers teach (Witkin, 1977b). For example, field-independent teachers lecture, use questions to introduce topics, emphasize standards and principles, and provide both positive and negative feedback. Field-dependent teachers, on the other hand, design student-centered learning experiences, teach facts, use questions to check student learning after instruction, and link what is taught to life experience.

Mesoff (1979) identified differences in field-dependent and field-independent learning styles in research studies with groups. Field-dependent individuals were found to be participant observers, emphasize cooperation and collaboration, facilitate group process, conform to peer pressure, look for feedback, and be motivated by the other group members. Field-independent individuals were shown to be active participants, test out opinions and ideas, assume group leadership (especially in a vacuum), be less affected by peer pressure and feedback, and be motivated by meeting challenges. Table 16-8 summarizes the differences in field-independent and field-dependent learners, teachers, and group members.

The Kolb model is based on experiential learning theory (ELT) developed from the works of Jung (1971), Dewey (1938), Lewin (1951), and Piaget (1970), all of whom emphasized both the process of learning, especially active participation, and the environmental influences of learning. Kolb's Learning Style Inventory (LSI) is designed to identify an individual's learning style preference as one of the following: (1) *accommodator* (active doer and risk taker), (2) *assimilator* (abstract conceptualizer and reflec-

Table 16-8   Comparison of Field-Dependent and Field-Independent Learners, Teachers, and Behavior in Groups

Field-Dependent Learning Style	Field-Independent Learning Style
Learners	
Global (wholes; gestalts)	Analytical (reflective; complex)
Relational	Idea or concept oriented
Short attention span (speed skater)	Long attention span (distance skater)
Views teacher as facilitator	Views teacher as information giver
Prefers discussion method	Prefers lecture method
Teachers	
Design student-centered learning experiences	Lecture
Teach facts	Emphasize standards and principles
Use questions to check student learning after instruction	Use questions to introduce topics
Link what's taught to life experience	Give both positive and negative feedback
Behavior in Groups	
Participant observers	Active participants
Emphasize cooperation, collaboration, and participation	Test out opinions, ideas, and hypotheses
Facilitate group process	Take on group leadership
Conform more to peer pressure	Less affected by peer pressure
Look for feedback	Less influenced by feedback
Motivated by group members	Motivated by meeting challenges

tive observer), (3) *converger* (problem solver and decision maker), and (4) *diverger* (active doer and reflective observer). A sample of the LSI can be found in Kolb (1984).

Nursing research on learning styles. A few studies have been conducted examining nurses' learning styles. Garity (1985a, 1985b) used Witkin's tool and found that head nurses had field-dependent learning styles, and Sherbinski (1994) used Kolb's tool and found that the predominant learning style of nurse anesthetist students was the assimilator style, which emphasizes reflective observation and abstract conceptualization. The assimilator learning style also was predominant in a study of diploma nursing students (Rakoczy & Money, 1995). In a sample of 93 home health aides, however, 56% were divergers and preferred instructional processes that present materials or information in a concrete learning style (Colucciello, 1993). No studies were found that addressed client learning styles. In a recent critical review, Thompson and Crutchlow (1993) supported the use of Kolb's model and recommended that nurse researchers conduct studies investigating the influence of learning style on the learning environment.

THE TEACHING-LEARNING PLAN

The steps in the teaching-learning plan parallel those of the nursing process and include assessing the learner, developing learner objectives, selecting teaching-learning strategies, implementing the teaching plan, and evaluating outcomes.

Assessing the Learner

There are some key elements that should be explored when assessing the learning needs of clients. These include (1) knowledge level, (2) developmental characteristics (e.g., age, reading ability), (3) preferred sensory channel (i.e., auditory, kinesthetic, visual), (4) motivation or readiness to learn, (5) anxiety level, (6) health values, and (7) health status. An effective way to gather some of this information is through questioning. An assessment tool based on questioning that I have used successfully with clients on both a cardiac surgical and a neurological unit is shown in Fig. 16-1.

Characteristics of the learner can serve as enhancers or barriers to learning and influence the outcome of the teaching-learning experience. A partial list of enhancers and barriers to learning is presented in Table 16-9.

Assessing Special Groups

Clients who are from an unfamiliar culture or who are challenged in some way often have complex and unique learning needs. Assessing the special characteristics of these learners will aid in identifying learning needs and choosing teaching strategies that are appropriate and effective.

Cultural considerations. According to Ferguson (1994), by the year 2000, 85% of new entrants to the nation's workforce will be members of minority groups and

---

Learner Assessment Tool

Things I know about my health problem are:

Today I'd like to learn these three things about my health problem from you, nurse...

1._____

_____

2._____

_____

3._____

_____

_____

I would like to know or ask the doctor/nurse...

If I were teaching a patient like me, I would...

Fig. 16-1   Learner assessment tool. (Modified from Bell, D.F., & Bell, D.L. [1979]. Effective evaluation. *Nurse Educator, 4*[6], 6-15.)

Table 16-9   **Learner Characteristics That Influence Learning**

Enhancers	Barriers
Moderate anxiety	Fear
Trust in caregiver	Denial of health problem
Motivation	Fatigue
Perceived threat or seriousness of illness	Pain or physical discomfort
Health-oriented beliefs and practices	External demands (job, family, other responsibilities)

women, 45 million Americans will be over age 65, and African-Americans and His-
panics will constitute 47% of schoolchildren (up from 25%). Among those over age
65, four out of five will have a chronic health problem. These statistics will have considerable impact on health care in general and on client teaching in particular. Nurses
caring for diverse populations must be culturally sensitive to the traditions, taboos,
and values that might interfere with the teaching-learning process. For example, in
the Asian population it is important to "save face"; therefore these clients may not indicate a lack of understanding about how to change a dressing, or they may be uncomfortable answering questions about sexual functioning. Because Africans prize authority, they may be reluctant to ask questions about their care if the questions seem
to challenge the caregiver. Various cultures respond differently to pain. African-American and Italian clients often display an expressive response to pain; Irish clients tend
to be stoic; Puerto Rican clients show intense psychological distress (Lipton & Marbach, 1984).

When a learner from an unfamiliar culture is being assessed, a systematic appraisal
of the client's beliefs, values, and health-care practices is essential. Barriers to communication and preferred methods of learning must also be identified, since both may be
culturally based (Tripp-Reimer & Afifi, 1989). Consulting sources that describe ethnicity and its potential implications for client teaching is highly recommended.

Challenged populations. The reading ability of the client is a critical consideration
when printed materials are used for teaching. In 1984 it was estimated that many
Americans read at the tenth grade level, and an estimated 20% of the population read
at the fifth grade level (Bartlett, 1984). In contrast, Redman stated at national work-
shops on client education that many pamphlets and educational materials designed by
health care providers are written at the level of a first year medical student! Therefore
it is important to carefully assess the client's reading level and ability to understand the
written word if printed teaching materials are used. When developing or selecting
teaching materials, one must take care that the reading level is appropriate for the target audience. The reading level of printed materials can be determined by using one of
the formulas offered by Rorden (1987) or Redman (1993b).

Individuals who are visually or hearing impaired may require adapted educational
materials. Reading materials in large print or audiotapes can be used with the visually
impaired, and sign language or closed-captioned videos can be used with the hearing
impaired. For those with a language barrier, an interpreter may be needed. Individuals
who have impaired mobility may require adaptations in the teaching plan to accommodate their level of functioning.

Developing Learner Objectives

It is sometimes difficult for new teachers to develop concise and measurable learner
objectives. The purposes of learner objectives are to (1) communicate what the learner
is to know and do, (2) guide in the selection and use of teaching materials, and (3)
evaluate whether the learner learned what the teacher tried to teach. For example, "to-

day we'll watch a video of patients giving their own insulin injections (media), tomorrow we'll practice drawing up insulin together (demonstration and return demonstration), and the next day you'll have the opportunity to give your own insulin injection (evaluation)."

Bloom divided learning objectives into two categories: (1) cognitive (Bloom, 1956) and affective (Krathwohl, Bloom, & Masia, 1964). *Cognitive objectives* are concerned with the learner's mastery of different levels of cognition along a continuum from simple to complex: (1) knowledge, (2) comprehension, (3) application, (4) analysis, (5) synthesis, and (6) evaluation. Examples of cognitive objectives include the following:

- Lists correct signs and symptoms of health problem (knowledge)
- Describes relationship between exercise and weight loss (comprehension)
- Schedules 30 minutes of exercise three times weekly (application)
- Calculates amount of hidden fat in restaurant offerings before ordering (analysis)
- Prepares and cooks meals for self and family with more low-fat choices (synthesis)
- Revises exercise and dietary choices as needed (evaluation)

Affective objectives describe changes in the learner's interests, attitudes, appreciations, values, and emotional sets or biases. Levels of affective objectives include (1) receiving, (2) responding, (3) valuing, (4) organizing a value system, and (5) characterizing a value complex. Examples of affective objectives include the following:

- Accepts that present weight is unhealthy (receiving)
- Shows willingness to comply with health belief of increased exercise to decrease weight (responding)
- Desires to attain optimum weight (valuing)
- Forms judgment about the responsibility of the individual for maintaining optimum weight (conceptualization of a value)
- Revises health beliefs about weight, diet, and exercise as new information becomes available (value complex)

Much more has been written about cognitive objectives than about affective ones in the general educational and nursing literature. Present changes in society, the global economy, and health care would seem to indicate the need to pay as much, if not more, attention to the affective domain of learning.

Selecting Teaching-Learning Strategies

Primary considerations in effective teaching and learning are setting the climate and selecting appropriate strategies. Some obvious ways to facilitate a climate conducive to learning include attention to room size, temperature, noise level, seating arrangements, and availability of supplies. The degree of formality or informality that sets the "tone" of the teaching-learning experience is also important. For example, teaching about dietary and activity recommendations to recovering stroke patients may involve a more formal and serious presentation. In contrast, a class for new parents on how to bathe the baby may be more informal and relaxed.

Cognitive capacity, psychosocial development, and physical maturation and abilities of the learner are important considerations when one is choosing a teaching strategy. (Whitman et al., 1992). Selection of appropriate strategies is also influenced by cultural and environmental factors. Many individual strategies are available for designing effective teaching-learning situations. Some of these are described here.

Questioning techniques. Teacher questioning that enhances critical thinking has a positive impact on meeting learner needs (King, 1994). Two types of questioning practices have been reviewed extensively: phrasing the questions and probing the responses. Clearly phrased questions are stated simply, use words that are easily understood, focus on the content, and stress specific thinking skills (Dantonio & Paradise, 1988). For example, "Why is a blood sugar of 70 abnormal for you, although it is within the normal range?" Or, "How do you plan to increase your physical activity without jeopardizing your cardiac status?"

Borg et al. (1970) identified four ways to probe:

1. Seeking clarification "What do you mean?"
2. Increasing awareness "Why do you think so?"
3. Refocusing "How does this relate?"
4. Cueing "Let's get you started"

Question-and-answer sessions. Learners ask questions of the resource person(s). The leader has the opportunity to get further information, examples, or clarification.

Demonstration. The teacher shows an individual or group how to perform a particular task. Materials must be well prepared beforehand.

1. Analyze everything to be done.
2. Be ready to begin without delay.
3. Arrange group around you so that they can all see.
4. Explain ahead of time what will happen and what to look for.
5. Demonstrate slowly and deliberately.
6. Explain each step.
7. Allow time for questions after each step.
8. End with final summary and more questions.
9. Let learner return the demonstration.

Group discussion. A purposeful conversation and deliberation on a topic of mutual interest is carried out under the guidance of the leader. Discussion enables participants to express opinions and to learn about topics of mutual interest. This technique provides maximum opportunity for the acceptance of personal responsibility for learning and sharing experiences and opinions with others.

Role-playing. Selected members of a learning group spontaneously act out specific roles. This technique is used to bring participants into the closer experience of feeling and reacting to a problem. It promotes understanding of own and others' feelings and viewpoints. Types of role-playing:

1. *Drama*—helps participants gain insight into other people (Plot, characters, and scenes are developed previously.)
2. *Exercise*—larger, more complex and prolonged version of role-playing, where groups are interacting
3. *Psychodrama*—directed primarily at therapeutic treatment of individuals with deep personal problems

Simulation games. Learners act out their understanding and insight in handling "live" problems or "critical incidents" using gaming techniques.

Film forum. The leader explains the purpose of the film, things to watch for in the film, etc. After the film has been shown, the audience may comment or raise questions. It is essential to preview the film beforehand and to make preparations to prevent mechanical failure.

• • •

Different media can also enhance teaching and learning. Questions to ask in choosing and using media, as well as their individual differences and special considerations, are summarized in Table 16-10.

Evaluating the Teaching-Learning Experience

Evaluation consists of determining the worth of a thing. It includes obtaining information for use in judging the worth of a program, product, procedure, or objective, or the potential utility of alternative approaches designed to attain specified objectives (Worthen & Sanders, 1975). In planning, designing, implementing, and validating teaching-learning experiences, knowledge of the theories and methods of evaluation is extremely important.

There are three evaluation methods that can be used concurrently in teaching and learning: formative, summative, and peer (Garity, 1982). *Formative evaluation* takes place while the teaching-learning experience is in progress. Its purpose is to identify needed changes in material, content, or teaching style in order to better meet overall program learning objectives. *Summative evaluation* occurs at the end of a teaching-learning episode and may focus on learner satisfaction, the level of learner performance, the incidence of occurrences related to the subject area (e.g., fewer episodes of hyperglycemia secondary to testing blood sugars more frequently), improved self-care skills documented through a home visit, or satisfaction with a lifestyle change (e.g., change in diet or exercise documented through a follow-up phone call). Information from summative evaluations is used to judge the superiority of the present teaching-learning experience compared with alternative methods or experiences.

While learners are certainly important evaluators of teacher effectiveness, teachers should also be evaluated by peers, particularly if they are novices and are expected to

Table 16-10 Choosing and Using Audiovisuals

Assessment questions:
1. Is the material accurate and current?
2. Is the age/learning level appropriate?
3. Is it interesting?
4. Is it the best available in the price range?
5. Is it an acceptable time length?
6. Is it worth the time and money?
7. Are the appearance and quality satisfactory?
8. Is it appropriate for the size audience?
9. Is the equipment available; can I operate it?
10. Is a different medium a better choice?

Media	Advantages	Considerations
Audiotapes	Useful for individuals and groups; involves auditory learners Economical, easy to prepare Can be used independently	Assess hearing with individuals, room size with groups Make backups or use good-quality tapes Review mechanics, check batteries or power
Books/pamphlets	Useful for individuals; involves visual sense Easy to use Allows client to self-pace	Assess reading ability and level of material Cost; must obtain permission to copy Texts go out of date rapidly
Computer programs	Allows self-pacing, multisensory involvement Sequential programs can be used by all learner levels Entertaining	Requires added time to learn computer use Equipment expensive Professional programming required
Films	Suitable for groups; involves sight, hearing Can stimulate emotions, build attitudes May be available from a public library Useful for compression of time and space	Does not permit self-pacing Difficult to produce Expensive to buy; allow time for order Requires darkness, special equipment
Flipchart/chalkboard	Suitable for groups; involves sight Allows step-by-step buildup Inexpensive	Bulky to transport Back to audience while writing Not reusable
Models/real objects	Useful for individuals/small groups Multisensory involvement Permits demonstration and practice	May not be easy to obtain Models costly Models often easily damaged
Posters/overheads	Useful for individuals/small groups; involves sight Easy to produce, inexpensive May be reused, easy to store	Requires viewing space and/or equipment Avoid crowding; consider color, size, and space For best appearance, have professionally done
Slides	Suitable for large groups Inexpensive, easy to produce/duplicate Easy to add/subtract material	Need partial darkness Test equipment, have extra light bulb Duplication of color slides expensive

---

Sample Evaluation Questions

Formative Evaluation of a Parenting Class

1. Things I know about my parenting are . . .
2. I learned these three things about my parenting from tonight's class . . .
3. I would like to know or ask about parenting . . .
4. If I were teaching a parent like me, I would . . .

Summative Evaluation of a Series of Classes on Parenting

1. What was the most effective part of the parenting classes for you?
2. Give one example of a new concept, fact, skill, or attitude you have added to your knowledge or experience.
3. How do you expect to apply this new knowledge to your parenting practices?
4. Explain briefly how you believe this knowledge will improve your parenting practices.

Peer Evaluation of a Parenting Class

1. Emphasized major points of the teaching-learning presentation
   ___ Very well   ___ Well   ___ Satisfactorily   ___ Not very well
2. Selected appropriate content
   ___ Highly evident   ___ Evident   ___ Somewhat evident   ___ Little evidence
3. Able to ask and/or answer difficult questions
   ___ Very well   ___ Well   ___ Satisfactorily   ___ Not very well
4. Interacted effectively with learners
   ___ Very effective   ___ Effective ___ Somewhat effective ___ Not effective

---

grow and develop. *Peer evaluation* conducted by a colleague or an outside observer offers a different perspective on the effectiveness of the entire teaching-learning episode. An evaluation of this type calls for an experienced teacher who can evaluate against more sophisticated criteria, such as selection and organization of content, utilization of the literature, evidence of learning needs assessment, ability to ask and/or answer difficult questions, and quality of teaching style. Sample questions from each of these types of evaluations are provided in the box above.

• • •

The sample teaching plan for the prevention of HIV infection presented in Fig. 16-2 illustrates the components of the teaching-learning process discussed in this chapter.

FUTURE TRENDS IN TEACHING AND LEARNING

Several trends are predicted in both teaching and learning. According to Oermann (1994) and Alspach (1990), future teaching will emphasize:

- Content that focuses on information management, problem solving, and decision making rather than memorization
- Teaching methods that center on more experiential learning, such as interactive videos, simulations, games, and computers
- More computer-assisted instruction and self-directed learning methods

---

Teaching Plan for Prevention of HIV Transmission

Assessment of the Learner

Eighteen-year-old woman who denies sexual activity but has boyfriend who wants to have a sexual relationship. Boyfriend has a history of intravenous drug use. Unable to answer questions on basic knowledge of human immunodeficiency virus (HIV) and acquired immunodeficiency syndrome (AIDS). States she wants to learn about HIV and how to prevent infection.

Nursing Diagnosis

Lack of sufficient knowledge about HIV and AIDS to maintain health when sexually active.

Long-Term Goal

Client will remain free of HIV.

Intermediate Goal

Client will practice safe sex with partner 100% of the time.

Short-Term Goal

Client will gain sufficient knowledge to protect self from HIV infection as measured by correctly answering questions and accurately returning demonstration after instruction.

Behavioral Objectives	Content Outline	Teaching Methods
By the end of the teaching and learning session, the client will:		
Identify HIV as a precursor of AIDS.	Describe HIV and its effects on the immune system.	Film on transmission of HIV; question-and-answer session to follow.
Describe ways to determine if one is infected with HIV.	Method of screening for HIV; stress lack of overt symptoms.	Film, printed materials, questions and answers.
Describe the potential physiological changes following seroconversion from HIV infection to AIDS.	Potential bodily effects are flulike symptoms, destruction of helper T cells, depression of the immune system, Kaposi's sarcoma, pneumocystis pneumonia, diarrhea, yeast and other opportunistic infections, death.	Lecture and discussion.

Fig. 16-2   Teaching plan for prevention of HIV transmission.

Behavioral Objectives	Content Outline	Teaching Methods
State four ways HIV can be transmitted.	Modes of transmission: direct contact with HIV-infected blood or body fluids, unprotected sex with an infected partner, sharing contaminated needles during intravenous drug use, passing from infected mother to fetus and to breast-feeding infant, blood transfusions given before screening for HIV began.	Pamphlets and discussion about modes of transmission.
Identify two rules to prevent the transmission of HIV.	1. Don't exchange any body fluids during sexual activity. 2. Don't share needles.	Pamphlets and discussion about methods of prevention.
Demonstrate, on an anatomical model, the correct way to wear and remove a condom.	Emphasize that there is a correct method for using and removing a condom.	Demonstration and return demonstration. Assemble all supplies, anatomical model of penis, different types of condoms, HIV-effective spermicidal foam or jelly, written directions, and illustrations of steps.
Formulate a dialogue with partner to convince him of the importance of wearing a condom.	Suggestions for dialogue with partner.	Role-play.
List five safe, intimate activities.	Safe activities include safe kissing (no open-mouth kissing or kissing if lesions on mouth or bleeding gums), giving blood, hugging, shaking hands, using toilets, eating and drinking with someone who has AIDS.	Printed information followed by questions and answers. *Review key points.*

Expected Learner Activities

Ask questions, add comments, discuss feelings and fears, participate in role-play, return demonstration on correct application and removal of condom, transfer learning to real situations.

Evaluation Activities

Ask questions and observe return demonstration to determine the amount of knowledge gained; reteach as necessary. Arrange telephone contact for follow-up evaluation and support.

Fig. 16-2, cont'd   For legend see opposite page.

Similarly, future learning will emphasize:

- Learning to learn, which focuses on the development of a continuous lifelong learner who acknowledges deficits in understanding or skill, and through additional learning overcomes these deficits
- Teaching learners how to think critically, how to accept the need to relearn, and how to deal with the constancy of change
- Computer links that allow learners to access and interact with the world's literature

Teaching remains an important component of the professional nurse's role. To effectively implement the teaching role, a thorough understanding of the teaching-learning process is vital. Nurses must take into account variations in client health status, risk factors, cultural considerations, and a myriad of other factors to develop effective teaching-learning experiences. Adapting teaching and learning to new practice environments and changing health values of the nation are the challenges facing us.

 ## Key Points

- Behaviorist theories are based on the premise that learning occurs through a stimulus-response sequence, followed by consistent feedback.

- Cognitive theories propose that learning is related to an internal change in perception that is influenced by both internal and external variables.

- Humanistic theories state that learning is self-initiated and should promote the development of insight, judgment, values, and self-concept.

- Andragogy and pedagogy are based on different assumptions and design elements of the teaching-learning experience.

- Characteristics of adult learners influence the teaching-learning process.

- The field-dependence versus field-dependence model and the experiential learning model are two paradigms that focus on learning styles and preferences of the learner and teacher.

- The teaching-learning process parallels the steps of the nursing process, beginning with assessment, followed by planning, implementation, and evaluation.

- Assessment of the learner is multifaceted and includes demographic, psychosocial, cultural, physical, behavioral, and cognitive factors.

- Planning the teaching-learning experience focuses on developing learner objectives and selecting appropriate teaching-learning strategies.

- For successful implementation of the teaching plan, the environment must be conducive to learning,

- Evaluation of the teaching-learning experience includes the level of achievement of learner objectives and the effectiveness of the teacher.

- Among the future trends in teaching and learning are a reliance on information management, the development of critical thinking and problem-solving skills, and a focus on experiential learning for the continuous lifelong learner.

Critical Thinking Exercises

1. Evaluate the effectiveness of the teaching-learning process in your own area of clinical practice. What are the typical activities of the teacher and the expected outcomes of the learner? What evaluation methods are used to determine whether learning objectives are achieved? What changes would you make in the teaching-learning process to improve its effectiveness?

2. Select a learning theory and health deviation of your choice (e.g., behavioral theory and diabetes). Develop learning objectives in the cognitive and affective domains. What teaching strategies would be effective in achieving those objectives with an adolescent client? With an older adult?

3. For each characteristic of the adult learner presented in Table 16-5, identify a *specific* strategy you would incorporate in the design of an effective teaching-learning situation.

4. Analyze teaching materials (care plans, pamphlets, audiovisuals) in use at your clinical facility for evidence of educational, gender, or cultural bias. Select two of these and describe the changes needed to make them culturally acceptable.

References

Alspach, J. (1990). Critical care nursing in the 21st century. *Critical Care Nursing, 10*(9), 8-16.

Ashley, J. (1976). *Hospitals, paternalism, and the role of the nurse.* New York: Teacher's College Press.

Astin, A. (1985). *Achieving educational excellence: A critical assessment of priorities and practices in higher education.* San Francisco: Jossey-Bass.

Bandura, A. (1971). Analysis of modeling processes. In A. Bandura (Ed.), *Psychological modeling.* Chicago: Aldine.

Bartlett, E.J. (1984). Anaphoric reference in written narratives of good and poor elementary school writers. *Journal of Verbal Learning and Verbal Behavior, 23*(4), 540-552.

Bell, D.F. (1978). Assessing educational needs: Advantages and disadvantages of eighteen techniques. *Nurse Educator, 3*(5), 15.

Bell, D.F., & Bell, D.L. (1979). Effective evaluation. *Nurse Educator, 4*(6), 6-15.

Bloom, B. (1956). *Taxonomy of educational objectives: Handbook I. Cognitive domain.* New York: David McKay.

Borg, W., et al. (1970). *The mini-courses: A microteaching approach to teacher education.* Beverly Hills, CA: Collier-Macmillan.

Carper, B. (1978). Fundamental patterns of knowing in nursing. *Advances in Nursing Science, 1*(1), 13-23.

Chinn, P.L., & Kramer, M.K. (1995). *Theory and nursing* (4th ed.). St. Louis: Mosby.

Colucciello, M. (1993). Learning styles and instructional processes for home healthcare providers. *Home Healthcare Nurse, 11*(2), 43-50.

Combs, A. (1965). *The professional education of teachers.* Boston: Allyn & Bacon.

Dantonio, M., & Paradise, L. (1988). Teacher question-answer strategy and the cognitive correspondence between teacher questions and learner responses. *Journal of Research and Development in Education, 21,* 71-76.

Davis, T., & Murrell, P. (1993). *Turning teaching into learning: The role of student responsibility in the collegiate experience.* Washington, DC: George Washington University Press.

Dewey, J. (1938). *Experience and education.* New York: Macmillan.

DeYoung, S. (1990). *Teaching nursing.* Redwood City, CA: Addison-Wesley.

Ferguson, V. (1994). The future of nursing. In O.L. Strickland, & D. Fishman (Eds.), *Nursing issues in the 90's* (pp. 3-12). New York: Delmar.

Gagne, R. (1974). *Essentials of learning for instruction.* Hinsdale, IL: Dryden Press.

Gagne, R. (1977). *The conditions of learning* (3rd ed.). New York: Holt, Rinehart, & Winston.

Garity, J. (1982). Program evaluation. In C. Stetler (Ed.), *A staff education manual.* Reston, VA: Reston Publishing.

Garity, J. (1985a). An investigation of the relationship between field dependent-independent cognitive style, interpersonal orientation, and learning preference among head nurses, and a selected group of staff nurses (Doctoral dissertation, Boston University, 1985). *Dissertation Abstracts International, 46*(9), 2521.

Garity, J. (1985b). Learning styles: basis for creative teaching and learning. *Nurse Educator, 10*(2), 12-16.

Glasser, W. (1965). *Reality therapy.* New York: Harper & Row.

Heinrich, K.T., & Scherr, M.W. (1994). Peer mentoring for reflective teaching. *Nurse Educator, 19*(4), 36-41.

Jenks, J. (1993). The pattern of personal knowing in nurse clinical decision making. *Journal of Nursing Education, 32*(9), 399-405.

Jung, C. (1971). *Psychological types.* Princeton, NJ: Princeton University Press.

Kemerer, R. (1991). Understanding the application of learning. In *New directions for adult and continuing education* (No. 49, pp. 67-80). San Francisco: Jossey-Bass.

King, A. (1994). Inquiry as a tool in critical thinking. In B.F. Halpern & Associates, *Changing college classrooms: New teaching and learning strategies for an increasingly complex world.* San Francisco: Jossey-Bass.

Knowles, M. (1970). *The modern practice of adult education.* New York: Association Press.

Knowles, M. (1980). *The modern practice of adult education: From pedagogy to andragogy* (Rev. ed.), Chicago: Follett.

Knowles, M. (1984). *The adult learner: A neglected species* (3rd ed.). Houston: Gulf Publishing.

Kogan, N. (1971). Cognitive learning styles. In G.S. Lesser (Ed.), *Psychology and educational practice* (pp. 242-291). Glenview, IL: Scott, Foresman.

Kolb, D. (1984). *Experiential learning: Experience as the source of learning and development.* Englewood Cliffs, NJ: Prentice Hall.

Krathwohl, D.R., Bloom, B.S., & Masia, B.B. (1964). *Taxonomy of educational objectives: Handbook II. Affective domain.* New York: David McKay.

Lewin, K. (1951). *Field theory in social science.* New York: Harper & Row.

Lipton, J. & Marbach, J. (1984). Ethnicity and the pain response. *Social Science and Medicine, 19,* 1279-1298.

Marsick, V., & Watkins, K. (1990). *Informal and incidental learning in the workplace.* New York: Routledge.

Maslow, A. (1970). *Motivation and personality.* New York: Harper & Row.

Mesoff, B. (1979). *Cognitive style and interpersonal behavior: Implications for human relations training settings* (ERIC Document Reproduction Service No. ED 185 442). East Lansing, MI: National Center for Research on Teacher Learning.

Oermann, M. (1994). Professional nursing education in the future: Changes and challenges. *Journal of Obstetrics, Gynecologic, and Neonatal Nursing, 23*(2), 153-157.

Pace, R. (1984). *Measuring the quality of college student experiences* (ED 255 099. 142, pp. MF-01). Los Angeles: UCLA Center for the Study of Education.

Partridge, R. (1983). Learning styles: A review of selected models. *Journal of Nursing Education, 22*(2), 243.

Pascarella, E. (1985). College environmental influences on learning and cognitive development: A critical review and synthesis. In J. Smart, editor: *Higher education: Handbook of theory and research* (Vol. 1). New York: Agathon Press.

Pavlov, I. (1927). *Conditioned reflexes* (G.V. Anrep, Trans.). London: Oxford University Press.

Piaget, J. (1954). *The language and thought of the child* (3rd ed.). London: Routledge & Kegan Paul.

Piaget, J. (1970) *Genetic epistemology.* New York: Columbia University Press.

Rakoczy, M., & Money, S. (1995). Learning styles of nursing students: A 3-year cohort longitudinal study. *Journal of Professional Nursing, 11*(3), 170-174.

Redman, B.K. (1993a). Patient education at 25 years: Where we have been and where we are going. *Journal of Advanced Nursing, 18,* 725-730.

Redman, B.K. (1993b). *The process of patient education* (7th ed.). St. Louis: Mosby.

Reeve, M. (1994). Development of an instrument to measure effectiveness of clinical instructors. *Journal of Nursing Education, 33*(1), 15-20.

Reverby, S. (1987). *Ordered to care: The dilemma of American nursing, 1850-1945.* New York: Cambridge University Press.

Rogers, C. (1969). *Freedom to learn.* Columbus, OH: Charles E. Merrill.

Rorden, J. (1987). *Nurses as health teachers: A practical guide.* Philadelphia: W.B. Saunders.

Sherbinski, L. (1994). Learning styles of nurse anesthetist students related to level in a master of science in nursing program. *Journal of the American Association of Nurse Anesthetists, 62*(1), 39-45.

Sherman, T., Armistead, L., Fowler, F., Barksdale, M., & Reif, G. (1987). The quest for excellence in university teaching. *Journal of Higher Education, 48,* 65-84.

Skinner, B. (1953). *Science and human behavior.* New York: Macmillan.

Tanner, C. (1994). On clinical teaching. *Journal of Nursing Education, 33*(9), 387-388.

Thompson, B.L. (1991). Ready, aim, train. *Training, 28*(2), 53-59.

Thompson, C., & Crutchlow, E. (1993). Learning style research: A critical review of the literature and implications for nursing education. *Journal of Professional Nursing, 9*(1), 34-40.

Thorndike, E. (1913). *The psychology of learning.* New York: Teachers College.

Tinto, V. (1987). *Leaving college: Rethinking the causes and cures of student attrition.* Chicago: University of Chicago Press.

Tripp-Reimer, T., & Afifi, L.A. (1989). Cross-cultural perspectives on patient teaching. *Nursing Clinics of North America, 24*(3), 613-619.

Whitman, N.I., Graham, B.A., Gleit, C.J., & Boyd, M.D. (1992). *Teaching in nursing practice* (2nd ed.). Norwalk, CT: Appleton & Lange.

Witkin, H., Moore, C., Goodenough, D., & Cox, P. (1977). Field-dependent and field-independent cognitive styles and their educational implications. *Review of Educational Research, 47,* 1-64.

Witkin, H. (1977a). Field dependence and interpersonal behavior, *Psychological Bulletin, 84,* 661.

Witkin, H. (1977b). *Review of Educational Research, 47,* 1-64.

Wolpe, J., & Lazarus, A. (1966). *Behavior theory techniques: A guide to the treatment of neurosis.* Oxford: Pergamon Press.

Worthen, B., & Sanders, J. (1975). In T. Wentling & T. Lawson (Eds.), *Evaluating occupational education and training programs.* Boston: Allyn & Bacon.

Interpersonal Communication *17*

Sandra J. Sundeen

 Objectives

At the completion of this chapter, the reader will be able to:

- Identify and describe the components of the communication process.
- Discuss the characteristics of each of the four phases of the nurse-client relationship.
- Analyze interpersonal relationships by applying theories of communication.

Profile in Practice
Ann Cain, PhD, RN, CS-P
Private Practitioner,
Annapolis, Maryland

As an undergraduate student, I was often drawn to helping people in psychological distress. It seemed to me that there had to be some way for them to get a handle on their lives. Therefore I was very challenged by the field of psychiatric nursing. After some experience as a graduate nurse working with people with complex emotional problems at a university psychiatric intensive treatment hospital, I realized that I needed more education. In order to be really good at working with these clients, I needed to learn how to use myself in a therapeutic way. I decided to get my master's degree in psychiatric nursing.

Psychotherapy is primarily a teaching or retraining process. By focusing on the clients' lives and helping them understand what they can control and change, therapy teaches a new model for living with more choices and options. The primary goal of therapy is to facilitate clients' efforts to change maladaptive behavior, to become independent, to think, and to act for themselves. Clients learn that the only persons they can change are themselves, and that growth implies letting go of things that are destructive. Clients learn that they can alter past influences and make different choices in their current and future lives.

All this was very challenging to me! I was excited enough that I wanted to share my knowledge with others. I began a very satisfying teaching career but always maintained a part-time psychiatric nursing practice either in community mental health centers or, since 1972, in my own private practice. I also continued my specialized training by getting a doctoral degree and by taking advanced professional training in the subspecialty of family therapy. In my opinion, that's the greatest challenge in the field of psychiatric nursing and in the role of nurse psychotherapist. One never gets bored! It's a diverse field that involves assessment, diagnosis, planning, intervention, and evaluation. It requires learning to listen in a thoughtful, objective way, responding to clients' special needs, and refraining from rushing in to solve people's problems for them. It requires recognizing that clients must do the work for themselves and that your role is that of an objective, caring consultant.

Nurse psychotherapists are advanced practice psychiatric nurses. Many practice autonomously and are eligible for certification, prescriptive authority, hospital admission privileges, and third-party reimbursement. Certified specialists can offer direct services in solo private practice, in group practices, or through contracts with numerous other employers. They work in community mental health centers, private and public hospitals, day care centers, and various other service delivery settings.

From birth until death, the ability to communicate enables humans to acquire sustenance, support, and survival techniques for the many challenges of life. The growth of skill in communication is a lifelong process. Its culmination is reflected in the wisdom that is associated with advanced age. People interact with others at many levels: one-to-one, with their families, in various groups, and on an international level. The outcome of an effort to communicate may be positive or negative; it may be expected or a total surprise. It is certain, however, that constant involvement in communication is inevitable. One cannot *not* communicate (Watzlawick, Beavin, & Jackson, 1967).

The potential for communication rests in one's biological heritage. This is a capacity that is shared with many other species. Human beings are different from other species in their ability to understand and send complex messages. People also have the ability to develop backup systems for communicating if the primary channel breaks down. For instance, although hearing is considered to be very important for accurate communication, hearing-impaired individuals can learn to compensate for their disability by focusing on other senses, such as vision.

The ways that people communicate have evolved throughout recorded history and continue to change and develop today. Ancient cave paintings and hieroglyphics are studied by scientists so that we may understand the thoughts and feelings of our ancestors; other scientists are busy inventing new ways to transmit messages. Just in the last century, we have witnessed the invention of the radio, television, computer, and communication satellites. Consider how quickly we can receive messages from people on the other side of the world or even the moon. The accomplishments that allow us to do this were motivated by a desire to communicate.

Communication is also essential for successful nursing practice. Florence Nightingale (1859) recognized this when she wrote, "He (the patient) feels what a convenience it would be, if there were any single person to whom he could speak simply and openly; . . . to whom he could express his wishes and directions without that person persisting in saying 'I hope that it will please God yet to give you twenty years,' or, 'You have a long life of activity before you'" (p. 55). She went on to advise that platitudes and empty advice were not needed by the sick. Rather, the nurse should focus on listening to the concerns of the patient and on keeping him apprised of current events.

Contemporary nursing theorists are equally concerned that nurses be aware of the importance of the interpersonal nature of patient care. The caring nature of nursing is known through the experience of a gentle touch or an understanding word. This chapter explores the various ways in which communication skills may be used to enhance nursing practice.

DEFINITIONS

A general definition of communication is found in Webster's New Collegiate Dictionary: "A process by which information is exchanged between individuals through a common system of symbols, signs, or behavior." Theorists who have studied communication have developed their own definitions. Ruesch (1972) has described it as "all those processes by which people influence one another." An additional observation has been made by Watzlawick, Beavin, and Jackson (1967). They state that all behavior is communication and, conversely, that all communication is a form of behavior. The emphasis on behavior and influence is important to the consideration of communication within the context of nursing. Through the conscious use of communication skills, nurses can have an influence on the health-related behavior of their clients.

LEVELS OF COMMUNICATION

The levels of communication include verbal, nonverbal, and metacommunication. *Verbal communication* includes all aspects of communication that depend on speech. All other communications are nonverbal. In general, much more information is communicated nonverbally than is communicated verbally. *Nonverbal communication* includes the study of body language or kinesics, territoriality, and personal space. Written language relies on the use of words but is considered to be nonverbal, since it does not involve speech. Table 17-1 describes the types of nonverbal communication.

Metacommunication

Metacommunication refers to the covert messages that are transmitted directing how to interpret or decode an overt message. For instance, a parent may scold a child in the presence of an adult friend, simultaneously winking his or her eye. The child receives the message, "What you did is wrong, but not serious. I'm doing this for the benefit of this outsider." The parent may then say, "Let's have some ice cream," which

Table 17-1   **Types of Nonverbal Communication**

Type	Characteristics	Examples
Action	Sending a message by body activity; does not include signs or symbols	Jumping, hitting, skipping
Sign	Symbolism	Applauding; exchanging "high fives"
Object	Messages given by personal possessions	The car that one drives; the books in a bookcase

Data from Ruesch, J., & Kees, W. (1956). *Nonverbal communication.* Los Angeles: University of California Press.

is a verbal metacommunication that reinforces the message given by the wink. Meta-communication depends on the relationship between the participants for success. The better they know each other, the more successful the metacommunication. Cultural similarity also helps in decoding metacommunications.

Crowther (1991) points out that the client talks more than the nurse in a helping relationship. Therefore the nurse must pay careful attention to the client's metacommunication. At the same time, the nurse must use nonverbal metacommunication to convey caring and understanding. This could include the use of silence, interjections, and other nonverbal messages.

CHARACTERISTICS OF A HELPING RELATIONSHIP

Peplau (1952) has described nursing as "a significant, therapeutic, interpersonal process." By using good communication skills, the nurse establishes and maintains a helping nurse-client relationship. Carl Rogers (1961), a psychologist who based his helping theory on the interpersonal relationship, asked the following questions designed to describe the characteristics of the helping relationship:

- Can I *be* in some way that will be perceived by the other person as trustworthy, as dependable, or consistent in some deep sense?
- Can I be expressive enough as a person that what I am will be communicated unambiguously?
- Can I let myself experience positive attitudes toward this other person—attitudes of warmth, caring, liking, interest, and respect?
- Can I be strong enough as a person to be separate from the other?
- Am I secure enough within myself to permit that person separateness?
- Can I let myself enter fully into the world of his or her feelings and personal meaning and see these as he or she does?
- Can I be acceptant of each facet that clients present to me? Can I receive them as they are? Can I communicate this attitude? Or can I only receive them conditionally, acceptant of some aspects and silently or openly disapproving of others?

- Can I act with sufficient sensitivity in the relationship that my behavior will not be perceived as a threat?
- Can I free them from the threat of external evaluation?
- Can I meet this other individual as a person who is in the process of becoming, or will I be bound by his or her past and by my past?

A nurse who can give a positive response to each question should be able to establish nurse-client relationships that enhance nursing care. A negative or uncertain response indicates an area that the nurse needs to address through exploration of personal attitudes and beliefs or with the help of a nurse-mentor.

THE COMMUNICATION PROCESS

The process of human communication has been examined by theorists from many fields, including psychology, sociology, anthropology, linguistics, and cybernetics. A study of these theories can help the nurse clarify a personal conceptual model of communication applied to nursing practice.

Structural Components of Communication

The structural components of communication include the sender, receiver, message, feedback, and context. A structural model of communication is illustrated in Fig. 17-1. The *sender* is the person who initiates communication by transmitting a *message*, verbal or nonverbal, to the *receiver*. *Feedback* refers both to the verbal or nonverbal response from the receiver and to the internal evaluation of the communication that occurs within the sender. The effective communicator constantly monitors how accurately the message was perceived by observing nonverbal responses and listening to verbal ones. The *context* in which communication takes place also affects the process. For instance, an intimate conversation is awkward in a crowd. A noisy classroom interferes with the student's ability to concentrate (Sundeen et al., 1994).

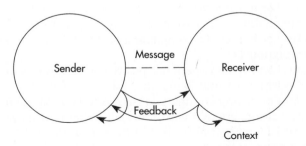

Fig. 17-1 Components of the communication process. (Redrawn from Sundeen, S.J., et al. [1994]. *Nurse-client interaction: Implementing the nursing process* [5th ed.]. St. Louis: Mosby.)

Communication Processes

Three processes of communication have been identified by Ruesch (1972). These are perception, evaluation, and transmission. *Perception* refers to the use of the senses to recognize the presence of a message. Perception usually takes place through auditory, visual, or tactile channels. It is affected by many factors. These may include the person's past experiences, his or her emotional state, the setting in which communication takes place, and the relationship between the people involved. *Evaluation* is the internal assessment of the message. This includes recognition of the overt message, comparison of the message to past experiences, and the emotional reaction to the message. *Transmission* is the conscious and unconscious, verbal and nonverbal, response to the message. This is then perceived by the original sender as a new message, and the cycle continues.

COMMUNICATION THEORIES

Selected theories of communication further illustrate the communication process.

Transactional Analysis

Transactional analysis is an approach to analyzing the communication process that was developed by Eric Berne. It was popularized when he published *Games People Play* (1964) and *What Do You Say After You Say Hello?* (1970). Berne viewed communication as a series of transactions between people. Transactions may be open and clear, but they are often clouded because the participants are playing interpersonal games. These games are related to roles that are learned as a result of life experiences. As people go through life, they learn to assume roles in various situations. In other words, they live out life scripts. The role that a person assumes in a particular transaction represents an ego state. If the person is authoritarian and directive, the ego state is that of "parent." *(P)*. If the response is submissive or playful, the "child" *(C)* ego state is operational. The "adult" *(A)* ego state is characterized by being objective and rational. No ego state is considered to be the "best" one. Each may be functional, depending on the situation. For instance, the child allows a person to have fun and to see the humor in life; the adult is helpful when there is a need to be productive at work; the parent is effective when a crisis must be handled quickly and efficiently. The well-balanced person is able to move among ego states as needed. It should also be noted that the ego states are not usually entered consciously. They occur spontaneously in response to the situation. However, it is possible, with training, to analyze the ego states that are present in personal interactions and to work to change these patterns. This is the purpose of therapy based on transactional analysis.

Berne (1964) has classified transactions according to the combination of ego states that are operating in a particular interaction. A *complementary* transaction is one in which the response corresponds with the sender's expectation. For instance, a parent message receives a child's response:

P: Pick up your clothes.
C: Do I have to?
P: Yes, You have to.
C: Okay, if I have to.

Adult-to-adult transactions are also complementary. These transactions encourage the continuation of communication. *Crossed* transactions take place when the response is not congruent with the sender's expectation. Examples of crossed transactions would be a parent-to-child or a child-to-parent response to an adult-to-adult message. For example:

A: We need to leave soon or we'll be late.
C: Why is it always my fault when we're late?

Crossed transactions tend to cut off communication and cause frustration. The third type of transaction is called *ulterior.* In this case the message is directed toward more than one ego state. The response may be in terms of one or both of the ego states addressed in the message. Paradoxical communications are examples of ulterior transactions. An example of such a transaction follows:

A/P: You probably shouldn't come home for the holidays. The weather could be bad.
C: Why are you saying that? You know I always come home.

Ulterior transactions are at the core of interpersonal games. Within families, members may rely on games so much that it is very difficult for an outsider to understand their communication. It may even be hard for a family member to be sure that the real message is understood. Transactional analysis often takes place in groups. When group members interact, they tend to use the same patterns of communication they use in their families. Games can then be identified and ulterior transactions replaced with complementary ones. Sometimes when a nurse is confused by a client's communication, it can help to review the interaction in terms of transactional analysis theory. Ulterior transactions may be taking place; the nurse may be trying to respond to the verbal message while unconsciously recognizing the conflicting nonverbal one.

Erickson's Theories

Milton Erickson is another communication theorist whose work can be helpful to nurses. He is known best for his work as a hypnotherapist, but his theories of hypnosis are actually based on communications concepts. Lankton (1985) has described the elements of Erickson's approach to interpersonal interaction, several of which are particularly pertinent to nursing practice. *Communication should be positive and individualistic.* Erickson believed that people who are given encouragement and support will usually choose the best course of action available to them. However, their options may be limited based on past learning. The caregiver's role is to help the person learn new options for behavior and to use problem-solving resources that are already available. *In-*

terventions should be active and goal oriented. A thorough understanding of human needs and development is more important than labeling behavior. The helping relationship is based on working together with the client to promote goal accomplishment by changing behavior. *Approaches need to be systems oriented.* Any change that is undertaken must occur within the context of the social system in order to mobilize support for the client.

Applications of Erickson's theories can be very complex and require specialized training. Some aspects of neurolinguistic programming, an interpersonal approach that is based on Erickson's theories, may be applied in nurse-client situations and are addressed later in this chapter.

SELF-AWARENESS AND COMMUNICATION

Since communication is interactive in nature, the nurse must function as a participant-observer. This can be difficult. It requires the nurse to be aware of personal responses, feelings, preferences, prejudices, and attitudes that might influence interactions with clients. Consider the following clinical vignette:

> *Ms. E. is a 45-year-old nurse who works for a community health agency. One of her responsibilities is to teach a health education course at the local high school. While she is teaching the unit on substance abuse, one of the students challenges her statement that the use of illicit drugs is not a healthy behavior. She becomes extremely defensive and is aware that her credibility with the students has been compromised. After class, she examines her response and realizes that it is related to her fear that her own adolescent son will experiment with drugs.*

Awareness of the underlying reason for a response can help a person put it into perspective. Varied life experiences can facilitate successful communication with clients if the nurse is in touch with the effect of the past on the present.

Influence of Feelings on Communication

Self-awareness also helps the nurse to be sensitive to subtle messages that are received from clients. Feelings, in particular, may be transmitted nonverbally. Nurses who pay attention to their own feelings in response to the client may receive clues about the feelings of the client.

Anxiety. Anxiety is known to be contagious. It spreads from one person to another because it is communicated nonverbally. Those who are near an anxious person will perceive clues about his or her state. For instance, he or she may be fidgety, tense, flushed, and/or perspiring and have loud and rapid speech. This person does not need to verbalize anxiety. It is apparent to anyone.

A nurse who feels anxious while caring for a client needs to analyze the origin of the feeling. It could be that the nurse is anxious because of something about the clinical situation or because of a personal matter unrelated to work. It is important for the nurse to recognize that he or she is anxious, because this will be communicated to the patient. It the nurse cannot identify a personal reason for feeling anxious, it is likely that the feeling is being communicated by the client. This perception needs to be validated by assessing the client's feelings verbally and through observation.

Anger. Another feeling communicated interpersonally is anger. Anger that is unconsciously perceived in another person will not necessarily make the receiver angry; it might result in anxiety. This is why it is important to validate the client's emotional state when one becomes aware that feelings are having an impact on the relationship. It is also useful to be aware of one's own usual reaction to anger. A defensive or rejecting response will not allow the client to feel secure enough to express anger or to describe its perceived cause. Invalidation of anger usually makes the feeling more intense. A fearful response may complicate the anger with anxiety that the situation could get out of control. Most people will respond positively to an opportunity to talk about their anger if they are reassured that they have a right to their feelings. This can be followed with a discussion of ways to express angry feelings in a healthy way. It should also be noted that a nurse who is angry at work will communicate this feeling to others. If the anger is related to the work situation, the nurse should deal with it before interacting with clients if this is at all possible. If the anger is unrelated to work, or if it cannot be overcome, it is best for the nurse to explain that he or she may seem preoccupied because of personal issues unrelated to the client. This avoids having the client assume that the nurse is angry at him or her. Of course, the nurse still takes care not to take the anger out on the client or to use the client as a counselor.

Caring. The profession of nursing is built around the fact that caring is also communicated interpersonally. Benner and Wrubel (1989) say that caring "means that persons, events, projects, and things matter to people." They emphasize the need to be "connected" in order to be able to care. Watson (1979) focuses on the interpersonal nature of caring. She identifies the relationship of caring to growth and health promotion and describes caring as being complementary to curing. The carative factors identified by Watson are listed in Chapter 7.

Human caring is first experienced in the parent-child relationship. A loving environment in infancy and childhood leads to the capacity to be a loving adult. Many of the clients who are in need of nursing care were deprived of a caring childhood. Nurses have an opportunity to mend some of the damage that this causes. When nurses speak of "caring for" someone, they are usually thinking of the totality of nursing interventions. An important part of "caring for" is "caring about." This refers to the emotional aspect of caring, or becoming involved with the client as one person to another. This is the type of caring that Rogers (1961) described as characteristic of the helping relationship. Some nurses are hesitant to care about clients because they fear "overinvolvement." Self-awareness is again the key to caring about the client while retaining a professional relationship. Caring in the nurse-client relationship is for the purpose of meeting the needs of the client for human relatedness. The nurse correctly seeks to meet personal needs for caring in other contexts. However, when the nurse is cared about as a person outside of the nurse-client context, a capacity is developed to relate to clients in an unconditionally caring way.

APPLICATIONS TO CLINICAL PRACTICE

The principles of communication are applied to nursing practice through the establishment of the helping nurse-client relationship.

The Nurse-Client Relationship

The nurse-client relationship has four phases: preorientation, orientation, maintenance, and termination. The phases of the relationship may be aligned with the stages of the nursing process. Preorientation and orientation are related to assessment. Planning is the bridge between the orientation and maintenance phases. Implementation and maintenance occur simultaneously. Evaluation occurs throughout the relationship but is particularly prominent during termination.

In many settings, the course of the relationship may be abbreviated because of short hospital stays or brief episodes of outpatient care. However, it is important to understand the characteristics of the relationship so that the nurse may plan realistically for the interpersonal aspects of patient care. In general, the maintenance phase of the relationship will be most affected by short-term contacts.

Forchuk and Brown (1989) developed an instrument to help community mental health nurses measure the progress of nurse-client relationships by describing the behaviors of the nurse and the client during each phase of the relationship (Table 17-2). They based their work on Peplau's (1952) model of the nurse-client relationship. In this model, the maintenance phase is called the working phase and is subdivided into two parts—identification and exploitation. The resolution phase is the same as the termination phase.

Preorientation phase. The *preorientation* phase begins before there is an encounter between the nurse and the client. During this phase, the nurse reviews available information about the client and plans for the first meeting. In particular, the nurse looks for information about the client's response to earlier contacts with the health care system, as well as identifying the circumstances that have led to the current contact. Information may be limited and should be used as background. Any impressions that are formed at this stage need to be validated with the client later. Care should be given to planning for the first contact with the client. If at all possible, a private area should be found. Distractions should be kept to a minimum. Anything that can be done to create a relaxed environment is very helpful. Most people are anxious when they encounter a health care provider, and this can inhibit communication.

Orientation phase. The first phase of the relationship that involves both the nurse and the client is the *orientation* phase. This begins with introductions.

Table 17-2   Community Mental Health Promotion Program Phases of Nurse-Client Relationship*

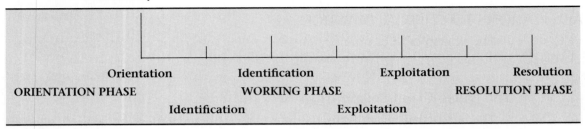

Orientation	Identification	Exploitation	Resolution
ORIENTATION PHASE	WORKING PHASE		RESOLUTION PHASE
	Identification	Exploitation	

Client

Seeks assistance.	Participates in identifying problems.	Makes full use of services.	Abandons old needs.
Conveys educative needs.	Begins to be aware of time.	Identifies new goals.	Aspires to new goals.
Asks questions.	Responds to help.	Attempts to attain new goals.	Becomes independent of helping person.
Tests parameters.	Identifies with nurse.	Rapid shifts in behavior; dependent—independent.	Applies new problem-solving skills.
Shares preconceptions and expectations of nurse due to past experience.	Recognizes nurse as a person.	Exploitative behavior.	Maintains changes in style of communication and interaction.
	Explores feelings.	Realistic exploitation.	Positive changes in view of self.
	Fluctuates between dependence, independence, and interdependence in relationship with nurse.	Self-directing.	Integrates illness.
	Increases focal attention.	Develops skills in interpersonal relationships and problem solving.	Exhibits ability to stand alone.
	Changes appearance (for better or worse).	Displays changes in manner of communication (more open, flexible).	
	Understands purpose of meeting.		
	Maintains continuity between sessions (process and content).		

Nurse

Respond to emergency.	Maintain separate identity.	Continue assessment.	Sustain relationship as long as patient feels necessary.
Give parameters of meetings.	Exhibit ability to edit speech or control focal attention.	Meet needs as they emerge.	Promote family interaction.
Explain roles.	Decrease testing maneuvers.	Understand reason for shifts in behavior.	Assist with goal setting.
Gather data.		Initiate rehabilitative plans.	

Modified from Forchuk, C., & Brown, B. (1989). Establishing a nurse-client relationship. *Journal of Psychosocial Nursing and Mental Health Services, 27*(2), 30.
*NOTE: Phases are overlapping.

Table 17-2   **Community Mental Health Promotion Program Phases of Nurse-Client Relationship—cont'd**

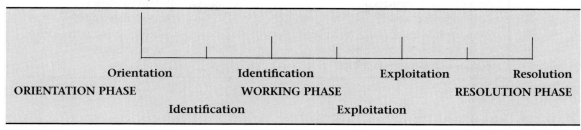

Orientation	Identification	Exploitation	Resolution
ORIENTATION PHASE	**WORKING PHASE**		**RESOLUTION PHASE**
	Identification	Exploitation	

Nurse—cont'd

Help client identify problem.	Accept client unconditionally.	Reduce anxiety.	Teach preventive measures.
Help client plan use of community resources and services.	Help express needs, feelings.	Identify positive factors.	Utilize community agencies.
Reduce anxiety and tension.	Assess and adjust to needs.	Help plan for total needs.	Teach self-care.
Practice nondirective listening.	Provide information.	Facilitate forward movement of personality.	Terminate nurse-client relationship.
Focus client's energies.	Provide experiences that diminish feelings of helplessness.	Deal with therapeutic impasse.	
Clarify preconceptions and expectations of nurse.	Do not allow anxiety to overwhelm client.		
	Help client to focus on cues.		
	Help client develop responses to cues.		
	Use word stimuli.		

Introductions. The nurse's introduction should include name, title, and function. For example, "I am Mary Smith. I'm a staff nurse on this floor, and I will be your primary nurse. That means that we will plan your nursing care together, and I will provide your care whenever I am working." A wealth of information has been given. Since the client may be anxious, this may need to be repeated at the beginning of the next contact. The nurse should then inquire about how the client would like to be addressed. Following the client's preference in this regard helps establish a helping relationship. The preferred mode of address should be recorded in the nursing care plan. It is extremely important to identify oneself to every client at each encounter unless it is absolutely certain that the client knows the identity of the nurse. Most identification badges are impossible to read and cannot be relied on for orienting clients to their care providers.

Elements of a Nurse-Client Contract	
Names of individuals	Meeting location
Roles of nurse and client	Time of meetings
Responsibilities of nurse and client	Conditions for termination
Expectations of nurse and client	Confidentiality
Purpose of the relationship	

Interpersonal contract. Following introductions, the nurse needs to orient the client to the parameters of the relationship. The elements of the nurse-client contract are listed in the box above. Contracts will vary a great deal. Some nurses may encounter clients for a brief time in a clinic or an emergency room; others may engage in long-term relationships in nursing homes or home care settings. However, in each case the basic types of information described above should be communicated. The client may need an opportunity to react to the nurse's description of their relationship. For instance, the nurse may describe a long-term series of meetings when the client expects only a brief contact with the health care setting. Clarification is necessary to prevent a barrier to communication from occurring because of conflicting goals. Agreement on the purpose, frequency, and duration of the relationship constitutes the interpersonal contract. The information about the nature of the relationship should be repeated at the end of the first contact and as often as necessary to be sure that the client understands it.

Data collection and goal setting. Following the establishment of the contract, the nurse and client are ready to move forward to data collection and goal setting. Data collection will lead to the formulation of a nursing diagnosis. Some North American Nursing Diagnosis Association (NANDA) diagnoses that may be applied to the communication process or the interpersonal relationship include:

Impaired verbal communication
Impaired social interaction
Social isolation
Altered role performance
Altered parenting
Altered family processes
Caregiver role strain
Parental role conflict
Ineffective individual coping
Defensive coping
Ineffective denial
Ineffective family coping: disabling
Ineffective family coping: compromised

Family coping: potential for growth
Decisional conflict (specify)
Self-esteem disturbance
Personal identity disturbance
Hopelessness
Powerlessness
Knowledge deficit (specify)
Altered thought processes
Dysfunctional grieving
Anticipatory grieving
Risk for violence: self-directed or directed at others
Post-trauma response
Rape-trauma syndrome
Anxiety
Fear

The nurse needs to identify the client's expectations about the episode of care. Feedback should be given about whether or not the client's goals are realistic in relation to what the nurse has to offer. Openness about realistic expectations avoids later disappointment when unrealistic goals are not met. As the nurse proceeds with the nursing assessment, additional information will be provided, leading to mutual goal setting. The establishment of mutually agreed on goals marks the end of the orientation phase of the relationship. As goals are identified, they also become part of the contract between the client and the nurse.

Maintenance phase. The maintenance phase of the relationship is sometimes called the working phase because it is the time during which the nurse and the client work on accomplishing the identified goals of the relationship. The nurse uses the relationship with the client to assist in addressing the identified health care needs by using interpersonal skills. These might include such techniques as interviewing, empathizing, listening, nondirective interventions, and elements of neurolinguistic programming. The particular technique used depends on the needs of the client, the focus of the relationship, and the abilities of the nurse. It is helpful to develop a variety of relationship skills so that they may be adapted to meet the needs of various clients.

Interviewing. Interviewing skills are needed during all phases of the relationship. The interview may be structured or nonstructured. In a *structured interview,* the nurse follows a set format to elicit information from the client. An example of this is the use of a standardized assessment tool to collect health data on admission to a health care program. This is an efficient way to collect information but may be limited depending on the adequacy of the instrument or format that is used. It is also useful for the collection of data for research purposes. A strictly structured interview may lead the nurse to use "tunnel vision," with more attention focused on the completion of the data collection form than on the interpersonal clues that are being communicated by the client.

Nondirective therapeutic communication techniques. The *unstructured interview* allows the nurse to use nondirective therapeutic communication techniques to enable the client to explore areas of concern. Skillfully employed nondirective techniques do not hamper the relationship; rather, they indicate to the client that the nurse is interested in clarifying his or her messages. Practice is needed in order to feel comfortable with these approaches. Several common nondirective techniques as described by Sundeen et al. (1994) are summarized in Table 17-3.

Nontherapeutic communication techniques. As the nurse conducts the interview, it is also necessary to be careful not to use *nontherapeutic communication techniques.* Sundeen et al. (1994) have described several of these. They are usually signals that the nurse feels uncomfortable addressing the issues that the client is trying to discuss. Clients may bring up difficult subjects indirectly or with hesitation. Then it is easy for the nurse to avoid confronting these messages, allowing the interaction to shift to more comfortable themes. Nontherapeutic communication techniques are summarized in Table 17-4.

Active listening. To communicate effectively with others, it is essential to engage in *active listening.* This means that the nurse gives full attention to the client. This is communicated verbally and nonverbally. Eye contact conveys interest and involvement (Fig. 17-2). Head nods and facial expressions also indicate understanding. These should be used consciously. Unconscious nodding may indicate unintended agreement.

A particular type of active listening is the use of *neurolinguistic programming* (NLP), described by Richard Bandler and John Grinder. This communication technique is based on the work of such experts in the field of communication as Virginia Satir, Fritz Perls, and Milton Erickson. This is a complex approach to communication that requires specialized training. Two concepts that are part of NLP are discussed here. They may help the nurse to enhance assessment and interaction skills. They are pacing and representational systems.

According to King, Novik, and Citrenbaum (1983), *pacing* involves sending a message to the client that is reflective of his or her current experience. For instance, the nurse might say, "You made a face when I gave you this medicine. I guess it tastes pretty bad." Pacing is used to establish lines of communication with the client. It is then possible to lead the client to a desired behavioral change. In the preceding example, the nurse might go on to say, "This water will take the bad taste away." Of course, this would not work if water were not effective for overcoming the taste of the medicine. The communication is used to enhance the effect of the intervention and to indicate to the client that the nurse is in tune with his or her feelings.

Another approach to pacing is described by Knowles (1983). She describes a process called *mirroring.* In this case the nurse imitates the client's body position, gestures, or even breathing patterns. When this is done inconspicuously, it is a powerful way of communicating understanding, thereby facilitating the communication process. Once the nurse has succeeded in pacing the client's current behavior, it may be possible to lead the client toward behavioral change. For instance, if the client is anxious, the body position may be rigid, there may be loud and fast speech, and breathing may be rapid. After synchronizing his or her own body position, speech, and rate of breathing

Table 17-3   **Summary of Therapeutic Communication Techniques**

Technique	Definition	Therapeutic Value
Listening	An active process of receiving information and examining one's reaction to the messages received	Nonverbally communicates to client nurse's interest in client
Silence	Periods of no verbal communication among participants	Nonverbally communicates nurse's acceptance of client
Establishing guidelines	Statements regarding roles, purpose, and limitations for a particular interaction	Helps client to know what is expected of him
Open-ended comments	General comments asking the client to determine the direction the interaction should take	Allows client to decide what material is most relevant and encourages him to continue
Reducing distance	Diminishing physical space between the nurse and client	Nonverbally communicates that nurse wants to be involved with client
Acknowledgment	Recognition given to a client for contribution to an interaction	Demonstrates the importance of the client's role within the relationship
Restating	Repeating to the client what the nurse believes is the main thought or idea expressed	Asks for validation of nurse's interpretation of the message
Reflecting	Directing back to the client his ideas, feelings, questions, or content	Attempts to show client the importance of his own ideas, feelings, and interpretations
Seeking clarification	Asking for additional inputs to understand the message received	Demonstrates nurse's desire to understand client's communication
Seeking consensual validation	Attempts to reach a mutual denotative and connotative meaning of specific words	Demonstrates nurse's desire to understand client's communication
Focusing	Questions or statements to help the client develop or expand an idea	Directs conversation toward topics of importance
Summarizing	Statement of main areas discussed during interaction	Helps client to separate relevant from irrelevant material; serves as a review and closing for the interaction
Planning	Mutual decision making regarding the goals, direction, and so on of future interactions	Reiterates client's role within relationship

From Sundeen, S.J., et al. (1994). *Nurse-client interaction: Implementing the nursing process* (5th ed.). St. Louis: Mosby.

Table 17-4 **Summary of Nontherapeutic Communication Techniques**

Technique	Definition	Therapeutic Threat
Failure to listen	Not receiving client's intended message	Places needs of nurse above those of client
Failure to probe	Inadequate data collection represented by eliciting vague descriptions, getting inadequate answers, following standard forms too closely, and not exploring client's interpretation	Inadequate data base on which to make decisions; client care not individualized
Parroting	Continual repetition of client's phrases	The metacommunication is "I am not listening" or "I am not a competent communicator"
Being judgmental	Approving or disapproving statements	Implies that nurse has the right to pass judgment; promotes a dependency relationship
Reassuring	Attempts to do magic with words	Negates fears, feelings, and other communications of client
Rejecting	Refusing to discuss topics with client	Client may feel that not only communication but also the self was rejected
Defending	Attempts to protect someone or something from negative feedback	Negates client's right to express an opinion
Giving advice	Telling client what nurse thinks should be done	Negates the worth of client as a mutual partner in decision making
Stereotyped responses	Use of trite, meaningless verbal expressions	Negates the significance of client's communication
Changing topics	Nurse directing the interaction into areas of self-interest rather than following lead of client	Nonverbally communicates that the nurse is in charge of deciding what will be discussed; possible to miss important topics for individual client
Patronizing	Style of communication that displays a condescending attitude toward the client	Implies that the nurse-client relationship is not based on equality; places the nurse in a "superior" position

From Sundeen, S.J., et al. (1994). *Nurse-client interaction: Implementing the nursing process* (5th ed.). St. Louis: Mosby.

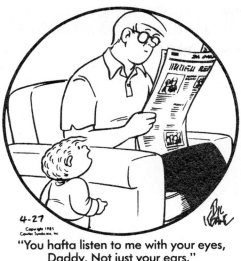

"You hafta listen to me with your eyes,
Daddy. Not just your ears."

Fig. 17-2 Communication involves all of the senses. (Reprinted with special permission of King Features Syndicate.)

with those of the client, the nurse can gradually relax, speak quietly, and breathe more slowly. If the pacing has been successful, the client is likely to do the same. Wichnoski and Kubick (1995) describe the use of pacing and leading techniques to develop rapport with the client and thus enhance compliance with the plan of care.

One may also gain access to the client by identifying and using congruent *representational systems*. Knowles describes the three sensory modalities that are included: auditory, visual, and kinesthetic. This theory is based on the premise that every person has a preferred sensory channel for communication. It is possible to identify and access the preferred channel in order to communicate in a way that is comfortable for the client. One way to identify the sensory modality that the person uses most frequently is to listen for the predicates in sentences. Individuals tend to use predicates related to one of the three modalities more often than those related to the other two. For instance, in response to the comment, "My husband and I are angry with each other," a person who uses the visual modality might say, "I see what you mean"; one who uses the auditory modality might say, "I hear what you're saying"; and one who uses the kinesthetic modality might say, "I feel that I understand what you mean." The box on p. 392 lists predicates related to the three sensory modalities (Knowles, 1983).

Empathy. The use of good communication skills, active listening, and the techniques of pacing and using representational systems all help the nurse develop empathy with the client. *Empathy* refers to the ability to relate to another person at a feeling level with a deep understanding of the other's experience, without losing the perspective of one's individuality. Empathy is often differentiated from sympathy, in which the individual reacts from the standpoint of past personal experiences, rather than trying to see the situation through the other person's eyes.

Preferred Predicates		
Auditory	**Kinesthetic**	**Visual**
listen	feel	see
hear	knock out	behold
gripe	turn	observe
hassle	thin-skinned	view
attend	tender	witness
give ear to	stir	perceive
get	excite	discern
listen in	arouse	spy
eavesdrop	whet	sight
hang upon every word	sharpen	discover
tip	sore spot	notice
take in	itch	distinguish
overhear	creeps	recognize
register	sting	imagine
reach	thrill	catch sight of
listening	tingle	take in
hearsay	shudder	look

According to the NLP communication model, most people's speech reflects a preference for one of three sensory categories. The lists above suggest typical word choices in each group.

From Knowles, R.D. (1983). Building rapport through neurolinguistic programming. *American Journal of Nursing,* pp. 1011-1014.

Ehmann (1971) has described four steps in the process of empathy. The first is *identification.* During this stage, the nurse becomes open to the other person's feelings by focusing on the verbal and nonverbal messages that are being received. The second step is *incorporation.* At this point, the nurse internalizes the feelings of the other person but does not take ownership of them. At the third step, *reverberation,* the nurse compares the perceived experience of the client with past personal experiences and the feelings that were associated with them. *Detachment* is the last step. The nurse moves back from the internal process and is able to share the perception that resulted with the client. Kalisch (1973) has developed an assessment tool that allows the nurse to evaluate the level of empathic response to a client (Table 17-5). Self-evaluation of this skill will help the nurse improve the ability to communicate meaningfully with clients. Fig. 17-3 presents a model of empathy in the nurse-client interaction developed by MacKay et al. (1990).

Trust. Purposeful application of all the techniques of communication will assist the nurse in working productively with the client toward goal achievement. It will also help the nurse establish trust as a solid foundation for the relationship. *Trust* is basic to

Table 17-5   **The Nurse-Patient Empathic Function Scale: A Schematic Presentation**

	Level of Patient's Feelings	
Categories of Nurse Empathic Functioning	**Conspicuous Current Feelings**	**Hidden Current Feelings**
0	Ignores	Ignores
1	Communicates an awareness that is accurate at times and inaccurate at other times	Ignores
2	Communicates a complete and accurate awareness of the essence and strength of feeling	Communicates an awareness of the presence of hidden feelings but is not accurate in defining their essence or strength; an effort is being made to understand
3	Same as category 2	Communicates an accurate awareness of the hidden feelings slightly beyond what the client expresses himself
4	Same as category 2	Communicates without uncertainty an accurate awareness of the deepest, most hidden feelings

From Kalisch, B. (1973). What is empathy? *American Journal of Nursing, 73*(9):1548.

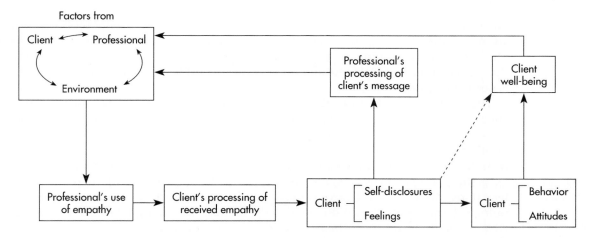

Fig. 17-3 Model of empathy in professional-client interaction. (Redrawn from MacKay, R.C., Hughes, J.R., & Carver, J.C. (1990). A model of empathy in the helping relationship. In R.C. MacKay, J.R. Hughes, and J.C. Carver [Eds.], *Empathy in the helping relationship.* New York: 1990, Springer.)

the success of all human relationships, beginning with the maternal-infant bond. Trust does not happen automatically. The nurse needs to work to build trust. An important element of trust is *reliability.* This refers to carrying out promises, to responding to requests promptly, and to keeping appointments. Another component of trust is *honesty.* Questions should be answered clearly and completely. If the nurse is unsure of the answer to a client's question, this should be communicated. The nurse then finds the correct information and provides it to the client as soon as possible.

Proper management of confidential information is also important to the maintenance of trust. Any information that is given to the nurse in the context of the professional relationship is confidential. This means that it may not be shared with anyone who is not directly involved in the client's health care. This should be explained to the client. It may also be necessary to tell the client that the nurse is obligated to communicate pertinent information to other members of the health care team. An element of judgment related to confidentiality is required. Clients sometimes give nurses information that is not relevant to the immediate health care problem. The nurse must decide whether it is in the client's best interest to share that information with other team members. For instance, a person who is being treated for stable diabetes may mention marital discord. The nurse may be concerned that the added stress could cause the diabetes to become uncontrolled. In this case it would be appropriate to inform the client that the nurse plans to share this information with the physician. On the other hand, the nurse could assess that the problem appeared to be transient and not particularly stressful. Then the nurse might decide not to share the information at that time. A good rule is, "When in doubt, communicate." All members of the health care team are bound by rules of confidentiality and a code of ethical behavior. The nurse should be particularly wary of a client's request to keep a secret as a condition for giving information. If the client shares information that is critical for the provision of safe health care, the nurse must communicate it to colleagues. Examples of such situations are threats of suicide or confessions of failure to take prescribed medications. The nurse should respond to requests for secrecy by explaining the need to be sure that the client receives safe care and that the nurse must be free to take whatever action is needed to ensure safety.

The trusting relationship with a nurse will help the client have a positive experience with the health care system. The maintenance phase of the relationship continues until the goals are accomplished or other conditions require termination. Examples of other conditions include discharge of the client from the health care agency, completion of a student learning experience, and resignation of the nurse from the agency.

As the nurse practices good communication skills, proficiency will increase and interactions with clients will become more rewarding. As health care becomes more technological and people feel more alienated, the need for caring relationships will increase. It is up to nurses to make sure that the health care system continues to be a caring system.

Termination. The last phase of the helping relationship is *termination.* Ideally, this occurs when the nurse-client goals have been accomplished and both participants feel satisfied with the outcome. However, the reality of the health care system is that sometimes termination must take place before goal accomplishment is completed. When this is the case, it is important to help the client identify additional resources for continued assistance. *Summarizing* the accomplishments of the relationship helps to identify the work that has been done and what needs to be done. Both the nurse and the client should contribute to the summary. This can also be an excellent learning experience for the nurse in terms of the success or failure of past interventions.

When two people terminate a meaningful relationship, it helps to be able to envision the other person in the future. It can be a time of sharing future plans. For instance, if the relationship is ending because of the end of a student experience, the client may like to know what experience the student will have next; or if graduating, what the student's job plans are. If a client is being discharged from the health care setting, it can be reassuring to know that the familiar staff will still be there if a problem recurs.

Sometimes clients wish to give the nurse a remembrance of the relationship. Most health care agencies prohibit the acceptance of gifts or gratuities from clients. The nurse needs to evaluate these offerings in the context of the relationship. If the client asks the nurse to accept a small token of little monetary value, such as a handmade trinket, it may be thoughtful to accept it. It is even better if the nurse has anticipated this event and is prepared to reciprocate. Items of value should never be given or received in a professional relationship. Also, the nurse must be careful not to use the giving of gifts to avoid confronting the feelings associated with termination of a relationship.

The ending of a close relationship can be difficult for both the client and the nurse. Terminations serve as reminders of past losses, and feelings associated with those losses may be reexperienced, especially if they were not resolved at the time. The nurse needs to analyze personal responses to termination in order to prevent interference with the helping relationship. It can be very helpful to clients to assist them in expressing their feelings in the context of termination and in learning to resolve feelings that may have been troublesome in the past. Anger is a feeling that is expected to accompany termination. It is frequently expressed indirectly by missing appointments or refusing to interact. If the nurse is alert to signs of anger, it can be acknowledged and accepted, and the nurse and client can move on to sharing the positive feelings they have for each other. Sadness is also typical of partings. The nurse may be able to facilitate the client's expression of sadness by sharing personal feelings. In this case the nurse's goal is not to receive help from the client in handling feelings, but to demonstrate that the relationship was meaningful and sadness is appropriate. Mutual expression of sadness often leads to sharing of the caring feelings that have developed between the nurse and the client. When a relationship has been terminated successfully, the participants will be left with feelings of warmth for each other and nostalgia for the relationship.

PROFESSIONAL COMMUNICATIONS

The professional relationship is unlike other relationships in life. Expectations of the participants are unequal. The client expects that the nurse will assume responsibility for the progress of the relationship. The nurse expects the client to participate in directing the goals of the relationship as much as possible but realizes that the primary responsibility rests with the nurse. Meetings are planned, formalized, and goal directed. The relationship itself is time limited, and termination is final. The promise, actual or implied, of continuation of the relationship after termination is unfair to the client because it blocks addressing the experience of loss. Participation is also not equal at the feeling level. Nurses encourage clients to share their most personal feelings and help them to learn to manage personal problems. The nurse, however, must find other resources for dealing with personal difficulties.

Because of the uniqueness of the professional relationship, an ongoing supervisory relationship with an experienced nurse colleague is highly advisable. The supervisor can help the nurse to analyze interactions and to identify the influence of personal needs and feelings on the nurse-client relationship. Peer supervision, with or without a designated group leader, can be very helpful for experienced nurses. The supervisory relationship is based on the same principles of trust and confidentiality as the nurse-client relationship.

COMMUNICATIONS RESEARCH

Communications and nurse-client interaction are fertile areas for nursing research. This is also a complex area of research. Descriptive research may assist with identification of the structural components of communication. Classic examples of this type of study include the work done by Birdwhistell (1970) in kinesics and by Hall (1959) in the use of personal space. Experimental studies in the application of communication theory are much more difficult to design. It is difficult to isolate the effect of a particular intervention when the client is being exposed to multiple health care providers and multiple therapeutic approaches, as well as interactions with relatives and friends. However, it is possible to find examples of research that has been completed and is useful in understanding the characteristics of communication and the helping relationship.

Extensive relationship research was conducted by Carkhuff, Truax, and their associates (1967, 1969). They identified the core dimensions of the helping relationship. These include accurate empathy, nonpossessive warmth, and genuineness. Aiken and Aiken (1973) built on this work in relation to the nurse-client relationship. They identified the dimensions of empathic understanding, positive regard, genuineness, and concreteness or specificity of expression. Nursing research has investigated the characteristics of empathy in the context of the nurse-client relationship. For example, Stotland et al. (1978) explored the relationship between ability to empathize and the amount of time spent with clients by nursing students. They found that early in the semester, the highly empathic students spent less time with clients than the other students did. They hypothesized that this was related to the empathic students' awareness of the disparity between the relationship needs of the clients and their ability to meet those needs. As they grew in confidence, they spent more time with the clients.

MacKay, Hughes, and Carver (1990) found that an empathic response by a nurse facilitated client self-disclosure. Another important finding of this study was that 98% of

---

Research Synopsis

Heifner (1993) has identified the elements of *nurse-client connectedness,* which is defined as "a therapeutic state of interaction that enhances the effectiveness of the relationship and benefits both the nurse and the patient" (p. 14). An exploratory, descriptive, qualitative design was used. The investigator interviewed eight experienced psychiatric–mental health nurses. The themes that emerged from the interviews included client vulnerability, commonalities between client and nurse, and the nurse's feeling of being valued by the client. From these, the essential elements of nurse-client connectedness were derived.

These elements are as follows: the nurse contacts the client; the nurse feels tense; the client seems vulnerable; the nurse's tension decreases; the nurse encourages the client to talk about the vulnerable area; the nurse recognizes commonalities with the client and may or may not choose to disclose these; the nurse feels reciprocity with the client; the nurse feels valued by the client; the nurse and client become more invested in the relationship and take risks, leading to connectedness.

---

nursing interventions were factual rather than affective. Other nursing studies have been conducted by Williams (1979), who investigated the relationship between empathic communication and self-concept and by Mansfield (1973), who looked at the verbal and nonverbal communication of empathy. Wheeler (1988) has published a summary of research on the subject of empathy, in which she emphasizes the need for a unified conceptual model.

Other nurses have investigated other aspects of communication. Topf (1988) has provided a model for studying communication characteristics and developing an assessment tool for nurses. Smith and Cantrell (1988) have explored the concept of distance in the nurse-client relationship. They applied the personal space theories developed by Hall and added the concept of "verbal distance," which has to do with the intrusiveness of the interaction. They found that physical distance was anxiety provoking only when accompanied by verbal intrusiveness. This was the case for all distances. The research synopsis presented in the box above describes another nursing study related to communication. These examples demonstrate the real need for nurses to investigate other aspects of relationships and communication between nurses and clients. Increased knowledge about these elements of nursing practice will help nurses to base more of their interventions on theory rather than intuition.

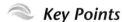 Key Points

- Communication is the process that people use to influence each other and encompasses all behavior.

- Levels of communication include verbal communication, nonverbal communication, and metacommunication.

- The structural components of communication include the sender, receiver, message, feedback and context.

- The processes of communication are perception, evaluation, and transmission.

- Important communication theorists include Eric Berne, who developed the theory of transactional analysis, and Milton Erickson, who applied his work regarding communication to hypnotherapy.

- Self-awareness and recognition of feelings are important elements of successful communication. The nurse should be skilled in recognizing and intervening in anxiety and anger and be able to communicate caring.

- Communication principles are applied to nursing practice through the establishment of the nurse-client relationship.

- The preorientation phase of the relationship is the time during which the nurse reviews existing client data and prepares for the setting of the contact.

- The orientation phase includes introductions, establishment of the interpersonal contract, data collection, and goal setting.

- The maintenance, or working, phase involves the nurse using interpersonal skills to address the client's identified health needs. The techniques used might include interviewing, empathizing, listening, nondirective interventions, and elements of neurolinguistic programming.

- The last phase of the relationship is termination. The nurse's responsibilities are to summarize goal achievement, help the client to express the feelings associated with loss, and help the client to discuss plans for the future.

- Professional communication differs from social communication in that the expectations of the participants are not equal in professional communication.

- Nurse-client communication and the professional relationship are topics that would profit from additional nursing research.

Critical Thinking Exercises

1. Compare and contrast the similarities and differences between your relationships with a close relative, a close friend, a casual acquaintance, a colleague at work or school, and a client. Consider the parameters of interpersonal closeness, openness, equality, responsibility, and anticipated duration.

2. Describe the nursing actions that you initiated in your last client contact that would support the development of trust. Did you do anything that would inhibit the development of trust?

3. It might be said that some therapeutic communication techniques, such as reflecting, restating, mirroring, and pacing, are contrived and manipulative. Do you agree or disagree? Support your opinion with examples.

4. Using theories of communication presented in this chapter, analyze the following interaction. If you think that the nurse has made a response that is nontherapeutic, substitute a therapeutic one.

> Situation: The client has come to the emergency room complaining of "pain in my head." The emergency room is very busy, with recent admissions of four victims of a serious automobile accident and two people with gunshot wounds. Two staff members called in sick. One was replaced with a nurse who had never worked in the ER. The other was not replaced.
>
> Nurse: (looking at the admission sheet): "I see you have a headache."
> Client: (softly) "I feel awful."
> Nurse: "How long have you had this headache?"
> Client: "I can't stand this feeling any longer."
> Nurse: (sounding impatient) "I can't help you if you don't tell me about your headache."
> Client: "What?"
> Nurse: (loudly) "You have to tell me about your headache."
> Client: (looks puzzled) "What headache?"
> Nurse: "It says here that you have a pain in your head."
> Client: "I guess you could call it that. I said my head was bothering me. I was dizzy, and I fell down and hit my head on a table. It *does* hurt where I hit it."
> Nurse: "I think we need to start over. Tell me how you're feeling."

5. Analyze the following interaction using concepts of transactional analysis and neurolinguistic programming:

> Client: "My foot feels funny."
> Nurse: "It looks all right to me."
> Client: "Why do you nurses always brush me off?"
> Nurse: "I'm not sure I see what your problem is."
> Client: "You're supposed to make me feel good. I don't feel good. Make me feel better."
> Nurse: "You have to help us help you."

References

Aiken, L., & Aiken, J. (1973). A systematic approach to evaluation of interpersonal relationships. *American Journal of Nursing, 73,* 863.

Benner, P., & Wrubel, J. (1989). *The primacy of caring: Stress and coping in health and illness.* Menlo Park, CA: Addison-Wesley.

Berne, E. (1964). *Games people play.* New York: Grove Press.

Berne, E. (1970). *What do you say after you say hello?* New York: Grove Press.

Birdwhistell, R. (1970). *Kinesics and context.* Philadelphia: University of Pennsylvania Press.

Carkhuff, R. (1969). *Helping and human relations* (Vols 1-2). New York: Holt, Rinehart & Winston.

Carkhuff, R., & Truax, C. (1967). *Toward effective counseling and psychotherapy.* Chicago: Aldine.

Crowther, D.J. (1991). Metacommunication: A missed opportunity? *Journal of Psychosocial Nursing and Mental Health Services, 19*(4), 13.

Ehmann, V. (1971). Empathy: Its origin, characteristics, and process. *Perspectives in Psychiatric Care, 9*(2), 77.

Forchuk, C., & Brown, B. (1989). Establishing a nurse-client relationship. *Journal of Psychosocial Nursing and Mental Health Services, 27*(2), 30.

Hall, E. (1959). *The silent language.* Garden City, New York: Doubleday.

Heifner, C. (1993). Positive connectedness in the psychiatric nurse-patient relationship. *Archives of Psychiatric Nursing, 7*(1), 11.

Kalisch, B. (1973). What is empathy? *American Journal of Nursing, 73,* 1548.

King, M., Novik, L., & Citrenbaum, C. (1983). *Irresistible communication: Creative skills for the health professional.* Philadelphia: W.B. Saunders.

Knowles, R.D. (1983). Building rapport through neurolinguistic programming. *American Journal of Nursing, 83*(7), 1011-1014.

Lankton, C.H. (1985). Elements of an Ericksonian approach. In S.R. Lankton (Ed.), *Elements and dimensions of an Ericksonian approach.* New York: Brunner/Mazel.

MacKay, R.C., Hughes, J.R., & Carver, E.J., editors. (1990). *Empathy in the helping relationship,* New York: Springer.

Mansfield, E. (1973). Empathy: Concept and identified psychiatric nursing behavior. *Nursing Research, 22,* 525.

Nightingale, F. (1859). *Notes on nursing.* London: Harrison & Sons.

Peplau, H. (1952). *Interpersonal relations in nursing.* New York: G.P. Putnam's Sons.

Rogers, C.R. (1961). *On becoming a person.* Boston: Houghton Mifflin.

Ruesch, J. (1972). *Disturbed communication.* New York: W.W. Norton.

Ruesch, J., & Kees, W. (1956). *Nonverbal communication.* Los Angeles: University of California Press.

Smith, B.J., & Cantrell, P.J. (1988). Distance in nurse-patient encounters. *Journal of Psychosocial Nursing and Mental Health Services, 26*(2), 22.

Stotland, E., Mathews, K.E., Jr. Sherman, S.E., Hansson, R.O., & Richardson, B.Z. (1978). *Empathy, fantasy, and helping.* Beverly Hills, CA: Sage Publications.

Sundeen, S.J., Stuart, G.W., Rankin, E.D., & Cohen, S.A. (1994). *Nurse-client interaction: Implementing the nursing process* (5th ed.). St. Louis: Mosby.

Topf, M. (1988). Verbal interpersonal responsiveness. *Journal of Psychosocial Nursing and Mental Health Services, 26*(7), 8.

Watson, J. (1979). *Nursing: The philosophy and science of caring.* Boston: Little, Brown.

Watzlawick, P., Beavin, J., & Jackson, D. (1967). *Pragmatics of human communication: A study of interactional patterns, pathologies, and paradoxes.* New York: W.W. Norton.

Wheeler, K. (1988). A nursing science approach to understanding empathy. *Archives of Psychiatric Nursing, 2,* 95.

Wichnoski, H.C., & Kubick, S. (1995). Improving your patient's compliance. *Nursing 95, 25*(1), 66.

Williams, C. (1979). Empathic communication and its effect on client outcome. *Issues in Mental Health Nursing, 2*(1), 16.

Critical Thinking 18

C. Fay Raines

Objectives

At the completion of this chapter, the reader will be able to:

- Define critical thinking.

- Identify components and characteristics of critical thinking.

- Understand the relationship of critical thinking to problem solving and decision making.

- Apply critical thinking in nursing practice situations.

Profile in Practice

Latrell P. Fowler, PhD, RN
Medical University of South Carolina,
RN-BSN Satellite at Francis Marion University,
Florence, South Carolina

I always wanted to be a role model for others like my big sister was for me. She set the stage by her example of excellence in nursing. Maybe this is why I first became a nurse and then a teacher-mentor. As a new BSN graduate, I wanted *all* that nursing had to offer. I loved the excitement of coronary care and hospital nursing, but I also asked myself, "What else can I do in nursing?" As a new challenge, I became an instructor in the staff development department of a growing medical center. In this position, I saw the need for graduate education and completed my master's degree in clinical nursing. I worked as a clinical specialist for a few years, combining both educational and administrative functions in a newly developed role. Five years later, I was still searching for my niche in nursing as I left hospital nursing practice to join the faculty of an associate degree program. The rewards came quickly as I saw students progress through their education. After 10 years in ADN education, I once again began seeking new challenges. I

---

moved to RN-BSN education, where my greatest satisfaction is helping nurses meet personal and professional goals.

Nurses have wonderful opportunities to continually explore new horizons, and as students progressed through the BSN program, they frequently spoke of their broadened perspectives. I noticed that a significant element of BSN education was critical thinking, and I was curious about how to best facilitate it. Recognizing that there was more I could learn and teach, I enrolled in a doctoral program, where my interest in critical thinking ultimately became my dissertation topic. Through my dissertation research, I learned that various terms are used to describe critical thinking in nursing, and I also noticed that nurses use these terms interchangeably (i.e., problem solving, decision making, scientific reasoning, and clinical reasoning). I learned that logical reasoning tests do not effectively capture the nurse's skill of making clinical judgments; therefore I designed a research project with home health nurses in new client situations where clinical reasoning about complex situations must occur daily. I found that nurses' "think-aloud" data from actual practice involved comparisons of cases with mental prototypes of similar cases. Neither problem solving nor the nursing process guided nurses' judgments. The critical thinking I discovered in my research was more holistic than linear. The challenges I see for nurse educators, then, is to teach a holistic case-based approach to clinical reasoning rather than focusing entirely on the nursing process. We must also continue to explore the nature of clinical reasoning rather than seeking measures of critical thinking.

Educators and practitioners alike are challenged to "think on their feet" or reason in a changing environment. I use several methods to build clinical reasoning skills in RN-BSN students: reflective verbalization, journaling, reflective clinical observations, and written self-evaluations. Through self-reflective exercises, nurses learn to stretch their limits. Nurses who enter the BSN program are usually eager to engage in active learning exercises where they can immediately apply concepts to their practice setting. Teaching offers endless opportunities to mentor individuals and guide their career development. I am most rewarded when I know that I have helped nurses develop new perspectives.

A cornerstone of professional nursing practice is the ability to process information and make decisions. Demands of clients from diverse backgrounds with multiple health care needs, coupled with the demands of a complex health care system, require higher-order thinking that is not solely content based. It is essential that professional nurses think critically in order to process complex data and make intelligent decisions in planning, managing, and evaluating the health care of their clients. Similarly, critical thinking is essential if nurses are to make productive contributions toward establishing the future direction of health care. To become a critical thinker, a nurse must understand the concept of critical thinking, identify the skills and internalize the dispositions of a critical thinker, and deliberately apply critical thinking principles to clinical situations.

THE CONCEPT OF CRITICAL THINKING

In recent years critical thinking has received considerable attention as an essential component of educational programs and of nursing practice. The underlying point of many of these discussions is that there is a need for higher-order thinking as the complexity of our world increases.

Defining Critical Thinking

Critical thinking is an evolving concept and one that is not easily defined. An early definition, proposed by Watson and Glaser (1964), described *critical thinking* as the combination of abilities needed to define a problem, recognize stated and unstated assumptions, formulate and select hypotheses, draw conclusions, and judge the validity of inferences. A less prescriptive definition was offered by Ennis (1989), who characterized *critical thinking* as "reasonable reflective thinking focused on deciding what to believe or do" (p. 4). Paul (1992) stated that *critical thinking* is a process of disciplined, self-directed rational thinking that "certifies what we know and makes clear wherein we are ignorant" (p. 47). Alfaro-LeFevre (1994) proposed that *critical thinking* is "careful, deliberate goal-directed thinking . . . and requires strategies that compensate for problems created by human nature (e.g., the powerful influence of personal perceptions, values, beliefs)" (p. 4). Critical thinking for nursing, as described by Bandman and Bandman (1995), is "the rational examination of ideas, inferences, assumptions, principles, arguments, conclusions, issues, statements, beliefs, and actions" (p. 7) and includes the following functions:

- Discriminating among use and misuse of language
- Analyzing meaning of terms
- Formulating nursing problems
- Analyzing arguments and issues into premises and conclusions
- Examining nursing assumptions
- Reporting data and clues accurately
- Making and checking inferences based on data
- Formulating and clarifying beliefs
- Verifying, corroborating, and justifying claims, beliefs, conclusions, decisions, and actions
- Giving relevant reasons for beliefs and conclusions
- Formulating and clarifying value judgments
- Seeking reasons, criteria, and principles that justify value judgments
- Evaluating the soundness of conclusions

Conclusions are drawn as a result of reasoning, and critical thinking is used to evaluate the reasoning process by analyzing the use of language.

There are conflicting viewpoints as to whether critical thinking is subject specific or generalizable (U.S. Department of Education, 1995). Meyers (1991) believes that before critical thinking skills can be developed, mastery of basic terms, concepts, and methodologies must occur. McPeck (1990) agrees, noting that only by immersion in the discipline can critical thinking skills be fully developed. Ennis (1987), on the other hand, suggests that there are principles of critical thinking that bridge many disciplines and can transfer to new situations, although some familiarity with the subject matter is necessary.

Delphi Report. An attempt to define critical thinking by consensus was begun in the late 1980s, and the results became known as the Delphi Report. The Delphi research project used an expert panel of 46 theoreticians representing several disciplines from the United States and Canada to develop a conceptualization of critical thinking from a broad perspective (Facione, 1990). The resulting work described critical thinking in terms of cognitive skills and affective dispositions. The outcome was a definition of *critical thinking* as the process of purposeful, self-regulatory judgments: an interactive, reflective reasoning process (Facione, Facione, & Sanchez, 1994). A critical thinker gives reasoned consideration to evidence, context, theories, methods, and criteria in order to form a purposeful judgment. At the same time, the critical thinker monitors, corrects, and improves the judgment. The Delphi project produced the following consensus definition from its panel of experts:

> We understand *critical thinking* (CT) to be purposeful, self-regulatory, judgment which results in interpretation, analysis, evaluation, and inference, as well as explanation of evidential, conceptual, methodological, criteriological, or contextual considerations upon which that judgment is based . . .CT is essential as a tool of inquiry. As such, CT is a liberating force in education and a powerful resource in one's personal and civic life. (American Philosophical Association, 1990)

The Delphi participants identified core critical thinking skills as interpretation, analysis, inference, evaluation, and explanation (Facione, Facione, & Sanchez, 1994; Pless & Clayton, 1993). These critical thinking cognitive skills and subskills are presented in the box below.

Critical Thinking Cognitive Skills and Subskills

Interpretation	**Inference**
Categorization	Querying evidence
Decoding sentences	Conjecturing alternatives
Clarifying meaning	Drawing conclusions
Analysis	**Explanation**
Examining ideas	Stating results
Identifying arguments	Justifying procedures
Analyzing arguments	Presenting arguments
Evaluation	**Self-regulation**
Assessing claims	Self-examination
Assessing arguments	Self-correction

Summary of Definitions of Critical Thinking

While there is not a universally accepted definition of critical thinking, there is agreement that it is a complex process. The variety of definitions help to provide insight into the myriad dimensions of critical thinking. The definitions presented earlier are summarized for comparison in Table 18-1, and characteristics of critical thinking are listed in the box below.

The activities involved in the process of critical thinking include appraisal, problem solving, creativity, and decision making. The interrelationships between these concepts are illustrated in Fig. 18-1. These activities are embedded in the critical thinking process in both nursing education and nursing practice.

Table 18-1   **Definitions of Critical Thinking**

Author	Definition
Watson & Glaser (1964)	Combination of abilities needed to define problems, recognize assumptions, formulate and select hypotheses, draw conclusions, and judge validity of inferences
Ennis (1989)	Reasonable, reflective thinking focused on deciding what to believe or do
Paul (1992)	Process of self-disciplined, self-directed, rational thinking that verifies what we know and clarifies what we do not know
American Philosophical Association (*Delphi Report*, 1990); Facione, Facione, & Sanchez (1994)	Purposeful, self-regulatory judgments resulting in interpretation, analysis, inference, evaluation, and explanation
Alfaro-LeFevre (1994)	Careful, deliberate, goal-directed thinking
Bandman & Bandman (1995)	Rational examination of ideas, inferences, assumptions, principles, arguments, conclusions, issues, statements, beliefs, and actions

Characteristics of Critical Thinking

Critical thinking:
Involves conceptualization
Is rational and reasonable
Is reflective
Is partially attitudinal
Is autonomous
Is creative
Is fair
Focuses on deciding what to believe or do

From Wilkinson, J.M. (1992). Critical thinking and the nursing process. In J.M. Wilkinson, *Nursing process in action: A critical thinking approach* (pp. 21-33). Redwood City, CA: Addison-Wesley.

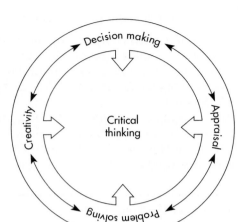

Fig. 18-1   Critical thinking model. (Redrawn from Strader, M.K., & Decker, P.J. [1995]. *Role transition to patient care management*. Norwalk, CT: Appleton & Lange.)

CRITICAL THINKING IN NURSING

In nursing, critical thinking is often portrayed as a rational linear process that is synonymous with problem solving and closely akin to the nursing process (Ford & Profetto-McGrath, 1994; Jones & Brown, 1991; Kintgen-Andrews, 1991; Klaassens, 1988; Malek, 1986; Nehring, Durham, & Macek, 1986). While the nursing process is one critical thinking competency that uses higher-order thinking to plan, provide, and evaluate nursing care, it is not all-encompassing. There is criticism that the nursing process constrains critical thinking because of its mechanistic approach (Allen, Bowers, & Diekelmann, 1989; Jones & Brown, 1991; Miller & Malcolm, 1990). Furthermore, equating critical thinking with problem solving implies that all critical thinking must be problem based. Models for critical thinking based on problem solving alone foster action according to predefined standards and objectives. The idea of pre-definition is inconsistent with many of the tenets of critical thinking. While critical thinking skills are important components of the nursing process and problem solving, they are not synonymous terms.

"The use of critical thinking . . .with whatever theory or process selected,
will enhance the validity, reliability, and worth of outcomes to clients,
patients, and practitioners."
Bandman & Bandman, 1995, p. 99

Two models for critical thinking in nursing focus on the curriculum and clinical judgment.

Curriculum Model

A nursing curriculum model for critical thinking that is an emancipatory model rather than a problem-solving one was proposed by Ford and Profetto-McGrath (1994). The emancipatory model requires the development of critical thinking skills beyond the level of problem solving. The model proposes that knowledge is more than information; it is composed of patterns, insights, interpretations, and deliberations. The emancipatory model requires a collaborative student-teacher relationship rather than a power-based one.

With a focus on critical thinking, nursing education is shifting from a purely problem-solving approach to one where critical reflection mediates the relationship between authentic knowledge and autonomous action. Knowledge is essential to critical thinking; however, the definition of knowledge depends on the cognitive intent of the situation. For example, knowledge of facts and rules that enable one to manipulate and control a situation constitutes a technical interest; understanding and meaning within a particular situation for the sake of doing what is right constitute a practical interest. In emancipatory interest the limits of a particular situation are expanded to include the larger sociopolitical, historical, and economic contexts to address the implicit fundamental power relationships. In this context having knowledge means being able to identify coercion and constraints within society and determine how these forces contribute to oppression or maintenance of the status quo; it means to take into account the larger social context of the situation, including revealing underlying assumptions and ideologies. An example of emancipatory interest in nursing practice is the hypertensive client who is not taking the prescribed medication. The nurse's knowledge of this fact is broadened to include factors in the client's larger social context (e.g., lack of money to buy medication) to understand the reasons and contributing factors for the lack of compliance.

Thinking critically and reflectively allows us to see new possibilities by going beneath the surface of a situation to examine underlying assumptions that constrain discourse and autonomous action. Critical reflection requires a disposition to listen; a tolerance for diversity, disagreement, and uncertainty; and an openness to new ideas. There are two components of critical reflection. First is a critical examination of one's own practices. This self-examination enables an understanding of the personal perceptions and assumptions of a situation that guide one's practice. The second component relates to the need for an understanding of a situation and of the way the system works to maintain the status quo. Action that is informed by critical reflection is emancipatory; "it is concerned with the empowerment of individuals as autonomous and responsible agents in the world" (Hedin, 1989, p. 81). This action involves risk taking and challenges the status quo.

Nursing Judgment Model

A model for nursing judgment described by Kataoka-Yahiro and Saylor contends that the *critical thinking* process is "reflective and reasonable thinking about nursing problems without a single solution and is focused on deciding what to believe and do"

(1994, p. 352). This model identifies the outcome of critical thinking as discipline-specific clinical judgments. While nursing judgment traditionally has been defined as clinical judgments made before or during the provision of direct client care, this model adopts a broader view. *Nursing judgment* involves decisions made in direct, semidirect, and indirect nursing roles based on their immediate relationship to client care. For example, a direct decision about client care may be made by staff nurses who provide that care. Decisions made by nurse managers about distribution of resources are semidirect nursing judgments. Decisions made by nurse educators about curriculum content are indirect nursing judgments.

Components of critical thinking. The critical thinking model for nursing judgment presents five components of critical thinking: specific knowledge, experience, competencies, attitudes, and standards of care.

Knowledge. Domain-specific knowledge is essential to successful clinical reasoning because knowledge provides the data for critical thinking processes. For example, one cannot identify appropriate actions for unexpected clinical symptoms without understanding the physiology involved. This example highlights the fact that for critical thinking to be productive, nurses must have a sound knowledge base.

Experience. The lack of practical experience and opportunity to make decisions can limit the development of critical thinking. Understanding complex situations comes through experience in analyzing similar and contrasting situations. The importance of experiential knowledge as a nurse moves from novice to expert clinician has been emphasized by Benner (1984).

Competencies. The nursing judgment model features cognitive rather than psychomotor competencies. Cognitive competencies are of three types: general critical thinking competencies, specific critical thinking competencies in clinical situations, and specific critical thinking competencies in nursing. *General critical thinking competencies* are common to other disciplines and nonclinical situations and therefore are not unique to nursing. Examples include the scientific process, hypothesis generation, problem solving, and decision making. *Specific critical thinking competencies in clinical situations* are used by nurses and other health care providers and include diagnostic reasoning, clinical inferences, and clinical decision making. *Specific critical thinking competencies in nursing* are unique to the discipline as, for example, the nursing process. According to Kataoka-Yahiro and Saylor (1994), the three types of cognitive competencies are not mutually exclusive, nor are they sufficiently encompassing by themselves to explain critical thinking.

Attitudes. *Attitudes* are "traits of the mind" and are central aspects of a critical thinker (Paul, 1992). According to Paul, critical thinking is impossible if one does not persevere at reasoning, does not fairly weigh evidence for an opposing viewpoint, or does not value curiosity or discipline. It is essential to cultivate independence, confidence, and responsibility and to acknowledge the limits of one's personal knowledge or viewpoint. Thus the critical thinking model for nursing judgment includes attitudes of confidence, independence, fairness, responsibility, risk taking, discipline, perseverance, creativity, curiosity, integrity, and humility.

Standards. Both intellectual and professional standards are important to the nursing judgment model. Critical thinking must meet the universal intellectual standards identified by Paul (1992) and presented in Fig. 18-2. Critical thinking also must be consistent with standards of professional nursing (e.g., American Nurses Association [ANA] Code for Nurses and ANA Standards of Professional Nursing Practice). That is, nurses engage in critical thinking for the good of individuals or groups rather than to cause harm or to undermine a situation. Professional standards include criteria for ethical nursing judgment, evaluation, and professional responsibility.

Levels of critical thinking. In addition to the five components of critical thinking described above, there are three levels of critical thinking included in the Kataoka-Yahiro and Saylor model: basic, complex and commitment. These levels are based on Perry's (1970) conceptualization of intellectual and ethical development as dichotomous, multiplicity, relativism, and commitment. In the first level of thinking, the in-

```
┌─────────────────────────────────────────────────────────┐
│  PERFECTION...............VS...............IMPERFECTION OF THOUGHT │
│                                                           │
│  Clear.........................vs...............Unclear   │
│                                                           │
│  Precise........................vs...............Imprecise│
│                                                           │
│  Specific.......................vs...............Vague    │
│                                                           │
│  Accurate.......................vs...............Inaccurate│
│                                                           │
│  Relevant.......................vs...............Irrelevant│
│                                                           │
│  Plausible......................vs...............Implausible│
│                                                           │
│  Consistent....................vs...............Inconsistent│
│                                                           │
│  Logical..........................vs...............Illogical│
│                                                           │
│  Deep...........................vs...............Superficial│
│                                                           │
│  Broad..........................vs...............Narrow   │
│                                                           │
│  Complete......................vs...............Incomplete│
│                                                           │
│  Significant...................vs...............Trivial   │
│                                                           │
│  Adequate for purpose...vs...............Inadequate       │
│                                                           │
│  Fair..............................vs...............Biased or one-sided│
└─────────────────────────────────────────────────────────┘
```

Fig. 18-2 Intellectual standards for thinking. (From Paul, R. [1992]. *Critical thinking: What every person needs to survive in a rapidly changing world.* Santa Rosa, CA: The Foundation for Critical Thinking.)

dividual views answers as dichotomous (dualism) and assumes that authorities have a correct answer for every problem. Also included in this level is acceptance that there is a diversity of opinions and values among authorities (multiplicity). In the next level, the individual continues to recognize the diversity of outlook and perception and has the ability to systematically detach, analyze, and examine alternatives. At the third level, the individual anticipates the necessity of making a personal choice after the relative merits of alternatives have been examined.

In the Kataoka-Yahiro and Saylor model, the basic level is adapted from Perry's dualism, with answers to complex problems seen as right or wrong—usually with one right answer for each complex problem. Although the goal is to move to higher levels of thinking, movement to higher levels can be restricted by a nurse's lack of knowledge and experience, in addition to inadequate competencies, inappropriate attitudes, and nonutilization of standards. The complex level of thinking is based on Perry's multiplicity and relativism positions, and here the best answer to a problem might be "It depends." Alternative, and perhaps conflicting, solutions are recognized. An example of complex thinking is deciding to deviate from standard protocols or roles in a specific complex client situation. At the commitment level, the nurse chooses an action or belief based on the alternatives identified at the complex level. If the chosen action is unsuccessful, alternative solutions are considered and used. These levels of thinking can be illustrated in the practice situation where a nurse receives a physician's medication order. Nurses functioning at each level of thinking will handle the situation as follows:

Dichotomous: "Since Dr. Jones wrote it, it must be correct."

Multiplicity: "Last week we had a client with the same problem, and Dr. Smith ordered a different medication. There must be two ways to treat this problem."

Relativism: "I wonder why we are treating an identical client condition in two different ways? I am going to explore this issue in more detail."

Commitment: "I have examined all the information I can find, and I think Dr. Jones made a mistake in the order. I am going to call and confer with her."

Creativity Thinking

Higher levels of thinking require a creative outlook. *Creativity thinking* is a process that leads to the development of ideas or products that are new and original. It is an essential component of critical thinking for health care providers, particularly as methods of health care delivery shift and demands for accountability increase. The environment in which students learn and nurses practice can either constrain or facilitate critical thinking. An environment that impedes critical thinking abilities is one that reinforces memorizing, retaining factual information, and following orders. An environment that is conducive to critical thinking is characterized by flexibility, creativity, support for change, and risk taking. An environment that demands perfection and reinforces the status quo constrains critical thinking. Such an environment leads to the attitude, "If it is not going to be accepted, why bother?"

*"A healthcare organization that functions within a bureaucratic
environment where new ideas are discouraged, anticipation of problems
frowned on, and adherence to rules, regulations and procedures stressed,
may not last through the changes necessitated by health care reform."*
Strader & Decker, 1995, p. 361

CHARACTERISTICS OF CRITICAL THINKERS

Seven interdependent traits of mind are essential to becoming a critical thinker
(Paul, 1992):

1. *Intellectual humility* is an awareness of the limits of one's knowledge and sensitivity to the possibility of self-deception.
2. *Intellectual courage* involves willingness to listen and examine all ideas, including those to which there is a negative reaction.
3. *Intellectual empathy* entails imagining oneself in the place of others in order to better understand them; it allows reasoning from the viewpoint of others.
4. *Intellectual integrity* refers to the application of rigorous and consistent standards of evidence and the admission of errors when they occur.
5. *Intellectual perseverance* consists of a willingness to continually seek intellectual insights over a period of time and in the face of difficulties.
6. *Faith in reason* reflects confidence in one's own ability to think rationally.
7. *Intellectual sense of justice* requires holding to intellectual standards without seeking one's own advantage.

Individuals who are critical thinkers have specific sets of characteristics. According
to Alfaro-LeFevre (1994), they are active thinkers who ask themselves questions such as
"Am I seeing things correctly?" "What does this really mean?" "Do I know why this
is?" and "How can I be more sure?" Other characteristics identified by Alfaro-LeFevre
include being:

- Knowledgeable about biases and beliefs
- Confident patient, and willing to persevere
- Good communicators who realize that mutual exchange is essential to understanding the facts and finding the best solutions
- Open-minded, listening to other perspectives, and withholding judgments until all evidence is weighed
- Humble, realizing that no one has all the answers
- Proactive, anticipating problems, and acting before they occur
- Organized and systematic in the approach to problem-solving problems and decision making
- Active thinkers with a questioning attitude
- Flexible, changing approaches as needed
- Cognizant of rules of logic, recognizing the role of intuition, but seeking evidence and weighing risks and benefits before acting

- Realistic, acknowledging that the best answers do not mean perfect answers
- Creative and committed to excellence, looking for ways to improve oneself and the way things get done

The Delphi Report's description of an ideal critical thinker also describes the attributes of a nurse with ideal clinical judgment:

> The ideal critical thinker is habitually inquisitive, well-informed, trustful of reason, open-minded, flexible, fair-minded in evaluation, honest in facing personal biases, prudent in making judgments, willing to reconsider, clear about issues, orderly in complex matters, diligent in seeking relevant information, reasonable in the selection of criteria, focused in inquiry, and persistent in seeking results which are as precise as the subject and the circumstances of inquiry permit. (American Philosophical Association, 1990, p. 3)

DISPOSITION TOWARD CRITICAL THINKING

Becoming a critical thinker involves more than developing a set of skills. It involves nurturing the disposition toward critical thinking to ensure the use of critical thinking skills outside of a structured setting, such as a classroom. Seven aspects of critical thinking disposition, based on the findings from the Delphi Report, are incorporated into the California Critical Thinking Disposition Inventory (CCTDI) (Facione, Facione, & Sanchez, 1994). These dispositional subscales, designed to be discipline neutral, have relevance for nursing practice:

- *Inquisitiveness* is intellectual curiosity and desire for learning even when there is not a readily apparent application for the knowledge. For nurses, a deficit here might signal a limited potential for developing expert knowledge and clinical practice ability. Nurses who routinely ask, "I wonder why...?" in the absence of a specific problem display inquisitiveness.
- *Systematicity* is the tendency toward organized, orderly focused, and diligent inquiry. Asking questions such as "In what order did the client's symptoms occur?" and "Is there more information we should consider?" are examples of systematic inquiry. Organized approaches are essential for competent clinical practice.
- *Analyticity* is "prizing the application of reasoning and the use of evidence to resolve problems, anticipating potential conceptual or practical difficulties, and consistently being alert to the need to intervene" (p. 346). An analytical nurse connects clinical observations with the theoretical knowledge base to anticipate clinical events.
- *Truth-seeking* is displayed as eagerness to seek the best knowledge in a given context, courage in asking questions, and objectivity and honesty, even if findings do not support self-interests or preconceived notions. Truth-seeking leads to continual reevaluation of new information. In nursing practice, the reason for why things are done a certain way is often given as "we have always done it that way." This response is contrary to truth-seeking behavior. Not being disposed to truth-

seeking can lead to nursing practice that is based on habit rather than on tested theory and may therefore hamper the development of more effective practice.

- *Open-mindedness* is tolerance of divergent views and sensitivity to one's own biases. This disposition is central to the goal of culturally competent care. Absence of open-mindedness might preclude provision of effective nursing care to populations that are different from the nurse.
- *Self-confidence* is trust in one's own reasoning processes. It permits trust in one's judgment and promotes leadership of others in resolving problems. The nurse who makes excellent assessments of client care situations but is reluctant to bring observations forward in interdisciplinary situations, especially if they differ from those made by the physician, shows a lack of self-confidence. Self-confidence to present the results of one's thinking is important in improving client care.
- *Maturity* is the disposition to be judicious in one's decision making. The critically thinking mature person approaches problems, inquiry, and decision making with the understanding that some problems are ill structured, some situations have more than one plausible option, and many judgments must be made based on standards, contexts, and evidence for which the outcome is uncertain. This trait has important implications for ethical decision making in nursing.

STRATEGIES TO BUILD CRITICAL THINKING SKILLS

Critical thinking is enhanced in environments that are caring, nonthreatening, flexible, and respectful of diverse points of view. Nurses who are familiar with the nursing process, the scientific method, and research methods already know much about critical thinking because they are based on some of the same principles.

Several strategies to enhance critical thinking are the following (Alfaro-LeFevre, 1994):

- Anticipate questions others might ask. This helps to identify a wider scope of questions that need to be answered to obtain relevant information. For example, "What will the client's family want to know?"
- Ask "what if" questions.
- Look for flaws in thinking for the purpose of evaluating assessments and solutions and making improvements. Ask, "What is missing?" and "How could this be made better?"
- Ask others to look for flaws in thinking.
- Develop good habits of inquiry—habits that aid in the search for truth, such as keeping an open mind, clarifying information, and taking enough time.
- Use phrases such as, "I need to find out" rather than "I don't know" or "I'm not sure."
- Turn errors into learning opportunities.

Persistent use of these strategies develops the skills and nurtures the disposition for critical thinking. Becoming a critical thinker is a lifelong process; we can all be better than we are if we work at it.

RESEARCH AND MEASUREMENT ISSUES ASSOCIATED WITH CRITICAL THINKING

While the concept of critical thinking is assuming a greater role in the design of instruction, the measurement of critical thinking remains difficult. There are few measures of critical thinking skills, and research with subjects other than students is quite limited.

Critical Thinking Measures

One of the most widely used measures of critical thinking skills is the Watson-Glaser Critical Thinking Appraisal (WGCTA). The test is composed of a series of objective items designed to measure five aspects of critical thinking: inference, recognition of assumptions, deduction, interpretation, and evaluation of arguments. Scores on the five subtests are equally weighted to derive a total score.

The Cornell Critical Thinking Test (CCTT) is a multiple-choice test. It assesses deductive reasoning, identification of faulty reasoning, judgment of reliability of statements, evaluation of evidence, choice of useful hypothesis-testing predictions, and finding assumptions.

The California Critical Thinking Skills Test (CCTST) is based on the Delphi Report's consensus definition of critical thinking. It provides an overall score on critical thinking skills and subscale scores on analysis, evaluation, inference, deductive reasoning, and inductive reasoning.

Research

Much of the research on critical thinking in nursing has been done with students rather than with practicing nurses. Thus information relative to critical thinking in clinical practice is sparse. The results of longitudinal studies that address the relationship between nursing education and critical thinking are mixed. Bauwens and Gerhard (1987), using the WGCTA, found no significant difference in critical thinking between entry to, and exit from, upper-division nursing study. Sullivan (1987) also used the WGCTA and found no significant differences between entry and exit among RN students in a baccalaureate program. Similarly, Kingten-Andrews (1988) found no significant gain over an academic year among practical nursing students, prehealth science freshmen, associate degree nursing students, and generic baccalaureate sophomore students. On the other hand, Berger (1984) and Gross et al., (1987) reported a positive relationship between education and critical thinking, with both associate degree and baccalaureate students scoring significantly higher at program completion than at entry.

Cross-sectional studies also report mixed findings. Baccalaureate senior students scored higher on critical thinking than did second-year associate degree student (Frederickson & Mayer, 1977). Baccalaureate seniors also scored higher on the WGCTA than did associate degree and diploma nursing students (Scoloveno, 1981). However, there were no significant differences between graduate and undergraduate students on the WGCTA (Matthews & Gaul, 1979).

A study of critical thinking ability of practicing nurses was conducted by Pardue (1987). Baccalaureate and master's prepared nurses scored higher on the WGCTA than did those with diplomas or associate degrees, but there were no significant differences in self-reported difficulty in making decisions.

None of these studies is definitive in its findings, particularly in light of variables other than the educational program that might have explained the results. The mixed findings in these studies also might be attributed to the fact that critical thinking is a complex process that is very difficult to measure or to other factors in the research design.

APPLICATION OF CRITICAL THINKING IN A CLINICAL SITUATION

> All disciplines have a logic and nursing is no exception . . . Nursing content is infused through, with, and continually shaped by nursing goals, nursing questions and problems, nursing ideas and concepts, nursing principles and theories, nursing evidence, data and reasons, nursing interpretations and claims, nursing inferences and lines of formulated thought, nursing implications and consequences, and a nursing point of view. (Paul & Heaslip, 1995, p. 47)

Nursing information and data are transformed into knowledge, which then becomes the basis of sound and critically monitored nursing practice.

The following example uses the elements of reasoning described by Paul (1993) and illustrated in Fig. 18-3, which work together to create a critical thinking environment.

Situation

Representatives of various agencies have come together to discuss the adequacy of health services for the elderly in their community. A registered nurse is selected as the leader of the group. Since the group is a loosely constructed one representing many different constituencies, the leader recognizes the potential for the lack of focus and the possibility of producing a product that does not meet the stated purpose or needs of the community. The nurse decides to consciously use the elements of critical thinking in leading the group through its task.

Identify the purpose. At the beginning of the first meeting, the leader states that their purpose is to analyze the adequacy of community health services for the elderly. During the course of subsequent meetings, the leader reiterates the purpose to keep the group focused. The major purpose often has to be distinguished from related purposes, such as expanding services for the elderly or assessing all health services in the community. Frequent reminders help in actually achieving the purpose and focusing thought and action.

Clearly and succinctly state the question being asked, the problem being solved, or the issue under discussion. In this situation, the major question is "Are

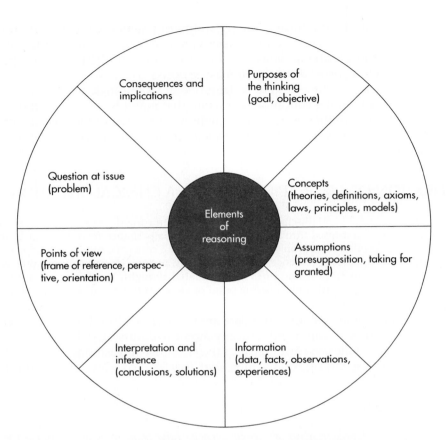

Fig. 18-3   Elements of reasoning. (Modified from Paul, R. [1994]. *Critical thinking: Transforming the quality of teaching, learning, and practice in the education of health professionals.* [Workbook for the Medical University of South Carolina College of Nursing, Charleston, SC.])

there adequate health services for the elderly of the community?" This question can be further broken into subquestions related to the type of services available, access to those services, the amount of use of the services, and unmet health needs of the elderly in the community. The questions should relate to the overall purpose and be answerable and relevant.

Recognize that all reasoning is done from some point of view. Because the group itself represents different constituencies, multiple points of view are expected to surface. In guiding the group, the challenge of the leader is to become aware of her own point of view and that of others, be fair in having all relevant points of view expressed, and allow evaluation of all perspectives while keeping the discussion focused on the purpose and relevant questions.

Understand that all reasoning is based on assumptions. Because assumptions are often embedded deeply in reasoning, it is sometimes difficult to identify them. However, not doing so places serious constraints on critical thinking and may distort the outcome. For example, the leader hears statements from one member of the group that health services for children are a greater problem than for the elderly. Another group member comments that because of their previous contributions to the community, health services for the elderly should have highest priority and no amount of service is adequate. The challenge to the nurse leader is to help the group to identify assumptions that influence the group's work, check the validity of the assumptions, and re-examine the questions being asked in light of the assumptions.

Clarify concepts and ideas that are necessary to explore the issue. The group should first define what is meant by "adequacy" and what is meant by "health services." These terms may have a wide range of meanings, depending on the points of view and assumptions of the group members. Clarifying these ideas may lead to further discussion and explication of assumptions stated earlier.

Examine the empirical data. At this point the group examines the available data. Examples of information that might be useful include the number and types of health services available in the community, whether or not there are elderly people who are unable to get access to those services, and the existence of health needs for which no services are provided. The challenge to the leader is to ensure that the data presented are complete and relevant to the question, to disregard information that is not relevant to the current issue, and to state the evidence clearly and fairly.

Draw inferences from the data. The leader must be sure that there is a link between the data and inferences, that they are reasonable given the data, and that they are consistent. In this situation, the group determined that institutional services are adequate for those elderly who can get to them. However, there is a lack of transportation services that prohibits many of the elderly from going to the settings where services are delivered. It was also determined that there is a lack of primary care and nutritional services.

Develop implications and consequences. At this stage the group must examine the conclusion of their reasoning and project the implications and consequences of that reasoning. Precise consequences for addressing or not addressing the issues must include both positive and negative consequences.

• • •

Today's health care environment requires nurses to solve complex problems, address complex questions, explore unique client situations, and evaluate the effectiveness of a wide range of interventions. Critical thinking is an integral part of effective nursing action. It is a complex process through which nurses can explore practice situations and search for effective outcomes. Conscious application of critical thinking principles can result in effective decision making and ultimately enhance the quality of care.

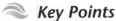 *Key Points*

- Critical thinking is an evolving concept that is not easily defined.

- Critical thinking skills are important components of the nursing process and problem solving, but critical thinking, the nursing process, and problem solving are *not* synonymous terms.

- Clinical judgments are outcomes of critical thinking.

- Appraisal, problem solving, creativity, and decision making are interrelated concepts in critical thinking.

- Nurses with expert clinical judgment display characteristics of high-level critical thinking.

- To think critically, nurses must be able to see connections; use logic; differentiate between fact, inference, and assumptions; evaluate arguments; consider many sides of an issue; be creative; and believe in their ability to think and reason.

- Becoming a critical thinker involves not only acquiring a set of skills, but also developing a disposition toward critical thinking.

- Becoming a critical thinker is a lifelong process.

- More work needs to be done to enhance and examine critical thinking embedded in nursing practice. Two areas needing particular attention are the development and refinement of instruments to measure critical thinking in practice and to further explore the relationship between clinical judgment and critical thinking.

 Critical Thinking Exercises

1. Differentiate between critical thinking, problem solving, and decision making.

2. Think about a patient care situation that you have recently encountered. What questions is your instructor likely to ask you when you present this situation?

3. Mr. Jones, aged 82, is admitted to your hospital unit. In conducting his initial assessment, you notice that he is somewhat confused. His admitting notes indicate that he takes Digoxin and Lasix. Describe the process that you will use to determine whether or not Mr. Jones is experiencing side effects from his medication. Focus on the questions you will ask yourself or others, *not* on the side effects themselves.

4. Describe the *best* and *worst* decision making you have seen by a nurse in a client care situation. Compare these two situations in terms of the thought process used, the underlying assumptions of the nurses, the accuracy of available information, the interpretation of information, and the soundness of the decision reached.

References

Alfaro-LeFevre, R. (1994). Teaching nurses critical thinking. *Academy of Medical-Surgical Nurses News, 4,* 8.

Allen, D., Bowers, B., & Diekelmann, N. (1989). Writing to learn: A reconceptualization of thinking and writing in the nursing curriculum. *Journal of Nursing Education, 28*(1), 6-11.

American Philosophical Association. (1990). *Critical thinking: A statement of expert consensus for purposes of educational assessment and instruction. The Delphi Report: Research findings and recommendations prepared for the committee of pre-college philosophy* (ERIC Document Reproduction Service No. ED 315-423).

Bandman, E.L., & Bandman, B. (1995). *Critical thinking in nursing.* Norwalk, CT: Appleton & Lange.

Bauwens, E.E., & Gerhard, G.G. (1987). The use of the Watson-Glaser Critical Thinking Appraisal to predict success in a baccalaureate nursing program. *Journal of Nursing Education, 26*(7), 278-281.

Benner, P. (1984). *From novice to expert: Excellence and power in clinical nursing practice.* Menlo Park, CA: Addison-Wesley.

Berger, M.C. (1984). Critical thinking ability and nursing students. *Journal of Nursing Education, 23*(7), 306-308.

Ennis, R.H. (1987). Critical thinking and the curriculum. In M. Heiman & J. Slomianko (Eds), *Thinking skills instruction: Concepts and techniques.* Washington, DC: National Education Association.

Ennis, R.H. (1989). Critical thinking and subject specificity: Clarification and needed research. *Educational Researcher, 18*(3), 4-10.

Facione, P.A. (1990). Critical thinking: A statement of expert consensus for purposes of educational assessment and instruction (executive summary). In *The Delphi Report.* Millbrae, CA: California Academic Press.

Facione, N.C., Facione, P.A., & Sanchez, C.A. (1994). Critical thinking disposition as a measure of competent clinical judgment: The development of the California Critical Thinking Disposition Inventory. *Journal of Nursing Education, 33*(8), 345-350.

Ford, J.S., & Profetto-McGrath, J. (1994). A model for critical thinking within the context of curriculum as praxis. *Journal of Nursing Education, 33*(8), 341-344.

Frederickson, K., & Mayer, G.G. (1977). Problem solving skills: What effect does education have? *American Journal of Nursing, 77*(7), 1167-1169.

Gross, Y.T., Takazawa, E.S., & Rose, C.L. (1987). Critical thinking and nursing education. *Journal of Nursing Education, 26*(8), 317-323.

Hedin, B.A. (1989). Expert clinical teaching. In National League for Nursing, *Curriculum revolution: Reconceptualizing nursing education* (pp. 71-89) (NLN Publication No. 15-2280). New York: The League.

Jones, S.A., & Brown, L.N. (1991). Critical thinking: Impact on nursing education. *Journal of Advanced Nursing, 16*(5), 529-533.

Kataoka-Yahiro, M., & Saylor, C. (1994). A critical thinking model for nursing judgment. *Journal of Nursing Education, 33*(8), 351-356.

Kintgen-Andrews, J. (1988). Development of critical thinking: Career ladder P.N. and A.D. nursing students, prehealth science freshmen, generic baccalaureate sophomore nursing students. *Resources in Education, 24*(1) (ERIC Document No. 297 153).

Kintgen-Andrews, J. (1991). Critical thinking and nursing education: Perplexities and insights. *Journal of Nursing Education, 30*(4), 152-157.

Klaassens, E. (1988). Improving teaching for thinking. *Nurse Educator, 13*(6), 15-19.

Malek, C.J. (1986). A model for teaching critical thinking. *Nurse Educator, 11*(6), 20-23.

Matthews, C.A., & Gaul, A.L. (1979). Nursing diagnosis from the perspective of concept attainment and critical thinking. *Advances in Nursing Science, 2*(11), 17-26.

McPeck, J.E. (1990). *Teaching critical thinking.* New York: Routledge.

Meyers, C. (1991). *Teaching students to think critically.* San Francisco: Jossey-Bass.

Miller, M., & Malcolm, N. (1990). Critical thinking in the nursing curriculum. *Nursing and Health Care, 11*(2), 67-73.

Nehring, W.M., Durham, J.D., & Macek, M.M. (1986). Effective teaching: A problem-solving paradigm. *Nurse Educator, 11*(3), 23-26.

Pardue, S.F. (1987). Decision-making skills and critical thinking ability among associate degree, diploma, baccalaureate, and master's prepared nurses. *Journal of Nursing Education, 26*(9), 354-361.

Paul, R. (1992). *Critical thinking: What every person needs to survive in a rapidly changing world.* Santa Rosa, CA: The Foundation for Critical Thinking.

Paul, R. (1993). The art of redesigning instruction. In J. Willsen & A.J.A. Binker (Eds.), *Critical thinking: How to prepare students for a rapidly changing world* (p. 319). Santa Rosa, CA: Foundation for Critical Thinking.

Paul, R. (1994). *Critical thinking: Transforming the quality of teaching, learning, and practice in the education of health professionals.* (Workbook for the Medical University of South Carolina College of Nursing, Charleston, SC.)

Paul, R., & Heaslip, P. (1995). Critical thinking and intuitive nursing practice. *Journal of Advanced Nursing, 22,* 40-47.

Perry, W.G. (1970). *Forms of intellectual and technical development in the college years: A scheme.* New York: Holt, Rinehart & Winston.

Pless, B.S., & Clayton, G.M. (1993). Clarifying the concept of critical thinking in nursing. *Journal of Nursing Education, 32*(a), 425-428.

Scoloveno, M. (1981). Problem solving ability of senior nursing students in three program types (Doctoral dissertation. Rutgers University, 1981). *Dissertation Abstracts International, 41,* 1396B.

Strader, M.K., & Decker, P.J. (1995). *Role transition to patient care management.* Norwalk, CT: Appleton & Lange.

Sullivan, E.J. (1987). Critical thinking, creativity, clinical performance, and achievement in RN students. *Nurse Educator, 12*(2), 12-16.

U.S. Department of Education. (1995). *National assessment of college student learning: Identifying college graduates' essential skills in writing, speech and listening, and critical thinking.* Washington, DC: U.S. Government Printing Office.

Watson, G., & Glaser, E.M. (1964). *Critical thinking appraisal.* Orlando, FL: Harcourt Brace Jovanovich.

Wilkinson, J.M. (1992). Critical thinking and the nursing process. In J.M. Wilkinson, *Nursing process in action: A critical thinking approach* (pp. 21-33). Redwood City, CA: Addison-Wesley.

Change, Complexity, and Chaos 19

Anne Griswold Peirce and Nathaniel W. Peirce

 Objectives

At the completion of this chapter, the reader will be able to:

- Discuss the various factors that influence change.

- Compare organizational development and transformation.

- Contrast the four models of planned change most commonly used in nursing.

- Apply the models of change to clinical situations.

- Discuss complexity in the change process.

Profile in Practice

Jeanette Lancaster, PhD, RN, FAAN
Sadie Health Cabaniss Professor of Nursing and Dean,
School of Nursing, University of Virginia,
Charlottesville, Virginia

I first became interested in the concept of "change" in the late 1970s when undergraduate nursing programs began redesigning their curricula to move toward an integrated rather than segmented model. I was struck by how differently people responded to the idea of change. Some became enthused and could hardly wait to move ahead; others supported the idea that change must and should occur and were willing workers in the process; in contrast, another group of people seemed reluctant to make any changes yet kept that perspective to themselves. The last group that I observed clearly wished to avoid change, and they made that fact known to all who would listen.

In studying the theories related to change, we know that people engage in change for a variety of reasons, including their personality, comfort with new ideas, ways of working, and anticipation about the future. People are also more likely to support change if they see some advantage in making the change—if

---

the expected new behaviors seem logical and not too complex, and if they can try out the new way on a small scale and make adjustments as needed. People with what is known as "hardy personalities" are more likely to engage willingly in change. These people believe they have control over their world and that they can make a difference. They also feel challenged by thinking that the change may be difficult but not impossible, and they commit to trying the new way in order to move the organization forward.

I cannot recall a time in my 20-plus-year career in nursing when understanding, enjoying, and surviving change has been more a part of daily life. As health care delivery changes, so must nursing education, practice, and research. The skills that will serve nurses and nursing well in a rapidly changing system are the following: Remember that change is everywhere, and this is not the time to lament how good the old days were—they are gone! Keep a sense of balance in your lives and a sense of perspective in what matters in your professional and personal roles. Understand the mission and goals of your organization and look for ways to support them. Realize that sometimes your goals conflict with those of the organization, and this may herald some soul searching about where you can best serve in order to meet your needs and those of your employer. Remember that change causes many to fear the present and the future; therefore, face your own fears and help colleagues confront their fears. Continue to listen, learn, and grow. Nursing is a knowledge profession; thus our contributions are crucial because of what we know, think, and understand about people, health care, and the practice of nursing.

"There is nothing permanent but change."
Heraclitus, 513 BC

Change is a process that transforms people, systems, organizations, cultures, and societies into new variations. The notion of change is promoted in both public and private organizations as an indicator of progress, efficiency, and survival; paradoxically, it is also vilified as a threat to the individual and society. Likewise, the human response to change can be accepting and welcoming, as well as chaotic, unpredictable, and resistant.

The omnipresent nature of change compels all professions to analyze and understand its ramifications for individuals and organizations. The nursing profession is no exception. The current debate over the delivery of health care has given the nursing profession the impetus to more closely examine what change means to the discipline. The debate on health care reform has already resulted in a multitude of changes, even if no legislative action ever occurs. Nursing's response will create further change in the profession and paradigms of practice. All these planned and unplanned changes are best dealt with by nurses who understand change.

Nurses today need to have the courage and conviction to bring about change to improve the quality of care for patients. While many changes in nursing practice and management are imposed by external forces, "nursing changes would be more efficient and effective if guided by internal, as well as external, change agents, because nursing experts have a greater understanding than outsiders of the manner in which various nursing system elements interact" (Gillies, 1994, p. 470).

Planning for change and reacting to unplanned change is part of nursing. For these reasons it is essential for nurses to not only become knowledgeable of planned change theory, but also to participate in the evolution of new change models and interventions. It is not enough to just use previously developed business models without considering how and why nursing is different.

The models of change used by nursing are based on systems theory. Systems theory is a linear cause-and-effect model that uses the analogy of machines or computers to explain how people react to change. Recent work in many different fields has shown that dynamic, adaptive systems, such as people, cannot be examined in the same ways as linear, nondynamic systems. Dynamic systems have an emergent nature; they change and evolve in ways that cannot always be predictable. Thus it seems that change should be examined within a dynamic framework, for change is basically about people. This chapter presents information about chaos and complexity theories as an alternative framework that may be used to develop more realistic models of change for the nursing profession. Common frameworks currently used to examine change are also presented.

DEFINING CHANGE

The dictionary defines change as both a noun and a verb. As a noun, *change* is defined as the act, process, or result of changing. It may also be defined as an alteration, transformation, or substitution. Other synonyms are mutation, permutation, variation, and vicissitude. As a verb, *change* means to make different in some particular, to modify, to make radically different, to transform, or to give a different position, course, or direction. Other synonyms for the verb form of change include switch, exchange, modify, or undergo loss, transformation, transition, or substitution. From the dictionary definitions, then, change can be described as both a process and an outcome.

The nursing literature is replete with articles and books about change and the change process. Yet there are relatively few conceptual or operational definitions of change. The definitions that are offered are often simplistic or overreaching. For example, change is "a dynamic process by which an alteration is brought about that makes a distinct difference in something" (Grohar-Murray & DiCroce, 1992, p. 201) or "change is any alteration, regardless how slight or how major, or how large or how small" (Bernhard & Walsh, 1995, p. 162). Such succinct definitions do not take into account the complexity of change. Instead, Sheehan (1990) suggests that change is "synonymous with conversion, innovation, novelty, metamorphosis, revolution, and transformation."

The current discourse in the nursing literature includes whether transition should be the organizing construct rather than change, and Meleis and Trangenstein (1993) differentiate between the two. According to them, *transition* occurs over time, and has a sense of movement and an internal orientation, in contrast to *change,* which implies a substitution, and has a faster or more abrupt movement, as well as a more external orientation.

It might appear that the use of transition would focus attention only on the human process during change. Transition instead may be imbedded in all changes. *If change is the movement from one state to the next, then transition may describe that movement.* Transition may also be a richer term for describing the movement of an individual or organization through change.

In the business literature, change is often defined in terms of the type or magnitude of change produced. For example, *transactional change* is concerned with the change of everyday occurrences, such as the way in which nursing care is documented or a procedure is accomplished. *Transformational change* is that which fundamentally alters a behavior or attitude (Burke & Litwin, 1992). An example of transformational change would be the recent movement of nursing care out of the hospital and into the community.

Change is an integral part of each aspect of life, and thus it is not surprising that religious and philosophical views also influence its definition. The contrasting views of Eastern and Western philosophy and religion have been used to explicate change as a process (Eastern) and as an outcome (Western).

Although integral to life, it is easy to appreciate that change is also subjective. As such, the view of change is influenced by the individual. Any individual who likes change will view it differently from one who does not accept or want change.

Thus change is not easily defined. It is a process and an outcome, a movement and a state, expected and unexpected, gradual and rapid, good and bad, and all states in between. Change is altered by the reaction and perceptions of involved individuals and is illuminated through patterns of behavior. As we endeavor to understand change, it is important to remember that change is universal but may not always be understandable or predictable.

ELEMENTS OF CHANGE

The elements important to change are the change itself, the context, the time, and the individuals involved (Davis, 1991). Lack of awareness of these elements can be disastrous to those who want to promote change. Several crucial elements of change are considered in this chapter, including attitudinal, behavioral, language, metaphorical, informational, rate, volume, and cross-cultural factors of change. These elements are illustrated in Fig. 19-1.

Individual-Attitude Change

Promoting change in people is difficult, since people are reluctant to give up old ways of thinking. Yet the promotion of organizational change, or any other type of change, is very dependent on a change in individual attitudes. For this reason, it is important to consider not only how to change structure when planning for change, but also how to change people.

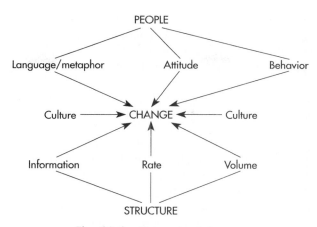

Fig. 19-1   Elements of change.

Psychological theory can be used to guide the change process. Since much of change is about people, it is beneficial to have any knowledge that helps one to deal more effectively with the people involved in innovation. One recommendation is that Gestalt theory be used in the plan for change (Stickland, 1992). *Gestalt theory* is based on the assumption that learning is a process of changing insights or thought patterns. An individual learns from using, perceiving, and receiving stimuli from the environment. Thought patterns change through a process of simultaneous, mutual interaction between the individual and the environment. For example, a nurse and client share the process and the experience of moving to optimal health. The interaction of their roles enables them to gain insights into each other, and this facilitates change.

A number of problems inherent in attitudinal change have been identified, and ways to effect attitudinal change have been proposed. The first step is to understand if an attitude is changeable and to what degree. According to Beer and Walton (1987), there are three types of attitudinal change. *Alpha change* occurs when there is a real change in a "measurement" of the concept but no change in the way it is conceptualized. To illustrate, individuals may change the value they place on the use of alternative medicine, but they still consider these therapies an adjunct to "real medicine." *Beta change* occurs when there is a real shift in expectations. For example, individuals might come to expect that *all* disease be treated with nutrition as part of an overall medical treatment regimen. *Gamma change* represents a complete and radical change, such as espousing the use of nutrition as the *primary* treatment for disease. Alpha change is the easiest to promote, and gamma is the most difficult.

Change in Behavior

While all three types of change—alpha, beta, and gamma—reflect changes in attitude, they do not ensure changes in behavior. When change can be viewed publicly, it is more likely to result in lasting behavioral change (Tice, 1992). Management should start a change process by requiring behavioral change of top executives. People believe in a change only when they see it work (Duck, 1993). Before that happens, it is just talk.

Involvement in the process of change can also facilitate behavioral change. How and what the individuals involved think about the change process affects their actions (Downey & Brief, 1986; Lowstedt, 1993). The more people are involved in the planning and implementation of the change process, the greater the chance of success (Armenakis, Harris, & Mossholder, 1993; Axelrod, 1992). For example, to improve the quality of working conditions on an obstetrical unit, a participation project to initiate needed change in scheduling practices was implemented. New models of the work schedule were developed with the staff, and the preferred schedule of the majority was implemented. After a trial basis, an evaluation of the new schedule was conducted, and adjustments identified by the staff were made. The overall satisfaction with the change was favorable, in part because of involvement in the process (Snell & Turner, 1991).

Language and Metaphor of Change

The use of metaphor and language may also be important, since language is the vehicle used to discuss and conceptualize change. Gioia and Chittipeddi (1991) suggest that "sensemaker" and "sensegiver" be used as descriptive metaphors for the people involved in promoting change. These metaphors suggest a different involvement in the change process than does the term "change agent," which is most frequently used in nursing. *Agent* suggests the external orientation of a manager, whereas *sensemaker* and *sensegiver* suggest the internal orientation of a guide to the change process.

The appropriate uses of metaphor can also help provide needed reference points during the change process. Listening to the metaphors of speech can give important clues to understanding change in context (Marshak, 1993). For example, two metaphors that could be used to describe change are "create a new vision" and "lay a good foundation." Each of these metaphors implies a different type of change. Their respective use by two persons to describe one change could signal a conflict in the rate and direction of change.

Changing the common vernacular, or metaphors, of an institution can even facilitate change as it occurs. For instance, the process of change in one psychiatric institution involved moving from a standard 28-day program for all patients to more fluid and individualized treatment plans. Simply changing the language from "treatment program" to "treatment process" helped the staff to better understand and accept the change of not rigidly adhering to 28 days of treatment (Hamm, 1992).

Information and Change

Information is a critical element in the change process. While some argument can be made about the amount of information required, all planned change must include the transfer of information. Different types of information may be needed. Stickland (1992) suggests that both factual and sensory data are needed if change is to be successful. An alternative view is that the repetition of the message is important. When persons promoting change have talked about it so much they cannot bear to think about it any more, the message is just starting to get through (Duck, 1993).

Rational strategies for change depend heavily on information (Rogers, 1983). In fact, communication is the focus in these models. It is thought that if the individuals involved understand the need for change, their behavior will change, be rational, and be logical. The quality and amount of information exchanged is critical to the success of planned change, for only information will convince the individual of the need to change.

Normative strategies also rely on the transfer of information by educating those participating in the change process. Learning and change must be considered together, since one cannot learn without changing the brain's neural network, and one cannot change without learning (Kosko, 1993). Again, the quality and type of information exchanged is important. Even with power-coercive strategies, where change comes from those holding power or seeking control, there is some need to explain change in order to implement the innovation.

The change process usually involves the collection of information through an evaluation, needs assessment, or survey. Although other methods are available, survey methodology is recommended as the most comprehensive way to assess change factors (Armenakis, Harris, & Mossholder, 1993). For example, before implementing change on a nursing unit, nurse managers should survey the staff to determine the need for change, in addition to assessing other important and previously identified factors, such as resistance, language, attitude, and behavior.

The type of information collected is important to understanding both the need for change and the factors involved. These change factors are termed the driving and restraining forces (Lewin, 1951). *Driving forces* are those that push the system toward the desired change, whereas *restraining forces* pull the system away. Only a very thorough analysis of the system can enable the person promoting change to understand those opposing forces. For example, driving forces for computerized documentation might include the perceived benefits of computerized charts being quicker and more accurate, whereas restraining forces could include lack of time, resources, and money to properly educate those involved.

Information is important to change, but correct information does not always ensure success, nor does more information always improve matters (Mawhinney, 1992). More information means more facts to consider and thus more variables to add to the equation. The problems encountered by adding more information are called *information-based complexity* (Traub & Wozniakowski, 1994). All information gathered in preparation for change contains a certain amount of inherent error. Thus more information by definition means more error. While more information may indeed add to an understanding of change, the increased amount of error must also be considered. Newsworthy events illustrate this point. Even though much information is reported by journalists, it is often inconsistent and sometimes incorrect. In reports of a natural disaster, for example, the number of people missing or dead varies among news sources and changes from day to day.

While not yet applied to change theory, it may be that *fuzzy logic,* which considers degrees of truth or correctness, can provide the best overall solution to a given problem of change (Kosko, 1993). Individuals and groups planning change could consider degrees of change in their evaluation of change rather than determining whether a situation is changed or unchanged. This way of thinking is more consistent with the real world, in which events are rarely black or white but rather shades of gray.

Rate and Volume of Change

The rate at which change or changes occur also influences the response to change. Many life changes are both expected and gradual, such as developmental changes of maturation. Even organizations have analogous developmental changes as they grow and mature. In many ways, these types of slow and gradual changes are easy to accept, and in some cases it may not even be obvious that a change has occurred. In part, this has to do with the predictability of the change.

However, other types of changes cannot and should not occur slowly. And while some change can be small in nature, many changes require large-scale alterations. Rapid change, large changes, or changes that are both rapid and large are not easily dealt with by most individuals (or organizations). There appears to be a natural preference for stability and/or control (Lewin, 1992). This resistance to change is influenced by habit; by selective attention to, and retention of, only confirming information; by fear of the unknown; and by fears related to the loss of security and income (Arnold, Capella, & Sumrall, 1987). That these real or perceived threats are directed to fundamental aspects of life may make the resistance to change more understandable (see box below).

Cross-Cultural Aspects of Change

Much of the theoretical work on change is deeply rooted within Western thought and thus may not be relevant to other cultures. In fact, planned change models that propose total system linearity and predictability may also not be realistic, even within some Western cultures. Marshak (1993) proposes that change theory based on Eastern thought, specifically Confucianism and Taoist, may present an alternative and important view.

Factors That Make It Harder to Change
Rapid change Large changes Multiple changes Unexpected changes

In Eastern thought, life is cyclical, and therefore so is change. The change process does not have an end point but rather is ongoing and in constant need of refinement. Equilibrium and harmony are critical and must be maintained. Change is expected; it is not an aberration but rather an accepted part of life.

PLANNED CHANGE

"When you know a thing, to recognize that you know it, and when you do not know a thing, to recognize that you do not know it. That is knowledge."
Confucius

The profession of nursing is undergoing massive change with the development of new practices, evolving health care policies, and the need to respond to organizational changes in the clinical setting. As a result, there has been extensive discussion in the nursing field on planned change theory and models. In a survey of the nursing literature from 1982 to 1992, 176 articles on planned change were identified. Excluding those that use only a nursing research utilization model, 155 remained for further examination. Twenty-two (14.4%) of these contain evaluations of planned change theories; however, only seven (4.5%) provide an in-depth evaluation of the theories (Tiffany et al., 1994). These authors have observed that "the high frequency of citation of inappropriate or incomplete change theories, combined with the low rate of evaluation of change theories, indicates a need for introduction of appropriate planned change theories" (p. 59). They further propose that practicing nurses need more understandable expositions and practical applications of planned change.

Defining Planned Change

Three of the most cited definitions of planned change in the nursing literature are those proposed by Chin, Bennis and colleagues, and Zajc. Chin (1976) views *planned change* as the way in which a practitioner analyzes and works out situations of change. "These ways are embodied in the concept with which they apprehend the dynamics of the client system they are working with, their relationship to it, and their process of helping with its change" (p. 90). Bennis, Benne, and Chin (1985) view *planned change* as a purposeful, conscious implementation of one's understanding and acquired skills to manage the course of change. Finally, Zajc (1987) looks at *planned change* as a form of theory that describes how the change agent plans to proceed toward a desirable goal.

Planned Change Theories and Models

Much of the nursing discourse on planned change emerges from the business fields of organization development (OD) and, more recently, organization transformation (OT). *Organization development* is a term that has been used in the business literature to explicate change within an organization. Most OD theorists view organizations as open systems reacting to the environment. In an open system the manager has to have the expertise to understand and interpret the environmental changes in order to manage change. Thus, as a field, OD is concerned with the "theory and practice of managing the continual adaptation of internal organizational arrangements to changes in the external environment" (Beer & Walton, 1987, p. 340).

Although OD encompasses more than just change, all development requires change. According to Porras and Silvers (1991), the field of planned change is still evolving as a result of rapid change in the environment. This places a burden on organizations to adapt quickly in order to progress and survive. The model illustrated in Fig. 19-2 summarizes the OT and OD models of change. The OD approach, the more traditional, has been synonymous with the term *planned change*. The OT approach is a second-generation OD and represents an emerging field. At this point, the definition of OT is rapidly evolving.

Organization development is defined as "(1) a set of behavioral science theories, values, strategies, and techniques (2) aimed at the planned change of organizational settings (3) with the intention of generating alpha, beta, and/or gamma cognition change in individual organizational members, leading to behavioral change and thus (4) creating a better fit between the organization's capabilities and its current environmental demands, or (5) promoting changes that help the organization to better fit predicted future environments" (Porras & Silvers, 1991, p. 54).

Organization transformation is "(1) a set of behavioral science, theories, values, strategies, and techniques (2) aimed at the planned change of organization vision and work

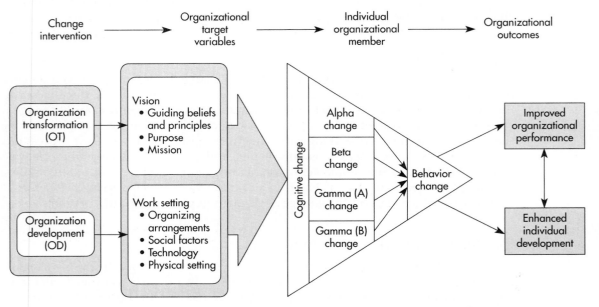

Fig. 19-2   Organizational change. (Redrawn from Porras, J.L., & Silvers, R.C. [1991]. Organization development and transformation. *Annual Review of Psychology, 45,* 51-78.)

settings (3) with the intention of generating alpha, beta, gamma cognition change in individual organizational members, leading to behavioral change and thus (4) promoting paradigmatic change that helps the organization better fit or create desirable future environments" (Porras & Silvers, 1991, p. 54).

Thus OT is distinguished from OD as being an approach to create a new vision for the organization. OD, on the other hand, is designed to help an organization adapt to a changing environment or improve its alignment with expected environments (Porras & Silver, 1991). OT draws from more recent developments in psychology, systems theory, and transpersonal psychology.

There are those that contend that the development of a third-generation theory would be more beneficial than either organizational development or transformation (Beer & Walton, 1987; Duck, 1993; Mawhinney, 1992). This third-generation theory could include all types of interventions as well as applications to the myriad of circumstances faced by organizations. Complexity theory, as described later in the chapter, may provide the framework needed for the newest approach to change theory.

In examining planned change, there are several theories and models that have been cited by nurses for application in the clinical setting. Four types of models are commonly discussed: rational, normative, paradoxical, and power-coercive. Table 19-1 illustrates the matrix of the four models and their relationship to persuasion and power as the forces for change.

Rational model. Rational models are proposed to be effective in a system that is universally ready for change (Armenakis, Harris, & Mossholder, 1993; Tappen, 1995). The premise of these models is that, with good information, most people will make the logical choice to change. The rational models are least dependent on power, as illustrated in Fig. 19-3. They assume that people behave rationally and that there is little need to force action. The models propose that communication is the key to the process.

Steps in the change process. The rational models generally present the following three steps as necessary to the change process: development of the change, communication about the change, and consequences (acceptance or rejection) of the change.

Table 19-1 **Models of Planned Change**

Model	Anticipated Resistance to Change	Amount of Force Behind Change Approach	Major Approach of Model
Rational	Low	Low	Education and communication
Normative	Moderate	Moderate	Persuasion and participation
Paradoxical	Moderate	Moderate	Rethinking
Power-coercive	High	High	Force

From Tappen, R.M. (1989). *Nursing leadership and management* (2nd ed.). Philadelphia: F.A. Davis.

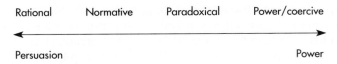

Fig. 19-3   Power-persuasion continuum of planned change.

Step 1: Development. In rational models of change, there is a critical need to fully develop the proposed change before its presentation to those involved. For instance, a nurse who wanted to develop a change in an institution's method of documentation would collect information about the existing methods of documentation. The nurse would evaluate this information and would choose the best documentation method to present to those involved in decision making.

Step 2: Communication. The method chosen for communication is critical to the success of the process. All individuals concerned must receive the information, understand it, and accept the reasoning that led to its choice. The person responsible for the proposed change must understand the characteristics of those who will experience the change and the characteristics of the change itself before deciding on the most appropriate method of dissemination. Various methods of communication might include booklets, memos, one-on-one discussion, and group discussions. Communication is most persuasive when it comes from a variety of different sources (Armenakis, Harris, & Mossholder, 1993).

In the rational model, a trial period or pilot study is often attempted before widespread implementation of the change. The trial period allows problems to be identified and worked out before full-scale implementation. Also, human nature is such that a partial commitment may be viewed more favorably by those involved in the change than forcing a full commitment. And, most important, a trial period allows for more communication.

Step 3: Consequences. Once the change is instituted, the expectation is that it will be accepted because it was the rational choice. Steps included in the model for development and communication are thought to ensure subsequent adoption of the change.

Example of a rational model. One of the best-known rational models is Rogers' (1983) diffusion of innovation process. This is a five-stage model and is summarized in the box below.

Rogers' Diffusion of Innovation Process

Stage 1	Knowledge
Stage 2	Persuasion
Stage 3	Acceptance or rejection
Stage 4	Implementation
Stage 5	Consequences

In this model, the first stage is knowledge, in which the individual becomes aware of the innovation and its function. The leader prepares for the proposed change by gathering all pertinent information related to the innovation. In the second stage, persuasion, the individual forms a favorable or unfavorable attitude toward the innovation. In the third stage, the individual decides to accept or reject the innovation. The fourth stage of implementation occurs when the individual puts the innovation into action. In the final stage, the individual considers the consequences of the change. In this stage, the change is either adopted or rejected.

The adoption of a change has three phases: trial, installation, and institutionalization. The trial phase is a pilot study of the change. If the pilot is successful, then in the second phase, the change becomes fully integrated into the system as a regular routine. Finally, in the third phase of adoption, the change becomes deeply rooted in the behavior pattern.

Introducing an innovation in an organization rests in the linkage of the change agent with the change agency and client (Rogers, 1983), as illustrated in Fig. 19-4. Seven roles can be identified for the change agent who is introducing a single innovation (see box below). The goal of the change agent is to develop self-renewing behavior and "shift the client from a position of reliance on the change agent to self-reliance" (Rogers, 1983, p. 317).

Critique of the rational model. Rational models are based on the assumption that if individuals know that the change is the rational choice, they will accept it. Rational models further assume that individuals know what each choice means and understand all the implications for each choice. Recent work by Langer (1989) has shown that much of human decision making is far from rational. Furthermore, even if it is the most rational choice, it may not always be the correct choice in a given situation. All decision making must consider numerous variables, and each variable has some uncertainty attached to it. It may be unrealistic to think that there is always one best solution or that the consequences of any decision can be predicted with certainty (Kosko, 1993).

Normative model. When the resistance to change is more pronounced, it is suggested that change agents consider a normative model. Normative models focus on the norms of individuals targeted for change and on the actions of the leader. The

---

The Change Agent's Seven Roles

1. Develops a need for change
2. Establishes an informational-exchange relationship with client
3. Diagnoses client's problem
4. Creates intent to change the client
5. Translates intent into action
6. Stabilizes adoption of innovation and presents discontinuances
7. Moves client to a self-reliant position

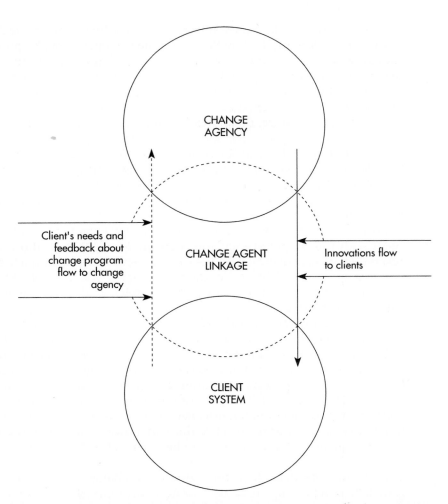

Fig. 19-4 Linkage of the change agent with the change agency and client. (Redrawn from Rogers, E.M. [1983]. *Diffusion of innovations* [3rd ed.]. New York: The Free Press.)

norms thought to be important to change are attitudes, needs, values, and feelings. One major assumption of this model is that if both the leader and the target group actively participate in the change process, resistance will be mitigated. Three major theorists have developed normative-type models.

Lewin's model (1951) consists of three stages labeled "unfreezing," "changing," and "refreezing." In the first stage (unfreezing), there is a careful assessment of the forces driving and restraining change. The leader conducts a detailed analysis of the environment, the characteristics of the change, and the potential responses to the change. After a careful analysis, the status quo is "unfrozen" by a deliberate introduction of disequilibrium to move the organization to a desired state. Once there is movement toward change, the leader can begin to implement the planned change process by introducing new information, encouraging new behavior, providing opportunities for feedback, clarifying goals, and maintaining open communication. In the final stage (refreezing), the goal is to stabilize and integrate the change so that it becomes internalized in the system.

Havelock (1973) and Lippitt's (1973) models center on the action of the leader rather than the environment, as in Lewin's normative change model. Their models use a participatory and democratic style of leadership for the planning and implementation of change. The models place the leader in the role of change agent and require the participation of those involved at the beginning of the planning phase.

The action of the leader follows five steps (see box below). First, the leader builds a relationship with those involved that is based on trust and respect. It is critical during this phase that the leader listens well, communicates clearly, and is very open. In the second step, the target group is very involved in diagnosing the problem and establishing the need for change. The leader guides the process. Generally, consensus for change is developed through collaboration between the leader and the group. In the third step, the resources (time, skills, money, commitment) that are needed for the planned change are assessed. After the assessment is completed, specific and attainable goals are set by the group (fourth step). In the last step, which is similar to Lewin's refreezing and Roger's institutionalization, the leader continues to provide support for the change, feedback on progress, and maintenance of the actions needed to continue the change.

Critique of the normative model. Normative models are proposed to work when there is low to moderate resistance to change and a consensus can be built. Even when conditions are appropriate, change is not that easily accomplished. In part, change is not easy because any attempt to isolate the relevant factors denies the real and complex nature of most problems. That is, any attempt to isolate causation for change or reactions to change is futile because most change events are multicausal (Duck, 1993).

The normative models do not consider the history or underlying culture of the organization. Schein (1985) and others have stressed the importance of organizational culture to the change process. Organizational culture tends to vary with an organization's life cycle. Therefore leaders and managers will be more successful in implementing change if "change problems, strategy, and tactics are tied to a life-cycle frame-

Steps of Normative Change	
Step 1	Build relationship.
Step 2	Establish need for change.
Step 3	Assess resources.
Step 4	Set goals.
Step 5	Support change process.

work" (Beer & Walton, 1987, p. 47) rather than a strict adherence to a normative model. Thus change attempted on a newly constructed nursing unit where change is expected may be easier to accomplish than change on a unit that is more mature and "set in its ways."

The normative models consider such norms as trust and individual feelings important to the change process, since change is thought to occur more easily when it focuses on feelings and when there is trust. Trust in the change process is based on the predictability of the events and the perceived capability of those involved (Duck, 1993). During change, individuals want to know the intentions of those promoting the change and the ground rules. People also want to understand who is responsible for the specific activities and what steps will need to be accomplished to bring about the change. Although trust and capability are the basis for the normative models, they are not easily obtained and should not be assumed. Instead, it should be remembered that the process of change by its very nature reduces predictability and, sometimes, capability.

Paradoxical model. The paradoxical model is rooted in the background of psychotherapy and focuses on the manner in which problems are viewed and solved (Westenholz, 1993). It has been noted in psychotherapy that an illogical plan or way of looking at a problem may succeed in changing a system or organization that cannot be changed by logic. Paradoxical thinking helps others to think in new ways about old problems. Sometimes only a very illogical plan is capable of forcing a new way of thinking (Westenholz, 1993). Remember, it may be human nature to work against the change in order to maintain a consistent frame of reference.

Much of this work comes from the observations of Watzlawick, Weakland, and Fisch (1974). In the paradoxical model there are two levels of change: first- and second-order changes. In a *first-order change,* the patterns of behavior and the nature of relationships remain the same despite attempts at change (Watzlawick, Weakland, & Fisch, 1974). The change "paradoxically" serves to reinforce the status quo. For example, following decentralization of a hospital, the managers were having difficulty relating to each other as peers. The communication pattern had been "top-down," or superior to subordinate in nature. Following the change, when one manager approached another as an equal and attempted to change the pattern of communication, the other manager retreated further into the previous mode of communicating only with the hospital president. Thus, even though an attempt was made to change the pattern, no real change occurred. In fact, the patterns of behavior that needed to change became more entrenched.

Second-order change may be needed to alter the former patterns of behavior. A *second-order change* requires reframing the problem from a new perspective. Watzlawick, Weakland, and Fisch (1974) suggest four steps:

- Clearly define the problem.
- List all solutions tried.

- Clearly define parameters of realistic change.
- Create a paradoxical, second-order change strategy.

In the final step, the selection of a new second-order strategy is usually in direct opposition to former attempts to bring about planned change. As such, in attempting to change communication patterns in the example given above, the leader may try the paradoxical move of not allowing managers to communicate during a selected meeting. This move might force managers to talk to one another outside of the meeting, thus setting up a new pattern of peer communication.

Critique of the paradoxical model. As with the other models, there are drawbacks to this change model as well. First, the leader who promotes paradoxical thinking has to be highly motivated and be willing to carry out what appears to be strategies that are at odds with the normal ways of doing things. Second, the strategy means taking a risk that can backfire. A leader who presents a paradoxical way of thinking can become so associated with that view that he or she is unable to talk to others about the original problem and solution and so loses credibility with those involved. Finally, reframing the problem requires imagination and creativity. It is not easy to look at a problem from a new point of view, and few individuals are able to think paradoxically.

Power-coercive model. The power-coercive model is promoted as a way to deal with both strong resistance to change and inability to reach consensus. In power-coercive models, direct force moves the target system toward change. "Although leaders recognize the influence of people's needs, feelings, attitudes, and values on change, they do not necessarily respect them" (Tappen, 1995, p. 351).

In the power-coercive model, six phases of the change process are initiated by the change agents (Tappen, 1995):

- Define the issue and identify the opponent.
- Organize a following.
- Build a power base.
- Begin action phase.
- Keep the pressure on.
- Use stronger tactics to overcome the resistance (the final struggle).

The person or group involved in the change (not necessarily the leader) assumes the risks of this strategy. These steps can be followed by people who are the "have nots" in a system and who want to use various forms of power (money, position, legal system, control of access to resources, public support, etc.) to bring about change (Alinsky, 1972; Haley, 1969).

Critique of the power-coercive model. The power-coercive model uses power to force change. There are times, of course, when this method may be necessary. However, most change situations probably do not require force. Forcing others to change against their will can lead to unforeseen consequences in an organization. When this method is employed, those involved must be prepared to deal with the resistance. With forced change, the unforeseen will occur.

UNPLANNED CHANGE

"Chaos is the law of nature; order is the dream of man."
Henry Adams

Change is not always planned. External events and crises may cause more changes than does planned change (Beer & Walton, 1987). Suffice it to say, events happen, people change, and life evolves in ways that cannot be known. Even planned changes can unfold in ways that are unpredictable.

The models of planned change are based on the assumption that organizations are predictable, linear systems. Yet many systems are far from that, especially systems that encompass human beings. *Complexity theory* is the study of nonlinear, dynamic systems, such as people and organizations. Within this theory, both order and disorder co-exist as natural parts of the system. Among the tenets of complexity theory are that (1) systems exhibit behavior that is more than the sum of their parts, (2) much behavior is nonlinear and irreversible, (3) uncertainty is a part of every system, and (4) systems can generate random, nonpredictable behavior. Rather than the world envisioned by Plato, where disorder is error and order is the norm, complexity theorists envision the world as Heraclitus did, in a perpetual state of flux where disorder is expected.

CHAOS AND COMPLEXITY

Underlying most work in the social sciences are implicit assumptions about cause and effect, and the predictability of events. Recent research in fields such as physics, anthropology, economics, biology, and even mathematics has revealed that absolute predictability and control may not be a realistic goal. It appears that dynamic systems, even simple ones, can generate random, unpredictable behavior. Consider, for example, the weather. Despite access to large-scale computers with which to calculate a vast knowledge base of weather predictors in combination with timely satellite pictures, weather forecasts are still not 100% accurate. Weather just does not represent a predictable linear model. Furthermore, if weather cannot be modeled as a linear system, human behavior, of which we know even less, certainly cannot.

One reason for the apparent inability to predict such phenomena as weather, disease progression, and response to change is the notion of sensitivity to initial conditions. In changing and evolving systems, small chance events or differences in conditions have the ability to lead to very different outcomes. As an example, any small shift in temperature, wind direction, or barometric pressure is enough to cause major differences in the weather. In part, this is due to the iterative effects of positive feedback; in other words, the small change becomes magnified as the system grows. Small errors do not always stay small (Kellert, 1993).

Unfortunately, chaos can appear in any stable system when the system is given the right push (Pool, 1989). *Chaos* has been defined as the unpredictable behavior that can arise from systems (Lipsitz & Goldberger, 1992). It appears that most systems have points where they are the most sensitive to disturbance. Rather than absorbing the effects of the disturbance, the system begins to respond in unpredictable ways. For example, electrical stimulation given at the right point in the cardiac cycle can cause the heart rhythm to show bifurcations and other abnormal rhythms. The point where a system exhibits change is known by many names, depending on the discipline. Periods of change are called "crisis points" by developmental psychologists, "hinge points" by archaeologists, "punctuations" by biologists, and "phase transitions" by physicists.

Familiarity with an organization or a person may reveal obvious points of weakness or concern. These points should be thought of as places where the person or system is vulnerable or even unstable. For example, a change of administration is probably not well thought out if it is scheduled to occur during a major holiday time.

Dynamic systems are remarkably resilient and show an ability to maintain order despite the surrounding disorder. The type of disturbance, the magnitude of the disturbance, the susceptibility of the system, and happenstance can all influence how a system responds (Cambel, 1993). Complexity theory tells us that it may not be possible to know all the points of vulnerability within a system despite careful analysis and planning. All plans regarding change should include discussions of how to recognize and deal with critical points. When unexpected change occurs, the system should be supported in order to avoid chaos.

 ## Key Points

- Change is a natural and unavoidable aspect of life.

- Change affects everything, including people, organizations, societies, and nations.

- While some change can be planned, much of change is unplanned, and even planned change does not always unfold as designed.

- Change has been viewed as a hypothetical linear system where each part of the system was thought to be understandable and controllable.

- The rational model of planned change is based on the assumption that with good information most people will make the logical choice to change.

- The normative model of change is based on the assumption that if both the leader and the target group participate in the change process, resistance to change will be reduced.

- The paradoxical model of change is based on the notion that an illogical plan or way of looking at a problem may succeed in changing a system where logic failed.

- The power-coercive model is useful when dealing with both strong resistance to change and inability to reach consensus.

- While all the models have valid aspects, none of the models has been shown to be effective in all situations.

- Recent work in many different disciplines has shown that more information or more structure does not always ensure smooth change.

- Systems under stress, such as those experiencing change, can act in a variety of strange and unpredictable ways called chaos.

- Complexity theory has shown that the behavior of a part of a system cannot be used to predict the behavior of the whole system.

- New models of change should take into account the dynamic nature of change, specifically patterns of behavior during change, areas of vulnerability during the change process, and the roles involvement and information play.

- The change process should be considered complex and not a process that can be reduced to a few rules or clichés.

Critical Thinking Exercises

1. Look at a recent change in your clinical area. Explain or evaluate the process of change according to one of the change theories discussed in this chapter. How was the change implemented, and what was the outcome?

2. If you were going to institute a major change in a home health agency, what would be your first step? How would this differ if you wanted to make a change in a hospital?

3. Describe a situation where an unexpected event occurred during the implementation of a change. Why do you believe the unexpected event occurred? How could this have been avoided?

References

Alinsky, S.D. (1972). *Rules for radicals: A practical primer for realistic radicals.* New York: Vintage Books.

Armenakis, A.A., Harris, S.G., & Mossholder, K.W. (1993). Creating readiness for organizational change. *Human Relations, 46*(6), 681-703.

Arnold, D.R., Capella, L.M., & Sumrall, D.A. (1987). Hospital challenge: Using change theory and processes to adopt and implement the marketing concept. *Journal of Health Care Marketing, 7*(2), 15-24.

Axelrod, D. (1992). Getting everyone involved: How one organization involved its employees, supervisors, and managers in redesigning the organization. *Journal of Applied Behavioral Science, 28*(4), 499-509.

Beer, M., & Walton, A.E. (1987). Organization change and development. *Annual Review of Psychology, 38,* 339-367.

Bennis, W.G., Benne, K.D., & Chin, R. (Eds.). (1985). *The planning of change* (4th ed.). New York: Holt, Rinehart & Winston.

Bernhard, L.A., & Walsh, M. (1995). *Leadership: The key to the professionalism of nursing* (3rd ed.). St. Louis: Mosby.

Burke, W.W., & Litwin, G.H. (1992). A causal model of organizational performance and change. *Journal of Management, 18*(3), 523-545.

Cambel, A.B. (1993). *Applied chaos theory: A paradigm for complexity.* San Diego, CA: Academic Press.

Chin, R. (1976). The utility of systems models and developmental models for practitioners. In W.G. Bennis, K.D. Benne, R. Chin, & K. Corey (Eds.), *The planning of change* (3rd ed.). New York: Holt, Rinehart & Winston.

Davis, P.S. (1991). The meaning of change to individuals within a college of nurse education. *Journal of Advanced Nursing, 16,* 108-115.

Downey, K., & Brief, A. (1986). How cognitive structures affect organizational design. In H. Sims & D. Gioia (Eds.), *The thinking organization.* San Francisco: Jossey-Bass.

Duck, J.D. (1993, November-December). Managing change: The art of balancing. *Harvard Business Review,* pp. 109-118.

Gillies, D.A. (1994). *Nursing management* (3rd ed.). Philadelphia: W.B. Saunders.

Gioia, D.A., & Chittipeddi, K. (1991). Using sensemaking and sensegiving in strategic change initiatives. *Strategic Management Journal, 12*(6), 433-448.

Grohar-Murray, M.E., & DiCroce, H.R. (1992). *Leadership and management in nursing.* Norwalk, CT: Appleton & Lange.

Haley, J. (1969). *The power tactics of Jesus Christ and other essays.* New York: Avon Books.

Hamm, F.B. (1992). Organizational change required for paradigmatic shift in addiction treatment. *Journal of Substance Abuse Treatment, 9*(3), 257-260.

Havelock, R.G. (1973). *The change agent's guide to innovation in education.* Englewood Cliffs, NJ: Educational Technology Publications.

Kellert, S.H. (1993). *In the wake of chaos.* Chicago: University of Chicago Press.

Kosko, B. (1993). *Fuzzy thinking: The new science of fuzzy logic.* New York: Hyperion.

Langer, E. (1989). *Mindfulness.* Redwood City, CA: Addison-Wesley.

Lewin, K. (1951). *Field theory in social science: Selected theoretical papers.* New York: Harper & Row.

Lewin, R. (1992). *Complexity: Life at the edge of chaos.* New York: Macmillan.

Lippitt, G. L. (1973). *Visualizing change: Model building and the change process.* La Jolla, CA: University Associates.

Lipsitz, L.A., & Goldberger, A.L. (1992). Loss of complexity and aging: Potential applications of fractals and chaos theory to senescence. *JAMA, 267*(13), 1806-1809.

Lowstedt, J. (1993). Organizing frameworks in emerging organizations: A cognitive approach to the analysis of change. *Human Relations, 46*(4), 501-526.

Marshak, R.J. (1993). Lewin meets Confucius: A review of the OD model of change. *Journal of Applied Behavioral Science, 29*(4), 393-415.

Mawhinney, T.C. (1992). Evolution of organizational cultures as selection by consequences: The Gaia hypothesis, metacontingencies, and organizational ecology. *Journal of Organizational Behavior Management, 12*(2), 1-26.

Meleis, A.I., & Trangenstein, P.A. (1993). Facilitating transitions: Redefintion of a nursing mission. Unpublished manuscript.

Pool, R. (1989). Is it chaos, or is it just noise? *Science, 242*(4887), 25-28.

Porras, J.I., & Silvers, R.C. (1991). Organization development and transformation. *Annual Review of Psychology, 45,* 51-78.

Rogers, E.M. (1983). *Diffusion of innovation* (3rd ed.). New York: Free Press.

Schein, E. (1985). *Organizational culture and leadership.* San Francisco: Jossey-Bass.

Sheehan, J. (1990). Investigating change in a nursing context. *Journal of Advanced Nursing, 15,* 819-824.

Snell, L., & Turner, D. (1991, May-June). A new master rotation on a labor and delivery unit. *Canadian Journal of Nursing Administration, 19.*

Stickland, G. (1992). Positioning training and development departments for organizational change. *Management Education and Development, 23*(4), 307-316.

Tappen, R.M. (1989). *Nursing leadership and management* (2nd ed.). Philadelphia: F.A. Davis.

Tappen, R.M. (1995). *Nursing leadership and management: Concepts and practice* (3rd ed.). Philadelphia: F.A. Davis.

Tice, D.M. (1992). Self-concept and self-presentation: The looking glass self is also a magnifying glass. *Journal of Personality and Social Psychology, 63*(3), 435-451.

Tiffany, C.R., Cheatham, A.B., Doornbos, D., Loudermelt, L., & Momadi, G.G. (1994). Planned change theory: Survey of nursing periodical literature. *Nursing Management, 25*(7), 54-59.

Traub, J.F., & Wozniakowski, H. (1994). Breaking intractability. *Scientific American, 266*(1), 102-107.

Watzlawick, P., Weakland, J.H., & Fisch, R. (1974). *Change: Principles of problem formation and problem resolution.* New York: W.W. Norton.

Westenholz, A. (1993). Paradoxical thinking and change in the frames of reference. *Organization Studies, 14*(1), 37-58.

Zajc, L.S. (1987). *Models of planned educational change: Their ideational and ideological contexts and evolution since the late 1950's.* Unpublished, Ann Arbor, MI: University Microfilms International.

Nursing Research

Audrey G. Gift

 Objectives

At the completion of this chapter, the reader will be able to:

- Define nursing research and how it has evolved over the past 40 years.

- Describe the process by which research can be implemented into practice.

- Compare and contrast the different approaches to nursing research and how they can be used to answer different nursing questions.

- Describe the research process and the parts of the research report.

- Describe the ethical considerations in conducting a nursing research study, such as protecting humans as subjects in a study and maintaining the integrity of the research.

- List the various sources for funding a research study.

Profile in Practice

Barbara Parker, PhD, RN, FAAN
Professor of Nursing;
Director, Center for Nursing Research,
School of Nursing, University of Virginia,
Charlottesville, Virginia

I became interested in research in 1975 when I was a master's student in psychiatric nursing. I was providing individual and family counseling at a community mental health center, and several women began to talk about the violence they were experiencing from their husbands. I looked in the literature for guidance and could find only theories of masochism to guide my practice. I decided to write my master's thesis on wife abuse and followed with a doctoral dissertation on the same topic. On completion of my doctoral degree, I founded the

Nursing Research Consortium on Violence Against Women. Consortium members have worked in a variety of configurations to develop research proposals, conduct joint studies, and publish the findings. I have worked primarily with Dr. Judith McFarlane from Texas Women's University in Houston. In our first study, we interviewed 1203 women entering prenatal clinics to determine the incidence of abuse.* Women were interviewed three times during their pregnancy. Following delivery, we conducted a chart review to determine the impact of abuse on birth weight and pregnancy complications. The results of this study have been published in several nursing and medical journals (McFarlane et al., 1992; Parker, McFarlane, & Soeken, 1994; Parker et al., 1993).

In the first study we provided women with information regarding the process of abuse and legal and shelter options. Surprisingly, on subsequent visits to the prenatal clinic, we found that many women reported no more abuse. The second study,* building on this chance finding, was designed to test whether a nursing intervention designed to empower abused pregnant women would be effective in stopping the violence both during and after pregnancy. The study is ongoing, and we will have the results in a few years.

The greatest challenge I have found as a researcher is how to convince nurses to use the results of research studies. Even though we have repeatedly shown that it is important and not difficult to assess for abuse, and that women are not offended by being questioned, many nurses are reluctant to include the simple screen (see Chapter 5) in routine assessment. To assist nurses in intervening, we developed an intervention protocol that is available to all nurses through their local chapter of the March of Dimes (McFarlane & Parker, 1994).

*Studies funded by the Intentional Injury Division of the Centers for Disease Control (R49/CCR603514; R49/CCR309832).

Nursing research is the systematic study of nursing phenomena. Its purpose is to develop a knowledge base that will guide practice. The National Institute of Nursing Research (NINR) has defined *nursing research* as research directed toward gaining an understanding of nursing care of individuals and groups. It focuses on the biological, physiological, social, behavioral, and environmental factors influencing health and disease. Nursing research includes basic and clinical studies associated with the diagnosis and treatment of human responses to actual and potential health problems (NINR, 1993).

From this definition it becomes obvious that the intent of nursing research is to provide high-quality patient care. It ensures that nursing care be scientifically based rather than based on tradition. For this to happen, however, nurses must be aware of research and use it in practice.

To fully cover nursing's role in research, this chapter is divided into three sections: the history of nursing research, reading and using research in practice, and finally, conducting a research study.

HISTORY OF NURSING RESEARCH

Nursing research has often been described as beginning with the detailed observations made by Florence Nightingale during the Crimean War. She observed and recorded details about the environment (ventilation, temperature, cleanliness, purity of water, and diet) and linked these observations to patient outcomes. She realized that providing a clean environment reduced mortality in soldiers. However, few who followed her engaged in these systematic recordings.

Studies of the effectiveness of public health teaching date back to before World War I. Then, in the 1920s case studies of patients first began to appear in the *American Journal of Nursing*. During the 1940s and 1950s the focus was on nursing services research, which includes the organization and delivery of nursing services. Time and motion studies were done, and state-wide surveys of personnel were conducted.

The 1950s saw increased activity supporting nursing research. In 1952 *Nursing Research*, the first journal devoted exclusively to nursing research, was published. In 1953 the Institute for Research and Service in Nursing Education was established at Teacher's College, Columbia University, and provided learning experiences in research for doctoral students. The focus of this program, however, was on nursing education (Burns & Grove, 1993).

In 1955 funding first became available for grants in nursing through the Division of Nursing within the Bureau of Health Professions in the Health Resources and Services Administration of the U.S. Public Health Service. The aim was to provide resources for faculty development, including nursing research.

Also in 1955 the American Nurses' Foundation was chartered as the research and education subsidiary of the American Nurses' Association (ANA). One of its main goals has been to raise funds and distribute grants to support beginning nurse scientists. From 1955 to 1993 a total of 459 nursing research grants were awarded. Future plans include support for more advanced researchers.

The first research institution to emphasize clinical nursing research was established in 1957 as the Department of Nursing Research in the Walter Reed Army Institute of Research (Stevenson, 1986). At this time also, specialty organizations began to appear, and the need for nursing research to provide the basis for nursing practice standards became evident.

Regional research organizations, such as the Southern Regional Education Board (SREB) and the Western Interstate Commission on Higher Education (WICHEN), were formed. Their goals were to provide opportunities for nurse researchers to meet and disseminate nursing research findings and techniques. These regional research societies have changed names and/or geographic boundaries, but they remain an important factor in nursing research today.

Nursing research in the 1960s included studies focusing on nursing education, nursing delivery systems, and clinical practice. The 1970s saw the development of models, conceptual frameworks, and theories to guide nursing practice. Nurses began to use models from a variety of sources to provide direction for clinical nursing research. By the late 1970s three additional research journals appeared in nursing: *Advances in Nursing Science*, which publishes nursing research that focuses on nursing theories, and *Re-*

search in Nursing and Health and *Western Journal of Nursing Research,* both of which publish nursing research studies. This expanded the forum for communication of nursing research findings. More recently, research-focused specialty journals have begun to appear for the communication of research findings.

The beginning doctoral programs in nursing focused on nursing education, with many of the graduates taking administrative positions in higher education. Few nurses established careers in nursing research. In the 1980s, however, there was a dramatic increase in the number of doctoral programs in nursing. In 1995 there were 62 doctoral programs in nursing graduating over 250 doctorally prepared nurses a year. This is in contrast to 1979, when there were only 22 doctoral programs in nursing. The percentage of graduates pursuing a research career is continuing to rise, with most being employed in educational institutions but an increasing number taking positions in clinical settings.

National Institute of Nursing Research

In 1986 the National Center for Nursing Research was established within the National Institutes of Health (NIH). The name was changed to the National Institute of Nursing Research (NINR) in 1993. Dr. Ada Sue Hinshaw was the first director and served from 1986 to 1994, followed by Dr. Patricia Grady from 1995 to the present.

The NINR is composed of both extramural and intramural programs. *Extramural programs* provide funding to researchers in universities, hospitals, and other research centers across the country. A major program priority is the integration of biological and behavioral research. At present, the NINR is organized into three dimensions: promoting health and preventing disease, managing the symptoms and disability of illness, and improving the environments in which care is delivered. These dimensions include research in the following broad science areas:

- Research in *chronic conditions,* including arthritis, diabetes, and urinary incontinence; and in long-term care and caregiving.
- Research in *health and risk behaviors,* including studies of women's health; developmental transitions, such as adolescence and menopause; and health and behavior research, such as studies of smoking cessation.
- Research in *cardiopulmonary health,* including prevention and care of individuals with cardiac or respiratory conditions. This area also includes research in critical care, trauma, wound healing, and organ transplantation.
- Research in *neurofunction and brain disorders,* including pain management, sleep disorders, symptom management in persons with brain disorders such as Alzheimer's disease, and rehabilitation following brain and spinal cord injury. This area also includes research on patient care in acute care settings.
- Research in *immune and neoplastic diseases,* including symptoms primarily associated with cancer and AIDS, such as fatigue, nausea and vomiting, and cachexia. Prevention research on specific risk factors is also included.
- Research in *reproductive and infant health,* including prevention of premature labor, reduction of health-risk factors during pregnancy, delivery of prenatal care, care of neonates, infant growth and development, and fertility issues.

The *intramural program* of the NINR consists of research conducted on the NIH campus by staff. It consists of two laboratories concentrating on research regarding symptom management and caregiving. The Clinical Therapeutics Laboratory conducts symptom management studies. Presently the focus is on symptoms in individuals with HIV infection and on symptoms associated with aging. The Laboratory for the Study of Human Responses to Health and Illness was established in 1992 to conduct studies focusing on the biophysiological and behavioral processes that influence health and illness. Current studies focus on quality of life, caregiving, and functional status (NINR, 1993).

One activity of the NINR is the setting of the *National Nursing Research Agenda*. The purpose of this is to provide structure, depth, and direction for nursing research. A subcommittee of the National Advisory Council for Nursing Research provides oversight for this activity. The first priorities were for 1989 to 1994, and the following seven areas were selected:

1. Low birth weight—mothers and infants
2. HIV infection—prevention and care
3. Long-term care for older adults
4. Symptom management—pain
5. Nursing informatics—support for patient care
6. Health promotion for children and adolescents
7. Technology dependency across the life span

The second conference identified the next priorities for 1995 to 1999. These are:

1. Community-based nursing models
2. Health-promoting behaviors and HIV/AIDS
3. Remediation of cognitive impairment
4. Living with chronic illness
5. Biobehavioral factors related to immunocompetence

These priorities serve as a guide for NINR funding and promote research that addresses these issues.

Federal funding for nursing research has increased over the years. For instance, there was a rise in obligated dollars from $16.2 million in 1986 to $44.9 million in 1992 (NINR, 1993). However, the NINR remains the smallest institute within the NIH, and the small budget constrains the development of the NINR's programs. There are inadequate funds for collaborative efforts for clinical trials, consensus conferences, and the like (NINR, 1993).

USING RESEARCH IN PRACTICE

It is vital that nursing base its practice on nursing research rather than tradition. Many practices are ingrained in nursing and have been allowed to continue because nurses have not questioned the rationale for the practice. The first step is to question routines by examining the research base. This requires nurses to read nursing research and include the findings in their practice. This is not easily done. Those who have examined the extent to which nurses use research findings in their practice have found them only moderately committed to the use of research (Champion & Leach, 1989). The situation appears to be improving, however, as nurses are increasingly being given more autonomy for their practice (Coyle & Sokop, 1990).

An important step in research utilization is learning about the research findings (see box below). Nurses report that they learn about research by reading the professional nursing literature, attending conferences and inservices, and observing the practice of others (Coyle & Sokop, 1990). When these activities are encouraged by administration, utilization of research increases. Nurses share research findings in their nursing practice committees as policies and procedures are updated. The role models displayed in these committees are a valuable asset for research utilization in nursing.

Another way to learn about research findings is through the use of standards and practice guidelines available from national agencies and organizations, such as the

---

Assistance With Research Facilitation

Research Summaries in Clinical Nursing Journals

Several clinical journals now have sections in which they summarize and evaluate recent research studies. They then have a section in which the implications of the research for nursing practice are included. Examples of journals that have these research summary sections are the *American Journal of Nursing* and *Heart and Lung*.

Nursing Practice Committee

Practice committees are charged with writing and reviewing nursing policies and procedures for a hospital. It is important to consider the current relevant research when writing or revising policies and procedures. The committee can be asked to share reviews of the current research when the policy is presented. Also, there may be a list of references used in establishing the policy that are printed at the end.

Journal Club

Many practice settings have journal clubs that meet to discuss recent research related to the patient population under their care. If your institution does not have a journal club, you might want to consider establishing one. This will attract nurses interested in reading, evaluating, and discussing research. Each person could be assigned a journal to read and report about each month. This saves each nurse from trying to read all journals each month.

Practice Guidelines

By definition, clinical practice guidelines are based on research. They are a summary and evaluation of the current research with recommendations made for clinical practice. Guidelines are put forward by specialty nursing organizations, as well as by the federal Agency for Health Care Policy and Research (AHCPR). The ANA has published a booklet describing how to evaluate and use guidelines (Ferrell et al., 1994). They have also published a manual to be used by specialty organizations indicating how to develop guidelines (Marek, 1994). Of particular note in this manual are the scoring sheets used by the various AHCPR guideline panels in evaluating research studies.

AHCPR. Research on selected topics, such as the management of acute pain, urinary incontinence, or pressure ulcers, is reviewed, and recommendations are made for clinical practice. The goal is for all health professionals to implement the recommendations in practice.

A number of models have been proposed to describe the application of research findings to clinical practice. Most, such as the Stetler/Marram model (Stetler, 1994), are based on the premise that nurses desire knowledge, and the model explains how and why it is sought out. Titler et al. (1994), however, have developed the Iowa model, which depicts a different type of model for research utilization (Fig. 20-1). They describe what they call problem-focused triggers to research utilization. This occurs when a clinical problem is repeatedly encountered in practice, risk management, or quality improvement programs and leads to the use of research in practice. They give the example of learning that 50% of critical care patients reported a mean pain intensity of 7.5 on a 10-point scale, which led to the implementation of a research-based pain management protocol (Titler et al., 1994). Quality improvement data are a rich source of areas for nursing research.

The decision to use research to enhance practice requires an evaluation of the available research on the topic. The quality, quantity, and applicability of the research to the practice setting are considered. If the research is absent or insufficient, conducting a research study should be considered. This is discussed in the next section. However, if there is a sufficient research base to suggest appropriate changes for practice, these would have to be tested in the practice setting before being adopted.

When a change in practice is to be implemented, Titler et al. (1994) recommend first setting criteria and selecting outcome measures for evaluating the effects of the change. Documentation of the current situation is necessary, so that it can be used as a comparison with an assessment made using the same outcome measures after the change is implemented. The nature of the practice change determines whether the intervention is developed from a multidisciplinary or independent nursing perspective. For example, a change in pain management would most likely require the cooperation of physicians, nurses, and perhaps anesthesiologists for a successful program to be implemented, whereas other activities fall solely within the domain of nursing.

Pilot testing the change on one or two units before implementing the change throughout the institution is advisable. This will allow potential problems to be corrected ahead of time. If the staff nurses on the pilot unit(s) are educated about the research base and evaluate the change as desirable, they can assist in orienting others and discussing the positive outcomes of the change (Titler et al., 1994).

Outcomes to be included in the evaluation of a practice change should include not only patient outcomes, but the financial implications of the change as well. A change in practice requires the orientation of staff, changing of forms, and/or changes in other areas of practice. This can be costly to the institution. Such changes are warranted, however, if they result in significantly better patient outcomes. Other outcomes to evaluate would be the satisfaction of the staff with the practice change. Increased staff satisfaction will contribute to staff retention and a reduction in the cost of orienting

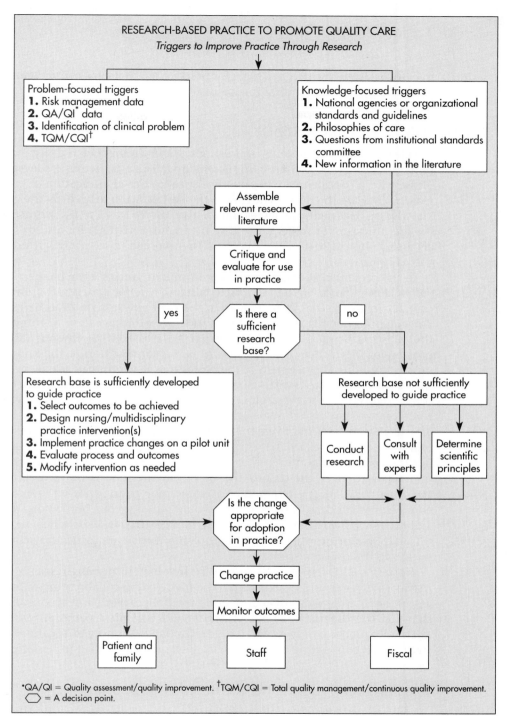

Fig. 20-1 Iowa model. (Copyright University of Iowa Hospital and Clinics. Redrawn from Titler, M.G., et al. [1994]. Infusing research into practice to promote quality care. *Nursing Research, 43*[5], 307-313.)

new staff. Using research as a basis for practice has as its goal improvement in patient, staff, and financial outcomes for the institution.

CONDUCTING A RESEARCH STUDY

While reading, evaluating, and using research in practice is every nurse's responsibility, involvement in conducting research varies with the nurse's level of education. Those with a baccalaureate degree are critical to the identification of problems for research. They are the nurses who are in the best position to identify the gaps in nursing knowledge. Baccalaureate degree nurses may also be asked to assist nurse researchers in the identification of subjects meeting the inclusion criteria for a study and in gaining access to clinical sites. They may also be involved in assisting with data collection (ANA, 1993).

In the present cost-containment environment, nurses' time has become even more valuable than before. When a nurse is hired to care for patients, that must remain the primary focus for the nurse. However, there are rewards that can be gained from involvement in nursing research. One of the most exciting can be learning the answer to the question being explored. This is particularly exciting when it results in an improvement in practice. Another reward is the contribution to the knowledge base of nursing and the advancement of the profession. Rewards may also be personal, such as increased knowledge, satisfaction with one's performance, or seeing one's name in print. Involvement in research is often a requirement for career advancement, but in some cases it may also provide other rewards.

These rewards for involvement in research are negotiated with the researcher on the basis of the time that will be required. For instance, if all that is required is the identification of subjects admitted with a certain diagnosis or the recording of routine data on a separate sheet, the reward may be simply the sharing of research findings. If, on the other hand, what is required is increased monitoring and/or the recording of more complex patient data, these activities would put more of a burden on the nursing staff and the reward would be expected to be more extensive. Nurses may be paid to collect research data or negotiate shared authorship if they are to make a significant contribution to the research study.

Nurses at all levels of practice may be involved in nursing research. Nurses with a master's degree would be expected to be involved by collaborating with other investigators, facilitating data collection, and providing expert clinical consultation. The design and coordination of research studies is a role most commonly reserved for the doctorally prepared nurse (ANA, 1993). Guidance on how to obtain assistance in designing and conducting a nursing research study is provided in the box on p. 451.

The Research Process and the Research Proposal

The *research process* involves planning the research, conducting the research, and then communicating the findings. Research begins with the question that is to be answered. This is often motivated by the nurse's desire to answer a clinical question or to

---

Assistance With a Research Study

Nursing Research Committee

These committees have been established in many hospitals to educate nursing staff about research and to inform potential investigators of institutional requirements for conducting nursing research. The objective is to facilitate nursing research while maintaining high-quality patient care (Vessey & Campos, 1992).

Nurse Researchers in an Academic Setting

Faculty in most universities are expected to conduct research. Nursing faculty are no exception to this expectation. Those prepared at the doctoral level have had the advantage of courses in research design and statistics. If they have had experience conducting clinical studies, they can be a valuable asset in designing a research study. In addition, many institutions have personnel who can assist with data entry or other aspects of statistical analysis. If the school has a nursing research center, this would be a good place to locate such personnel.

Nurse Researchers in a Hospital Setting

Many hospitals employ nurses to conduct independent research studies. The objective is to generate the data needed to maintain or improve high-quality patient care. Often these researchers direct a nursing research center with personnel hired to assist the nursing research enterprise.

Contacting Researchers From Published Studies

If researchers have used a particular measurement instrument or an analytical technique that you are interested in, contact them to learn of their experiences. Published studies indicate the institution where the researcher is employed, making it possible to contact them by phone or letter. Ask them to share any problems they may have had in using the instrument or technique. They may also be helpful in directing you to other recent literature on the topic.

---

find a better way to perform a nursing intervention, or by an interest in a particular phenomenon. When a research question is being formulated, the previous research done in the area is reviewed so that the study can be developed in a manner that will add to the body of knowledge. While reviewing, critiquing, and synthesizing the research literature, one should also note the details of the research. For instance, noting how variables are defined and measured in the studies will aid in the writing of the research proposal.

The *research proposal* is the plan for the research and is written to communicate what is to be done in the study. It will undergo many revisions as the plan evolves and becomes stronger. The research proposal begins with the *significance* section, which uses data to indicate why the research is important. This is a short section that ends by indicating the purpose of the study and the research questions or hypotheses that are to be examined in the study. The significance section is usually developed, along with the review of the literature.

The focus of the *review of the literature* section is to place the present study in the context of previous research. Research studies are described by indicating the focus of the study, the design, the number and type of subjects used, what and how variables were measured, and the findings. Strengths and weaknesses of studies are also included. The goal of this synthesis is to conceptually set the stage for the study. The conceptual framework used to guide the study is presented and indicates how the variables of the study are expected to be related to one another. As the literature is being reviewed, the details of the published studies are noted and plans for the methods to be used in the present study are developed.

The *methods* section of the proposal consists of several subdivisions that are usually planned at the same time but written in a standard order. It begins with the research design. The type of study to be conducted depends on the question being asked and what is already known about the particular phenomenon. The practical aspects of implementing the study in the clinical setting also need to be considered. A design should be chosen that will best answer the question and have the least impact on the clinical setting so that patient care is not compromised.

The next section describes the *sample* to be included in the study and the site of the study. The measurement subsection follows and describes the measures to be used in the study. The measurement section includes a description of the instrument's reliability and validity and the method by which it was established. In addition, measures need to be evaluated for their appropriateness to the study population, their appropriateness to the variable definition, and the feasibility of using them in the clinical setting, although this may not appear in the written report. Scoring techniques for the instrument are described and indicate the level of measurement for the instrument. For clinical or physiological measures, it is important to identify the exact instrument to be used to measure the variable, including its accuracy and precision. If the study involves the testing of different treatments, a section in which they are described must be included.

The *procedures* that will be followed for the study need to be decided. For instance, how will potential subjects be identified? The procedures section of the proposal states exactly what is to be done to the subjects in the study, including the times that all measures are to be taken and treatments given. A plan is then developed and indicated in the proposal for the analysis that will be used to answer each research question.

It is usually after the research question and design have been developed that the *title* is chosen, even though it appears on the first page of the proposal. The ideal title indicates the topic, the study design, variables of interest, and the population to be studied. The *abstract,* which is usually the last part of the study to be written, even though it becomes the first section of the proposal, is a brief but comprehensive summary of the research proposal.

The *reference* section goes at the end and lists all the journal articles or other sources of information cited in the text. The *appendix* is the section in which all supporting documents, such as data collection tools and letters of support, are contained.

Once the planning is completed and the proposal written, the forms required for human subjects' review or any other review (discussed later in the chapter), need to be written, submitted, and approved. Data collection can then begin. This is usually the most time-consuming phase of the research process and tends to take longer than expected. The data can be entered into a computer program as they are collected. This will allow analysis to proceed according to the research plan. Analysis, however, is not the final step in the research process. The study is not completed until the findings are communicated to the nursing community. This can be by verbal presentation, a poster session, or, most important, by publishing the findings.

CLASSIFICATION OF NURSING RESEARCH STUDIES

There are several ways to refer to nursing research studies. One way is to refer to the topics explored. Most commonly that involves characterizing studies that focus on nursing care as *clinical nursing studies* and those focusing on the delivery of nursing services as *nursing services research* or *systems research*. These are the focus of two of the three branches of the NINR's extramural programs, which further support this classification.

Another way to describe nursing research is according to how the knowledge that is generated will be use. This is most commonly referred to as basic research and applied research. *Basic research* involves the generation of knowledge for knowledge sake. Findings from these studies are not always directly useful in practice. Basic research is often considered synonymous with research conducted in a biological laboratory, sometimes using human tissues, blood, cells, etc., or animal models. An example would be the study of tissue response to pressure. *Applied research* on the other hand, is conducted to answer a clinical question or solve a nursing practice problem. It often uses the knowledge generated in basic research. An example would be the evaluation of pressure-relieving devices in improving skin integrity.

A third way to define nursing research is in terms of the type of questions asked in a particular study. These are considered to be hierarchical, with research at the lower or beginning levels being required before the higher or more advanced levels of research can be undertaken. It is essential to understand a phenomenon before attempting to change it. The first level of research is a study that focuses on describing a phenomenon of interest to nursing and is called a *descriptive study*. An example would be a study describing the nutritional requirements of respiratory patients. *Exploratory studies* are those that describe relationships, such as identifying the predictors of postoperative pulmonary complications. *Explanatory studies* are those that test a theory. A *theory* is an abstract conceptualization about interrelationships among phenomena. An explanatory study provides a richer understanding of relationships than does an exploratory study (Polit & Hungler, 1995). It will usually follow an exploratory study. The fourth level of research is that of *prescription*. The goal is to identify the results of actions, such as testing the effectiveness of nursing interventions. This labeling of nursing studies can be in addition to other ways of describing a particular study.

QUANTITATIVE AND QUALITATIVE APPROACHES TO RESEARCH

There are two major scientific approaches to nursing research, both of which are essential to nursing science. The most familiar category is the *quantitative approach*. This method requires that something be known ahead of time about the phenomenon of interest. A theory is chosen or formulated to explain relationships. The research methodology then involves a systematic, controlled collection and analysis of data. The goal is to offer support for the theory as an explanatory device for the phenomenon of interest.

Qualitative research is the other major approach to research. This involves the collection of data that are more holistic, contextual, and subjective, usually in the form of interviews and/or observations in a natural setting. The goal of this research is to understand the human experience. It results in the generation of theory, rather than the testing of theory. The appropriate research methodology is determined by the question being asked and the extent of the knowledge already established in relation to the phenomenon of interest.

Research Methods

Both research approaches are essential for the advancement of nursing knowledge. Some researchers combine the two approaches when studying a particular phenomenon and believe that this is the best way to gain a comprehensive understanding of complex nursing phenomena.

Quantitative research. Within each of these major approaches to research there are specific methodologies that can be used. Within the quantitative approach to research, the goal is most often to establish *cause*. Thus an approach is used that eliminates as many extraneous variables as possible, allowing the causal relationship between two or more variables to be examined. Three criteria are necessary to establish cause:

1. If an event is believed to cause an outcome, then the event must precede the outcome in time.
2. Whenever the outcome occurs, the event must always have been present before it.
3. There must be a theory or other explanation for the relationship between the event and the outcome.

In this research design, the cause, or the event, is called the *independent variable* and the effect, or the outcome, is called the *dependent variable.*

Experimental research. The quantitative research design that is considered the best for establishing cause is the *experimental design.* The three criteria that are necessary for a design to be considered experimental are that more than one group be used, that subjects participating in the study be randomly assigned to groups, and that the researcher have control over the independent variable (Cook & Campbell, 1979). The independent variable (commonly a treatment) is routinely administered to one group, with outcomes compared with those of a control group that does not receive the treatment or receives another type of treatment. This design is sometimes referred to as a *randomized controlled trial* (RCT). The goal is to remove all other possible explanations for the effect on the dependent variable except that contributed by the independent variable. An example is a study that tested the effectiveness of relaxation technique in reducing dyspnea and anxiety in outpatients with chronic obstructive pulmonary disease (COPD). Patients were randomly assigned to receive either taped relaxation instructions or to sit quietly in a room for 30 minutes. Patients who were taught to use relaxation techniques reported significantly less dyspnea and anxiety compared with those who sat quietly (Gift, Moore & Soeken, 1992).

Quasiexperimental research. When the research design includes having an independent variable that is manipulated but subjects not randomly assigned to groups, the study is labeled as a *quasiexperimental study* (Cook & Campbell, 1979; Polit & Hungler, 1995). An example of a quasiexperimental design would be the testing of an educational program in an acute care setting. To randomly assign patients to receive or not receive the teaching would mean that patients who did receive the teaching and patients who did not might be located in beds next to one another. They would be likely to talk, and the person not receiving the teaching might benefit from the information shared. There might also be resentment from those who were excluded from the teaching. To prevent this, the researcher would have to separate the treatment groups and experimental groups geographically or by time. The challenge to the researcher would be to separate the effect due to the teaching from the effect due to the initial noncomparability between groups. The ability to make causal claims is therefore more limited when a quasiexperimental design is used than when an experimental design is used.

Nonexperimental research. *Nonexperimental designs* include those in which the independent variable is not manipulated. Nonexperimental research designs are less expensive to implement and may be used for that reason. These designs need to be used when it is unethical or impossible to manipulate the independent variable, such as when studying the effects of smoking or widowhood. The *ex post facto* or *case-control* design is a type of nonexperimental design. Subjects are selected because of differences in the dependent variable, such as those with a particular condition and those without the condition, and their past history is examined in an attempt to determine differences that might have contributed to the condition. An example is a study by Skoner, Thompson, and Caron (1994) in which they selected women with stress urinary incontinence and those without it and found that the factors contributing to incontinence were a history of delivering a baby with a vaginal delivery, having an episiotomy or tear during delivery, and having a mother with stress urinary incontinence. High parity (four or more pregnancies) was not associated with increased risk. Another situation in which an ex post facto research design is frequently used is with research examining the factors contributing to nosocomial infections.

Surveys are nonexperimental research studies that obtain information from respondents using a self-report methodology. They usually ask people about their behaviors or what they plan to do. They tend to be broad in scope but superficial in nature because they are limited by the extent to which respondents are willing to report on the topic. Surveys can include a mailed questionnaire, telephone interview, or the like.

Other nonexperimental designs are *descriptive studies* in which the focus is to determine frequencies of occurrence of certain phenomena or to describe relationships among variables. No attempt is made to establish causal claims. Nonexperimental research can be used to describe the current state of practice and used as an incentive to change practice. After the change is implemented, it can be evaluated using research methods, such as an experimental design (see box below).

Qualitative research. Qualitative research also includes different research designs depending on the phenomenon being studied. The three types of qualitative research designs used most commonly in nursing are phenomenology, ethnography, and grounded theory research.

Use of a Descriptive Study to Improve Practice

Many advances have been made in surgery in the past 10 years. The use of fiberoptic technology and microsurgery has changed the detail work that can be accomplished in surgery, and this increased precision has resulted in the patient being on the operating room table for a much longer time than in the past. My colleagues and I began to notice that more patients who came in for elective surgery were experiencing skin breakdown a few days after surgery. Since these patients were healthy, we decided that the loss of skin integrity was likely to be preventable. However, we were not able to elicit support for a practice change. It was believed that before we could correct the problem, we needed to be more certain about the extent of the problem and the factors related to it. Was skin breakdown related to the length of time on the operating table, the positioning devices used, the type of surgery or the surgeon, the patient's age, the patient's individual risk of skin breakdown, or other factors?

To examine this problem more fully, a descriptive study was undertaken (Grous, Reilly, & Gift, 1995). The purposes of the study were to determine the incidence of skin breakdown in those undergoing prolonged surgery and to determine factors related to pressure ulcer formation. A proposal was written, and approval was obtained from the Institutional Review Board to conduct the study.

Subjects consisted of 33 adult patients undergoing operative procedures of 10 hours or longer. Fifteen (45%) were found to develop stage I or II pressure ulcers within 48 hours of surgery. No significant differences were found between those who did and those who did not develop pressure ulcers in relation to age, gender, preoperative Braden Scale score, position on the operating room table, or type or length of surgery. A significant difference was found in relation to the type of device placed on the operating room table under patients. A warming blanket was used more often on those who developed pressure ulcers (75%) than on those who did not. It was recommended that warming blankets be used in the operating room only when essential.

The results of the study were shared with the staff and other personnel in the operating room. There was then widespread support for a practice change. Criteria were developed to define situations where it would be essential to use a warming blanket. Otherwise, alternative warming devices were to be used. This change was simple to implement, since it had the support of the operating room personnel. We are presently involved in evaluating the effectiveness of the change by repeating the descriptive study. The incidence of pressure ulcer formation before and after the practice change will be compared.

Phenomenology. Phenomenology is used when the goal is to describe particular phenomena or experiences (Streubert & Carpenter, 1995). The focus is on the meaning ascribed to the phenomenon by the person. Therefore the primary method of data collection is to listen to the voices of the people experiencing the phenomenon. This usually takes the form of interviews.

An example of a phenomenological study is one in which audiotaped interviews were analyzed to determine what experiences children between the ages of 9 and 11 found stressful (Jacobson, 1994). The children indicated that experiences related to loss, such as the loss of a person, pet, or neighborhood, were infrequent but had the greatest consequences for their lives. Other stresses were related to feelings of threat to self, such as worry over having done something known to be disliked by an adult in their lives, and feelings of being hassled, such as forgetting their lunch or being told what to do by a sibling.

Another example of a phenomenological study is one in which a deeper understanding of the meaning of comfort was gained from the descriptions offered by patients who had experienced traumatic injuries or life-threatening illnesses (Morse, Bottorff, & Hutchinson, 1995). The researchers found that patients described comfort as relief, even if temporary, from the most demanding discomfort and did not describe it as the ultimate state of peace and serenity, as was expected.

Ethnography. Ethnography focuses on describing culture (Streubert & Carpenter, 1995). The basic question is "What is the nature of the group?" That which is implicit in a culture is made explicit. This requires an intimacy with the participants beyond simply talking to them. The researcher becomes a participant observer in the culture. This is accomplished by going to the location of the culture, observing their behaviors, and having them describe the meaning for the behaviors. This methodology is especially helpful in understanding complex cultures, such as a health care system, and is used extensively in anthropology.

An example of ethnography is a study by Wolf (1988) in which she describes therapeutic and occupational rituals of nurses. Therapeutic rituals are those that improve the condition of patients, whereas occupational rituals are symbolic actions that facilitate the transition of professional neophytes into their professional role. These rituals enable nurses to carry out their caring activities for ill or dying patients. They also help to reaffirm the values and beliefs of nurses.

Grounded theory. The third commonly used qualitative methodology in nursing is *grounded theory research,* which is the exploration of the processes of human interaction (Streubert & Carpenter, 1995). It explores the richness and diversity of human experience. A constant comparative analysis technique is used to generate themes or categories of the phenomenon of interest.

An example of a grounded theory study is one by Wilson (1989) in which the constant comparative method was used to describe the phases of coping used by those caring for relatives with Alzheimer's dementia. It was learned that much of the caregiving experience consisted of coping with negative choices when alternatives were undesirable. The first of the three stages described is "taking it on," which is when the caregiver accepts the responsibility of caregiving for a demented loved one at home because there does not appear to be any alternatives. The caregiver experiences uncertainty and unpredictability. The second stage, "going through it," is characterized by conflicting role demands that disrupt the family and fatigue the caregiver. Stage 3 is "turning it over," in which the caregiver reaches the breaking point and turns over the caregiving to others. Grounded theory research will often contribute to the development of middle-range theories.

ETHICS IN RESEARCH

In addition to selecting a research methodology, the researcher must be concerned with ethical issues. There are two main areas of ethical concern in nursing research: the use of humans as subjects and the maintenance of integrity within the nursing research process.

Protecting the Rights of Subjects

In planning a research study involving humans, one must consider the ethical principles of *beneficence* versus *nonmaleficence*. Researchers are obligated to consider the risks and benefits of their work—both the risks and benefits to the individual participating in the study and the risks and benefits to society as a whole. Research differs from the provision of therapy in that participation in research will often not be directly beneficial to the individual. The researcher often benefits more than the individual. However, even studies that pose little or no risk to the individual participating must show some benefit or the researcher will not be permitted to conduct the study.

Justice is the ethical principle considered when subjects are chosen for participation in a study. Those people who are unable to speak for themselves (such as children and those who are mentally deficient or otherwise incapacitated) are considered vulnerable. Such subjects should not be included in a research study simply because they are available. They should be included only if the researcher is interested in a study dealing specifically with that population. For instance, if one were studying nursing care of children, then children would be expected to be included as subjects.

It is essential that researchers also consider the diversity of research participants and protect against negative differentiation toward individuals or groups on the basis of their diversity (Silva, 1995). This principle directs the nurse researcher to be culturally sensitive in the frameworks chosen, the measurement instruments used, and the methodologies used to collect data. Analysis should examine the findings by intracultural subgroups.

The ethical principle of *autonomy* is most important when humans are asked to participate in a research study. Each individual is valued in our society, and each is therefore given the right to make decisions about his or her own life. The process by which individuals are provided with truthful information about a research study and invited to participate without coercion must be identified for each study. The researcher is expected to maintain the participants' confidentiality. Individuals also have the right to withdraw from a study at any time if they so desire.

Maintaining the Integrity of the Study

The second major area of ethical concern in research is that of maintaining the integrity of the research study. This involves the avoidance of scientific misconduct in the design, conduct, or reporting of the research. *"Misconduct in science* is defined as fabrication, falsification, plagiarism, or other practices that seriously deviate from those that are commonly accepted with the scientific community for proposing, conducting, or reporting research"* (NIH, 1994).

Fabrication is the making up of data for the purpose of deception, whereas *falsification* involves the changing or mutilation of data. These include the reporting of data that were not obtained according to the research protocol, the selective reporting of findings, and/or the omission of conflicting data. *Plagiarism* is defined as the representation of another person's work as one's own. Improprieties of authorship are often also included under plagiarism and involve the improper assignment of credit, such as the omission of others; presenting the same material as original in more than one publication; naming individuals as authors who have not made a definite contribution to the work; and submission of multiauthored publications without the concurrence of all authors (Prescott, 1989).

It is the responsibility of the principal investigator to maintain the integrity of the research. This involves monitoring not only one's own behavior but also that of others involved in the project. Ignorance is not an acceptable excuse for academic misconduct. Those involved in a research project must be taught proper techniques for carrying out the research in a timely, cost-effective, and ethical manner. The principal investigator needs also to monitor the activities of research assistants as the research is being conducted. This may involve scheduled meetings of the entire research team, having research assistants demonstrate the research protocol during announced and unannounced visits to the site, having another person verify data entry, and performing ongoing evaluation of all research staff (Gift, Creasia, & Parker, 1991).

While most nursing research ethical principles are written about research involving humans, it is also understood that researchers involved in animal research will conduct their research with the least possible harm or suffering to the animal. Animals are selected because they are the most appropriate species for the needs of the research (Silva, 1995). All research involving animals must be preapproved by an Institutional Animal Review Board.

REVIEW OF A RESEARCH PROPOSAL

There are several reasons why a research proposal is reviewed before a study is begun. There are those who review it for its *scientific merit*. This is to determine if the research question will make a contribution to science and if the proposed research design, sampling techniques, measurement, and analysis will answer the question in the best manner possible. This form of review is conducted in a variety of situations. One is in an academic setting when professors review a study to decide if a student researcher should proceed with the study. The goal is to have the student design the best study possible.

Researchers serving on review panels for funding agencies engage in scientific review of studies to decide which studies should receive funding. Often the results of this scientific review are then integrated into a decision about which studies are in line with the mission of the funding organization. Those with the most scientific merit and most in line with the mission of the agency receive the funding.

Another form of review is that done to gain access to subjects. This is usually necessary when the research is to be conducted in a setting where potential subjects are cared for by others. Those responsible for caring for the potential subjects will usually have a mission other than that of research, such as providing health care. The institution will want to be sure that a research study will not interfere with their primary mission or disturb their patients unnecessarily.

The only form of research review that is mandated by law is that which is done for the protection of human subjects or animals. The National Research Act of 1974, Title 45 Part 46 Code of Federal Regulations, and other related laws and regulations mandate the review of research involving humans. A review by an *institutional review board* (IRB) ensures that risks to subjects are minimal and reasonable in relation to the benefits of the investigation. It mandates that selection of subjects and informed consent be equitable and appropriate to the research.

Every research study involving humans must be reviewed by an IRB before data collection begins. If the proposal is written for the IRB, the researcher indicates the level and type of risk involved for subjects who participate in the study. How the subjects' confidentiality will be maintained, as well as how other federal guidelines for human subjects will be followed in the study, must be indicated. If a consent is required, it should be included in the appendix.

The level of review by the IRB, however, depends on the nature of the study and the potential risks to the subject. The levels of review include exempt review, expedited review, and full committee review. *Exempt review* is for those studies that are conducted in an educational setting and that involve normal educational practices or educational tests. Studies involving the collection or study of existing data, documents, records, or specimens would also receive an exempt review. Demonstration programs evaluating public benefit of service programs, as well as studies evaluating food taste, food quality, or consumer acceptance would also receive an exempt review.

The category of *expedited review* is for those studies involving no more than minimal risk to subjects. These include studies involving the collection of hair, nails or teeth, secretions, excreta, or other materials that would normally be removed from the body. Research involving the recording of data from noninvasive procedures routinely employed in clinical practice, as well as research focusing on drugs or devices that are not classified as experimental, would receive an expedited review by the IRB. Minor invasive procedures, such as the venipuncture removal of small amounts of blood or the collection of plaque and calculus, as well as voice recordings, moderate exercise of healthy volunteers, and research concerned with individual or group behaviors or characteristics, would receive an expedited review. All other research would require a *full committee review.*

All studies requiring a full committee review and most studies requiring an expedited review will involve the use of a written informed consent. A *consent form* is a succinct statement written in clear, understandable language. It gives information about the reason why the person was chosen to be included in the study, as well as the purpose, procedures, benefits, risks, and duration of the study. The name and telephone number of the responsible researcher and a 24-hour emergency number are provided. The consent form must indicate that the subject has the right to refuse to participate in the study or to withdraw from the study after it has begun without any penalty. Each adult subject or legal guardian who signs a consent must receive a written copy of the document. In some special situations permission is given to enroll subjects in a study using a verbal informed consent. The exact wording of the consent information is written and submitted to the IRB for approval along with the research proposal before the study can begin.

QUALITY IMPROVEMENT VERSUS RESEARCH

Often in a clinical setting it is difficult to decide where a quality improvement project ends and a research study begins. When quality assurance advanced to quality improvement, it became common to alter the practice environment and measure the benefits of that alteration. These activities often resemble research. One distinction, however, is mandated by law: a research study must be approved by the IRB before data collection can begin. Therefore, if a project begins as a quality improvement project, it cannot be turned into a research study afterward. Another factor dividing the two is the intended use of the project. If the findings were to be used only at a specific institution, it would be classified as a quality improvement project, whereas a project to be published in a research journal and shared with others would be classified as a research project. However, there are quality assurance journals in which quality assurance projects are published. To decide on the difference between the two, the relationship of the practice or product being studied to the routine standard of care needs to be examined. Quality improvement projects would involve only routine practices. The design of the project also influences the distinction, with the use of a randomized clinical trial most likely being a research project. The difference between research and quality improvement needs to be examined before data are collected for the project. That decision will affect how the results of the project can be used after it is completed.

SEEKING FUNDING FOR A RESEARCH STUDY

In seeking funding for a research study, the first consideration is the match between the researcher's idea and the funding mission of the agency. Funding for research can come from a variety of sources.

Funding Agencies

Nursing organizations. Nursing organizations, such as Sigma Theta Tau, The American Association of Critical-Care Nurses, and the Oncology Nursing Society, have research programs that allow them to fund small research projects. Information packets that contain guidelines indicating the focus of their particular research interests, what to include in a proposal, submission deadlines, and funding amounts can be obtained from the organization.

Businesses and corporations. If a research proposal involves the testing of a particular piece of equipment or a commercially available product, it is possible that the company producing the product will fund the research. The dollar amounts of research awards from these sources are often small, but many companies will also supply their products for the study.

Nonprofit agencies. These agencies, which include organizations such as the American Heart Association, American Cancer Society, and American Lung Association, have a focus for their research effort that is usually obvious from the title of the organization. Funding success is determined by how well the project and experience of the researcher meet their guidelines.

Foundations. A foundation is a nongovernmental, nonprofit organization with its own funds. Often these are from an individual, family, or corporation. A foundation usually has programs established to maintain or aid charitable, religious, educational, social, or other activities serving the common good. Those that have funded nursing research include The Robert Wood Johnson Foundation, American Nurses' Foundation, and W.K. Kellogg Foundation. Directories listing these funding opportunities are available.

Federal research agencies. The U.S. Public Health Service published *Healthy People 2000* in 1990, indicating a focus on health promotion and disease prevention. This document provides a guideline for research funding priorities for most federal funding agencies. The *National Institutes of Health* is the agency within the Public Health Service that funds research. Nurse researchers are eligible for funding from any institute; however, their research interests make them more likely to seek funding from the National Institute of Nursing Research and such institutes as the National Institute on Aging, the National Institute of Mental Health, and the National Institute of Child Health and Human Development. The Agency for Health Care Policy and Research (AHCPR) is another government agency that supports research. The focus of this agency is health care systems research. All federal funding for research is highly competitive and designed to support the experienced researcher.

Forms to Be Submitted

Funding agencies usually require a copy of the research proposal, as well as additional information. The funding agency requests these extra sections to evaluate the match between the proposed research and their funding mission, as well as to evaluate the competence of the researcher and the resources available to carry out the research.

A funding institution usually requires a budget and budget justification section. A *budget* consists of a listing of the money required to carry out the research proposal, and the *justification* section is an indication of how that money will be used. This is done to allow the funding agency to decide if the project is worth the expense.

Biographical sketches of key personnel, other sources of support, and a description of the resources and environment for research are sections that are required in most funding proposals. If a section indicating previous work of the principal investigator is required, it is usually called preliminary studies and is presented after the background of the study. It is essential that the researcher use these sections to indicate how the research study being proposed meets the funding objectives of the agency.

Key Points

- Nursing research has high-quality patient care as its ultimate objective.
- Research is a recent development in nursing.
- The National Institute of Nursing Research of the National Institutes of Health provides federal funding for nursing research.
- Using research to improve the quality of patient care is the responsibility of all nurses.
- Nursing research methods are most commonly divided into quantitative and qualitative approaches.
- The principal investigator in a nursing research study must protect the rights of the humans who are subjects in the study.
- The integrity of the research study protocol, data analysis, and publication are vital to conducting research studies.
- All research that involves humans must be approved by a federally mandated institutional review board before data collection can begin.
- Funding for nursing research can come from nursing organizations, businesses, non-profit agencies, foundations, or federal research agencies.

Critical Thinking Exercises

1. If you were to learn that a clinical procedure is not being performed in your institution according to the latest nursing research findings, what process would you

recommend for changing that practice? Who would be the supporters of this change, and who would need to be convinced of its merit?

2. Think of a clinical problem you are currently encountering. How would you design a research study to solve the problem? What questions would you need to answer before you began the study? What type of ethical issues would need to be resolved? What are the major barriers that would prevent you from conducting this study?

3. Describe the review procedures you would go through if you were to conduct a nursing research study in the clinical setting most familiar to you.

4. What would you do if you were asked to collect data for a research study on a patient who did not know he or she was part of the study? Would this ever be acceptable? Under what conditions?

References

American Nurses' Association. (1993). *Position paper: Education for participation in nursing research.* Washington, DC: The Association.

Burns, N., & Grove, S.K. (1993). *The practice of nursing research: Conduct, critique and utilization* (2nd ed.). Philadelphia: W.B. Saunders.

Champion, V.L., & Leach, A. (1989). Variables related to research utilization in nursing: An empirical investigation. *Journal of Advanced Nursing, 14,* 705-710.

Cook, T.D., & Campbell, D.T. (1979). *Quasi-experimentation: Design and analysis issues for field studies.* Chicago: Rand McNally.

Coyle, L.A., & Sokop, A.G. (1990). Innovation adoption behavior among nurses. *Nursing Research, 39,* 176-180.

Ferrell, M.J., DiCarlo, B., Anderson, J., Baker, C., Bell, D., Brunt, B., & Kelly, K.C. (1994). *Utilization of agency for health care policy and research guidelines.* Washington, DC: American Nurses' Association.

Gift, A.G., Creasia, J., & Parker, B. (1991). Utilizing research assistants and maintaining research integrity. *Research in Nursing & Health, 14,* 229-233.

Gift, A.G., Moore, T., & Soeken, K. (1992). Relaxation to reduce dyspnea and anxiety in COPD patients. *Nursing Research, 41,* 242-246.

Grous, C., Reilly, N., & Gift, A.G. (1995). *Skin integrity in patients undergoing prolonged surgery.* Manuscript submitted for publication.

Jacobson, G. (1994). The meaning of stressful life experiences in nine- to eleven-year-old children: A phenomenological study. *Nursing Research, 43,* 95-99.

Marek, K.D. (1994). *Manual to develop guidelines,* Washington, DC: American Nurses' Association.

McFarlane, J., & Parker, B. (1994). *Abuse during pregnancy: A protocol for prevention and intervention.* March of Dimes Birth Defects Foundation.

McFarlane, J., Parker, B., Soeken, K., & Bullock, L. (1992). Assessing for abuse during pregnancy: Severity and frequency of injuries and associated entry into prenatal care. *JAMA, 267*(23), 3176-3178.

Morse, J.M., Bottorff, J.L., & Hutchinson, S. (1995). The paradox of comfort. *Nursing Research, 44,* 14-19.

National Institute of Nursing Research. (1993). *Nursing research at the National Institutes of Health, fiscal years 1989-1992.* Washington, DC: U.S. Department of Health and Human Services, U.S. Public Health Service.

National Institutes of Health. (1994). Responsibilities of NIH and awardee institutions for the responsible conduct of research. *NIH Guide, 23,* 42.

Parker, B., McFarlane, J., & Soeken, K. (1994). Abuse during pregnancy: Effects on maternal complications and birthweight in adult and teenage women. *Obstetrics and Gynecology, 84*(3), 323-328.

Parker, B., McFarlane, J., Soeken, K., Campbell, D., & Torres, S. (1993). Physical and emotional abuse in pregnancy: A comparison of adult and teenage women. *Nursing Research, 42*(3), 173-178.

Polit, D.F., & Hungler, B.P. (1995). *Nursing research: Principles and methods* (5th ed.). Philadelphia: J.B. Lippincott.

Prescott, P.A. (1989). Academic misconduct: Considerations for educational administrators. *Journal of Professional Nursing, 5*(5), 283-287.

Silva, M.C. (1995). *Ethical guidelines in the conduct, dissemination, and implementation of nursing research.* Washington, DC: American Nurses' Association.

Skoner, M.M., Thompson, W.D., & Caron, V.A. (1994). Factors associated with risk of stress urinary incontinence in women. *Nursing Research, 43,* 301-306.

Stetler, C.B. (1994). Refinement of the Stetler/Marram model for application of research findings to practice. *Nursing Outlook, 42,* 15-25.

Stevenson, J.S. (1986). Forging a research discipline. *Nursing Research, 36,* 60-64.

Streubert, H.J., & Carpenter, D.R. (1995). *Qualitative research in nursing: Advancing the humanistic imperative.* Philadelphia: J.B. Lippincott.

Titler, M.G., Kleiber, C., Steelman, V., Goode, C., Rakel, B., Barry-Walker, J., Small, S., & Buckwalter, K. (1994). Infusing research into practice to promote quality care. *Nursing Research, 43,* 307-313.

Vessey, J.A., & Campos, R.G. (1992). The role of nursing research committees. *Nursing Research, 41,* 247-249.

Wilson, H.S. (1989). Family caregiving for a relative with Alzheimer's dementia: Coping with negative choices. *Nursing Research, 38,* 94-98.

Wolf, Z.R. (1988). *Nurses work: The sacred and profane.* Philadelphia: University of Pennsylvania Press.

Information Technology

21

Teresa L. Panniers

Objectives

At the completion of this chapter, the reader will be able to:

- Discuss the implications of information technology for nursing practice and health care.
- Evaluate technologies within the context of the technology assessment framework.
- Discuss the progress made by nursing in the integration of information into nursing practice.
- Outline, with examples, the growth and development of information technology in health care and the impact on nursing practice.
- Discuss the evolution of the specialty of nursing informatics.

Profile in Practice

Cheryl D. Parker, MSN, RN, CEN, INS
Management Consultant,
Superior Consultant Company, Inc.,
Farmington Hills, Michigan

My nursing career has been guided by two central themes, challenge and growth. These themes are demonstrated, both in my education leading from an associate degree in nursing through a post-master's certificate in nursing informatics, and in my practice beginning as an emergency department nurse to my latest challenge as an informatics nurse specialist (INS).

My decision to use my clinical knowledge and experience in a nontraditional nursing role grew from my love of computers as a tool and my frustration with the current state of clinical information systems in health care. Administrative data have been the traditional focus of health care information systems. However, as practitioners, we collect a large amount of clinical data from each patient that is virtually inaccessible to us the next time we encounter that patient. This problem is especially apparent in emergency care when we request a patient record and receive one that stacks several feet high, is handwritten and may be illegible, and from which data cannot be quickly extracted in any usable form. Furthermore, clinical information systems designed by persons without a clinical background are often lacking in areas that are important to health care practitioners. Since nurses are major providers of patient care and thereby record a significant amount of clinical data, it is important that nursing's needs be reflected in the design of clinical information systems. This is one of the many challenges for the informatics nurse specialist.

Meeting patient needs may occur in many different forums, and the practice of an informatics nurse specialist is just one example of the diversity in nursing practice.

As we enter the twenty-first century, the science and art of nursing will mature in concert with the rapid developments in information technology. Nursing will be challenged to standardize its nursing language so that it can be understood universally and incorporated into advanced information systems. Nurses will continue to define the scope and breadth of interventions used to promote health and prevent disease, and develop systems that support clinical decision making and critical thinking. Nursing will develop information systems that are integrated and can support the effective administration of nursing practice in a variety of settings. Nurses possess the innate abilities to actualize these goals. Our challenge is to employ the vast array of information technologies, in conjunction with the art and science of nursing, to meet the ultimate goal of promoting health and wellness for society.

Information technology pervades every aspect of nursing practice. This chapter addresses the application of the technology assessment framework to nursing practice. Ways in which nurses obtain data, process these data, and use the information and knowledge acquired through analysis and synthesis of data pertinent to the practice of nursing are explored. Examples of information systems used by nurses are highlighted. Finally, information resources that can be used to enhance nursing practice are illustrated.

INFORMATION TECHNOLOGY IN HEALTH CARE

Technology, the practical application of science, develops through interactions among individuals, instruments, and organizational structures (Pillar, Jacox, & Redman, 1990). In the field of health care, technology may be as simple as using a glass thermometer to record a temperature or as sophisticated as case management for overseeing the health care provided to individuals. These technologies, though differing in level of sophistication, are both aimed at achieving the human goals of preventing disease, maintaining health, and promoting wellness (Sandelowski, 1993).

Technology can be described as either therapeutic or information oriented in nature (Sandelowski, 1993). *Therapeutic technologies* include interventions such as pharmacotherapeutics, laser surgery, and massage therapy. *Information technologies* in health care can be categorized into two groups: information producing or information managing. *Information-producing technology* is used to diagnose disease or dysfunction, screen for pathogenic conditions, or monitor body functions. *Information-managing technology* includes the computerized systems for entering, storing, retrieving, and manipulating client data (Sandelowski, 1993). While therapeutic and information-oriented technologies are equally important adjuncts to providing health care, the focus of this chapter is on information-oriented technologies to enhance nursing practice within the health care field.

THE TECHNOLOGY ASSESSMENT FRAMEWORK

Technology is rapidly changing the way in which nursing is practiced. However, with a desire to enhance practice, many technologies have been implemented without examining their risks and benefits, as well as their cost-effectiveness. Recently, an analytical approach to the evaluation of technologies has emerged and has gained credence in the health care environment. The research framework, called *technology assessment,* provides guidelines for the systematic evaluation of health care technology (Pillar, Jacox, & Redman, 1990). Examination of the safety, efficacy, costs, and social impact of a technology constitute the elements of technology assessment and can be applied to any technology. *Safety* is measured in terms of the risk/benefit ratio and is a relative term. *Efficacy* is a determination of the probability that a technology will benefit individuals in a defined population. Efficacy is the benefit of a technology derived under ideal or laboratory conditions; in practice, researchers and practitioners critically examine a technology's effectiveness, otherwise referred to as "benefit under average conditions of use." An economic analysis is used to determine the cost/benefit ratio of a technology, as well as its *cost-effectiveness,* which is a measure of the benefits, not in dollars, but in some health-related effect such as added years of life. *Social impact* refers to the overall impact on society in terms of quality-of-life issues and the opportunity costs of the implementation and support of a technology (Pillar, Jacox, & Redman, 1990). Questions nurses should ask when applying the technology assessment framework are presented in the box on p. 469.

Issues Related to Information Technology

Marie Jones, a staff nurse in the critical care unit of a large medical center, has just arrived for work at 7 AM. As she enters the elevator with several other people, she bumps into her colleague, Steven, who says it's been a really busy night and he can't wait to get home to sleep. Marie agrees that it has been very busy lately and says she'll see him tomorrow. Just as Steven is leaving the elevator, he calls back to Marie that he has forgotten to record Mr. Sanford's medications that he gave earlier that morning. Steven asks Marie to record them for him and

Questions Nurses Should Ask When Applying the Technology Assessment Framework	
Safety	How safe is the device/procedure?
Efficacy	Does the device/procedure produce an acceptable outcome in the clinical setting?
Cost	How costly is the device/procedure to the individual, family, and society?
Social impact	What are the legal, political, and social ramifications of the device/procedure for the individual, family, and society?

shouts out his access code and password to the point-of-care clinical information system. Marie is taken aback momentarily, and when she has recovered her composure, she steps out of the elevator to speak to Steven about what has just transpired.

Safety in information handling is imperative as society relies more and more on automated data. Data integrity (i.e., data that are accurate and reliable) is an essential component in ensuring the safety of data. Steven violated this principle when he failed to update the client's record immediately in the point-of-care system. Mr. Sanford was placed in danger, since data that are not recorded leave open the possibility of an inadvertent medication error should another nurse mistakenly repeat the dose.

Data security refers to measures used to protect electronic client information. Since protecting client data is the most important objective, access codes are required to get into the system. An *access code* is a unique set of numbers and/or letters, usually chosen by the nurse, that is not shared with anyone else and that can be keyed in to allow the nurse access to a database. Multiple layers of codes may be used to access more sensitive client data. In the case scenario, Steven has compromised the security of his client's data by divulging his access code and password, not only to a colleague, but also to other individuals who overheard the conversation. Other methods of protecting client data include the development of policies to prevent unlawful access to data, the immediate removal of access codes of terminated employees, and the use of antiviral software to prevent data from being infected by a computer virus.

In addition to data security, safety also encompasses the prevention of accidental destruction of data by employing techniques to ensure that data are backed up and that the computer is protected against an electrical power surge by using a surge protector. The computer also must be protected from possible physical damage from water or chemicals.

Efficacy/effectiveness in information handling technology deals with the impact on processes of care. Computers can save time in indirect tasks, allowing more time for client care. Data can be collected once for use by all care providers (Zielstorff, Hudgings, & Grobe, 1993), and the information obtained from a clinical information system can be used to document care, determine positive outcomes, or assess the contribution of nursing care to the health and well-being of clients.

Economic considerations are important when assessing the level of technologic sophistication that is needed to handle information. The initial costs of hardware and software should be considered, as well as costs to maintain and upgrade the system, and to purchase software support contracts. The compatibility of systems within a health care institution and on wide-area networks should be considered, as should training costs associated with employing the system. An advantage of automated information handling is the cost savings in terms of human productivity that can be realized. Time can be saved in documentation, but the workload can increase as a result of the sophistication of computerized monitoring systems.

The social impact of information-handling technology also raises issues of privacy and confidentiality. The most serious concern is one of access to information of a sensitive nature. Simpson (1994) cites results from the *Harris-Equifax Health Information Privacy Survey* of 1993 showing that the American public is concerned about the maintenance of personal privacy and the procurement of informed consent before releasing any information contained in a computerized health care record. Nurses should collaborate with physicians, as well as laboratory and medical records personnel, to determine policies regarding authorized access to, and restriction of, data. Nurses also should provide physical privacy in a health care setting by placing terminals away from public areas and properly disposing of any printouts no longer required for documentation.

Legislation affecting privacy and confidentiality has been instituted. *The Fair Health Information Practices Act* of 1994 is designed to restrict the use of personal health information in an electronic health care record (Simpson, 1994).

INFORMATION TECHNOLOGY CONCEPTS IN NURSING

A definition of information and its relationship to knowledge and decision making serves as a conceptual basis for understanding the nature of information technology. *Information* is derived from data (basic facts or observations) that are organized in such a way as to have understandable meaning. Hadden (1986) considers information as meaningful data and distinguishes it from *knowledge,* which is an evaluation that can put the information to use. Table 21-1 provides an example of this distinction using an adaptation of Gordon's (1982) nursing diagnosis formulation exercises.

Table 21-1 Distinguishing Characteristics of Data, Information, and Knowledge

Term	Definition	Example
Data	Basic facts or observations	Pulse rate of 124
Information	Data organized to have meaning	Pulse rate of 124; blood pressure of 80/56; skin cool and clammy; client restless
Knowledge	Recognition of something with familiarity gained through experience	Client is experiencing initial signs of shock

In a hospital setting, client-specific data should permit nurses to identify each client, the interventions used to meet the client's needs, and the outcomes of client care (McCormick, 1991). With regard to fiscal considerations, nurses should be able to capture the amount and types of resources used and the income generated from care provided. Ideally, the data that describe the client's condition and progress, the care provided, and the outcomes of that care should be captured and analyzed across all settings in which the client receives care. The following hypothetical case provides a comprehensive view of a client's care captured in a computerized client record across a variety of settings.

Mr. Lazarus has been undergoing cancer chemotherapy for treatment of a lymphoma in an outpatient oncology center. In the past 24 hours, he has developed fever, chills, and pleuritic chest pain and is experiencing a productive cough. He has been admitted to the hospital for suspected pneumonia. On admission, the history of Mr. Lazarus' condition, as well as the treatment regimen at the outpatient center, are transferred electronically to establish an electronic client record.

On initial examination in the medical unit, the previous history and physical data are available to the resident physician, Dr. Cassidy, allowing him to update the client record with the information required to care for Mr. Lazarus during this acute episode of his illness. Following the initial workup, a chest x-ray film is taken, and blood is drawn. While Mr. Lazarus is being evaluated by Nurse Matthews, the radiologist is reading the x-ray film and, subsequently, enters the results of the chest film directly into the client care information system. At the same time, the technician in the clinical laboratory is entering the results of the sputum sample for culture and sensitivity directly into the system.

Nurse Matthews and Dr. Cassidy are able to retrieve these results at the client's bedside using the bedside computer terminal. Dr. Cassidy confirms the diagnosis and prescribes the appropriate antibiotic by entering it directly into the computer. The order is transmitted to the pharmacy, where it is immediately filled and transported to the unit, allowing Nurse Matthews to begin the antibiotic treatment. Nurse Matthews has been entering Mr. Lazarus' vital signs throughout the shift and is able to access a graphical depiction of the temperature, blood pressure, pulse, and respirations. She notes that his temperature is slowly returning to normal and his respirations are less rapid.

Mr. Lazarus has recovered enough to return home. Since he lives alone, he will be visited by a community health nurse for follow-up care. The visiting nurse has downloaded Mr. Lazarus' clinical record to her laptop computer and continues to document his care. When Mr. Lazarus no longer requires the services of the community health nurse, his record is uploaded to the clinical information system at the outpatient oncology center, where he continues to receive treatment for his lymphoma.

EVOLUTION OF INFORMATION TECHNOLOGY IN NURSING

Automated systems in health care have existed for 30 years. Hospital information systems (HIS) were the main systems used in the 1970s and were developed in response to a concern for reimbursement of the costs incurred by hospitalized individuals. Financial, charge-capture, and communication activities were carried out using mainframe computers that processed information in a centralized manner. In the 1980s with the advent of personal computers, information was able to be processed in a decentralized manner. Nurses found that data related to critical elements of care could be captured and entered at the point of service and that the information gleaned could be used to improve nursing practice. There was a greater emphasis placed on nursing information systems that defined and supported nursing care delivered at the bedside. Systems for care plans, documentation, and quality assurance were developed to support nursing practice. During the 1980s, systems also became more comprehensive, and attempts were made to integrate nursing data with data from other departmental systems.

The 1990s heralded the era of telecommunications, with the trend being one of open systems and communication over wide-area networks. The term *open systems* refers to the ability of different types of computers to communicate with one another. *Wide-area networks* (Fig. 21-1) enable computers located in different buildings in the same geographic area or, more broadly, across the country and around the world to be linked with each other. These technologies can assist nurses in tracking clients through

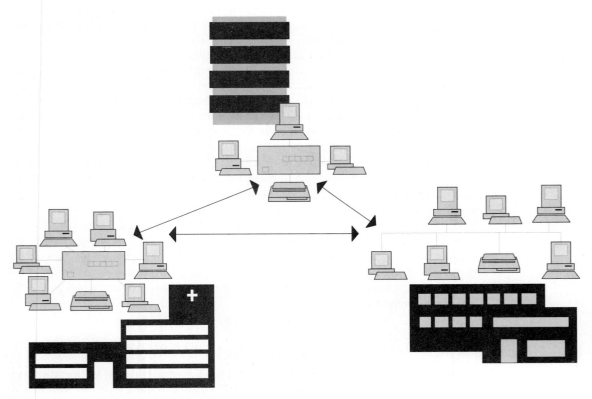

Fig. 21-1 Wide-area network: information flow.

each encounter with the health care system. The ultimate goal is to integrate information aimed at providing efficient and effective care.

THE STRUCTURE AND LANGUAGE OF NURSING DATA

While the data, information, and knowledge required to provide client care may be derived from a number of sources, nursing leaders have begun to distinguish those elements that describe the unique contributions of nursing to the promotion of health of individuals, families, and communities. The Nursing Minimum Data Set and established nursing taxonomies are examples of the progress made toward defining the diagnoses, interventions, and outcomes that are attributable directly to nursing.

The Nursing Minimum Data Set

The Nursing Minimum Data Set (NMDS), developed at the University of Wisconsin, Milwaukee, was generated to acknowledge the contribution of nursing to client outcomes. As the importance of nationwide health databases increases, it is important that a minimum number of essential nursing elements be included in those databases.

The *Nursing Minimum Data Set* is defined as "a minimum set of items of information with uniform definitions and categories concerning the specific dimension of professional nursing, which meet the information needs of multiple data users in the health care system" (Werley, 1988). The NMDS comprises a nursing diagnosis, nursing intervention, nursing outcome, intensity of nursing care measure, and health record number. The system also includes a unique identifier for the nurse provider and data elements in common with the *Uniform Hospital Discharge Data Set (UHDDS)*. Since this system is compatible with the UHDDS, there is great potential for documenting nursing's contributions to health care to insurers, hospital decision makers, nurse administrators, chief information officers (CIOs), chief nursing officers (CNOs), and informatics nurse specialists. A major purpose of the NMDS is to establish a comparison of client-centered data that can be used to evaluate the effectiveness of nursing care across practice settings and geographic boundaries. The NMDS recognizes personnel delivering care, the type of nursing care provided, the impact of that care on client outcomes, and the costs of nursing care. This system can enhance greatly the ability of nursing to conduct research and to create health policy.

Nursing Taxonomies

Nursing taxonomies have been developed to define nursing diagnoses and interventions. A *taxonomy* is "a method of classifying a vocabulary of terms for a specific topic according to specific laws or principles" (Zielstorff, 1994). Some of the major taxonomies developed include the *North American Nursing Diagnosis Association (NANDA) Taxonomy,* the *Nursing Interventions Classification (NIC),* the *Omaha Problem Classification,* and the *Home Health Care Classification (HHCC).*

North American Nursing Diagnosis Association (NANDA) Taxonomy. The *North American Nursing Diagnosis Association (NANDA)* classification system was developed to standardize nomenclature for nursing diagnoses. The work began initially in 1973 when a group of nurses met at the first national conference, and in 1982, following several conferences, the North American Nursing Diagnosis Association (NANDA) was formalized. The NANDA classification uses patterns of human response to categorize nursing diagnoses and further classifies the diagnoses by assigning specific labels within the broader structure of the patterns of human response (Fitzpatrick et al., 1989).

Nursing Interventions Classification (NIC). The Iowa Intervention Project has produced a taxonomy of nursing interventions called the *Nursing Interventions Classification (NIC).* The project is the outgrowth of years of collaborative work by scholars and clinicians headed by McCloskey and Bulechek at the University of Iowa College of Nursing. The taxonomy consists of three levels that classify nursing interventions initially as abstract domains, then as related sets of interventions, and, finally, as a very concrete set of 336 intervention labels. Examples include abuse protection, bathing, emergency care, and learning facilitation. This system is dynamic, with new labels being added as nurse researchers continue to study the phenomenon of nursing (McCloskey & Bulechek, 1996). An example of an intervention from the NIC that relates to nurses' processing and imparting information to clients is provided in the box below.

Example of a Nursing Intervention Using the Nursing Interventions Classification (NIC)

Nursing Intervention: Learning facilitation

Definition: Promoting the ability to process and comprehend information

Activities*

Provide information appropriate to developmental level.

Arrange the information in a logical sequence.

Arrange the information from simple to complex, known to unknown, or concrete to abstract as appropriate.

Adapt the information to comply with the client's lifestyle/routines.

Relate the information to the client's personal desires/needs.

Provide information that is consistent with the client's values/beliefs.

Provide information that is compatible with the client's locus of control.

Repeat important information.

Ensure that consistent information is being provided by various members of the health care team.

Correct information misinterpretations as appropriate.

From McCloskey, J.C., & Bulechek, G.M. (Eds.). (1996). *Iowa Intervention Project: Nursing interventions classification (NIC)* (2nd ed., pp. 365-366). St. Louis: Mosby.
*The activities listed above are an abbreviated list; see the NIC manual for the complete list.

Omaha Problem Classification. The *Omaha Problem Classification,* commonly referred to as the Omaha system, is a classification scheme used with clients treated in a community health setting. It consists of 43 health-related client problems that are categorized into four domains: environmental, psychosocial, physiological, and health behaviors. This scheme has been further developed to document expected outcomes. Since nurses provide the majority of community health care, this system has a direct impact on the provision of that care (Martin & Scheet, 1992).

Home Health Care Classification. Saba (1994) developed a *Home Health Care Classification (HHCC)* of nursing diagnoses and interventions. The HHCC uses a framework of 20 home health care components to classify and code nursing diagnoses and interventions specific to home health. Its major purpose is to classify clients, predict resource requirements, and measure outcomes. This system allows data to be computerized and uses the format of the ICD-10 classification scheme whereby the home health care component, the nursing service category, the subcategory, and actions are defined and coded.

In summary, once nursing has defined itself through the use of nursing diagnoses and interventions, nursing can begin to determine the resources required to provide client care in a variety of settings. The addition of a unique nurse identification code (i.e., a number that can be traced back to an individual nurse) will permit nursing to evaluate care by provider and determine the costs of care per nursing diagnosis and/or intervention. These data can be used within an agency as well as across settings to evaluate the quality of nursing care.

TECHNOLOGIES THAT SUPPORT THE DISSEMINATION OF NURSING DATA, INFORMATION, AND KNOWLEDGE

Once nursing diagnoses and interventions are defined, they can be coded and incorporated into information systems to evaluate nursing care, the resources required to provide care, and client outcomes directly attributable to nursing practice. The technologies available to transform or process data (e.g., nursing diagnoses, interventions, and resources used to provide care) continue to develop so rapidly that it is a challenge for nurses to keep abreast of innovations. Computers are smaller, increasingly more powerful, and more affordable. Networking technology allows nurses to enter data once and share these data repeatedly using relational databases. The most powerful database programs are called *relational,* because they allow separate databases to interconnect with each other. Several software innovations are making nurses' work easier and more efficient. Included in these are graphical user interfaces (GUIs) and voice recognition. Telecommunications are expanding the world of information sharing for nurses.

Networking Technology

Networking technology operates in a client/server environment. The *client* is a personal computer or computer terminal that receives shared services from a server. The *server* is a computer that provides network access to shared services (e.g., the use of word-processing programs and databases) from the nurse's personal computer or terminal (McDaniel, 1994).

Networks can be classified as local-area networks (LANs) or wide-area networks (WANs). A *local-area network* is a computer network in a hospital, a clinic, or an office. A *wide-area network* is a network that provides communication services to more than one hospital, clinic, or office. Through this technology, nurses are no longer subject to the limitations of stand-alone computers. Instead, they are able to share client data, as well as computer applications software, among computers.

While the network linking of entire hospitals or medical centers has yet to be achieved (Simpson, 1993), creative uses of networking technology have been demonstrated. For example, LANs have been used in operating rooms of hospitals for scheduling surgical procedures more efficiently and accurately. The LAN permits nurses in several locations to access the shared data from their individual workstations and, given the available resources, to develop the most feasible operating room schedule. In addition, the LAN is used to handle inventory control, supply orders, interdepartmental communications, staffing assignments, billing, intraoperative data control, paperless surgical reporting, case flow, and statistical analyses (Meikle, 1993).

Chapman and colleagues (1994) developed a LAN for the nursing service of a large urban teaching hospital, resulting in a network of 90 workstations linking 12 buildings. Through this network, nurses gained access to multiple programs that supported clinical, managerial, and research activities. Communications between departments were improved, and users had access to several software applications previously unavailable to them.

Relational Databases

Relational databases permit client-specific data to be stored independently of the programs that capture the data (Zielstorff, Hudgings, & Grobe, 1993), allowing for the efficient capture, storage, and retrieval of data needed by nurses. Relational databases can be queried to locate specific information from several separate tables, creating a subset of data that answers a specific question. For example, a relational database could be used to develop an incident-tracking system in a hospital setting. Nurses might create one table in the relational database that tracked medication errors and a separate table that tracked client falls. By using the common field of client identifier, such as the social security number, the database could be queried to produce a report that showed all clients for whom a medication error was reported and who also experienced a fall. This powerful aspect of relational databases provides quick, efficient, secure information processing at the user level (Simpson, 1993).

A nurse administrator might use a relational database to maintain records for a clinical laddering program for a hospital that employed, for example, 300 nurses spread across 15 nursing specialty units. All of the information about these nurses' specialty certifications, continuing education contact hours, and other honors and awards could be input into a computer under the control of a database management program for clinical laddering. While separate pieces of information, such as continuing education data and certification records, could be stored in different files, querying the relational database allows the nurse administrator to extract the information needed no matter where the data are stored. For example, information could be retrieved for all nurses who were certified in critical care, by date of expiration of certification. The system could then be queried for all nurses who were certified in critical care and had attended a specific series of continuing education programs.

Relational databases are also used to support point-of-care clinical information systems. Andrew (1994) provides an overview of point-of-care clinical information systems using integrated clinical databases. He discusses systems that are newly developed, as well as systems that are designed to enhance the capabilities of existing hospital information systems. Andrew evaluates the clinical systems according to the clinical environment in which they function, system specifications, potential applications, data entry capabilities, networking technology, and operational status. This listing is intended to provide nurses with general information and recognizes that follow-up with specific vendors is required for a comprehensive evaluation of the integrated database product.

Human-Computer Interfaces

GUIs are being used to make computers more user-friendly. Hannah, Ball, and Edwards (1994) describe the *graphical user interface* as dual purpose in nature: it shields the user from needing a great amount of technical knowledge and gives a consistent appearance to applications. The GUI creates a visual metaphor. For example, a nurses' station might be pictured on the computer screen, and, with the help of a device such as a mouse, a light pen, or a touch screen, the nurse would be able to access a program directly using icons depicting such things as clipboards and blood pressure cuffs. GUIs have been used by nurses to teach self-administration of insulin (Nashimoto et al., 1994) and to teach mothers how to care for their infants (Sweeney et al., 1994). Simpson (1993) credits GUIs as saving training costs for staff nurses and for eliminating the need for cumbersome manuals to support computer applications.

Voice recognition, also referred to as a speech-input interface, is the process of presenting input data to the computer through the spoken word (Capron & Perron, 1993). Voice recognition may be particularly useful for nurses who are at the bedside caring for clients and who would like the advantage of using normal speech to record patient data, leaving them free to provide "hands on" care. A study was conducted with 19 fourth-year nursing students to determine their acceptance of a prototype speech recognition interface system for entering cardiovascular assessment data (Dillon et al., 1994). The subjects displayed significant positive acceptance of the speech-input interface for entering client data into a computer system using speech as a method of data entry. The authors suggest that speech recognition technology may soon be common in hospitals and that as nurses' acceptance of computer technology increases, so, too, will their acceptance of speech recognition technology.

TECHNOLOGIES USED TO PROMOTE NURSING EXCELLENCE

At the most basic level, all professional nurses should be capable of using readily available tools with clinical data to assist in improving client care (Zielstorff, Hudgings, & Grobe, 1993). Accurate, timely, and effective presentation of data is a key to success in providing quality, affordable care. Nurses and other members of the health care team need access to the latest information on the appropriate assessment, diagnosis, treatment actions, and expected outcomes of care. In addition, nurses and other health professionals need access to standard care procedures. Nurses are challenged to use the information generated by automated systems to describe health care costs, accessibility, and outcomes of care (McCormick, 1991). Several promising methods of presenting data in a form useful to nurses are decision support systems, expert systems, computer-based learning systems, computer-adaptive testing, and on-line information sources accessed through the Internet.

Decision Support Systems

A *decision support system* (DSS) increases the nurse's decision-making effectiveness in semistructured situations characterized by uncertainty or risk (e.g., choosing among several pain management strategies) (Hadden, 1986). A growing number of analytical tools are being developed to support decision making, and Brennan (1988) provides a useful review with pertinent applications to nursing. *Bayesian analysis* (use of probabilities) to predict the outcome for one client based on the outcome from a larger population of similar clients is one area of major research activity in the application of a DSS to the health care environment. A DSS comprises three components: (1) a language component or interface that facilitates inquiries, (2) a database organized for use in decision making, and (3) a problem-processing component that contains the analytical models used to generate alternative solutions. It is the problem-processing component that distinguishes a DSS from an information-oriented system. A nurse using an appropriately designed DSS could enter client signs or symptoms (diagnostic cues or defining characteristics), and the computer would display the recommended nursing diagnoses, thus enabling more accuracy in the selection of a diagnostic label (Brennan, 1985). The recommended diagnoses are based on the computer program, which includes rules (problem-solving component) that link the defining characteristics to diagnostic labels. The rules are derived from nursing knowledge and research on the probabilities of linkage between the diagnostic cues and the diagnosis. While such systems for suggesting nursing diagnoses are experimental at present, the growing number of nurses with the technical expertise for such applications holds promise for further research and developments in the area of decision support in nursing. The HELP System, developed at the Latter Day Saints Hospital in Salt Lake City, uses decision analysis (Bayesian statistics) and its health care information system database to assist in clinical decision making. The system integrates client data from physiologic monitoring and the many other sources of data entry and allows decision making in the form of interpretations, warning alerts, or treatment protocols when abnormal conditions are recognized. Conditions for these alerts are defined in HELP sectors (e.g., likelihood of pleural fluid, hypoxia, renal failure, etc.). These sectors are considered knowledge frames that represent the data and logic to formulate a decision. Roughly 2000 such medically oriented knowledge frames are embedded in the HELP system, which is operational on clinical units throughout the hospital (Blum, 1986; Saba & McCormick, 1986).

Expert Systems

Expert systems are used to provide nurses with information and knowledge to support the provision of client care. Expert systems differ from decision support systems in that they use techniques associated with *artificial intelligence* (AI), a branch of computer science that uses predicate calculus and symbolic language to solve complicated problems (Brennan, 1988). Generally, an expert system consists of three major components: (a) a user interface, (b) a knowledge base, and (c) an inference engine. The *user interface* refers to the software program that nurses interact with as they query the expert system. The *knowledge base* comes from information obtained in the literature and from nurses who are experts in the field. The *inference engine* is a computer program that applies mathematical rules to the knowledge base to suggest an option to the nurse (e.g., a diagnosis or an intervention). An expert system mimics the clinical reasoning and judgment of human experts within one domain of practice. An example of an expert system is the Computer-Aided Nursing Diagnosis and Intervention (CANDI) (Chang et al., 1988), which is a knowledge-based system prototype to aid nursing diagnosis. The diagnostic engine compares signs and symptoms with its store of knowledge about problems and diagnoses and attempts to match the current client pattern with a pattern contained in its long-term memory.

Expert systems can be developed from scratch, using computer programming, or using an expert system shell (Saleem & Moses, 1994). An *expert system shell* is a commercial system that provides the tools or mechanisms necessary to perform the needed functions for building a knowledge base (Hannah, Ball, & Edwards, 1994). An example of a prototype system that uses programming language to build the system is one designed by Hanson and colleagues (1994) for use in a clinical simulation laboratory environment. This system provides nursing students with decision support in identifying and managing common postoperative complications. An example of an expert system that uses an expert shell is the system developed by Saleem and Moses (1994) to assess the conditions of hyperglycemia or hypoglycemia and cardiac disorders. Based on the signs and systems provided by the nurse in relation to a client's chest discomfort, the expert system suggests the likely cause of the chest discomfort. In addition, a user may invoke a special portion of the program to obtain further information to explain why the expert prompted the user with a specific question.

Computer-Assisted Learning System

Computer-assisted learning (CAL) refers to a wide range of educational techniques that use a computer to facilitate learning. Computer-assisted learning aids nurses in obtaining and transferring information and knowledge, provides feedback on the learning process, and frees teaching staff to extend the learning process to more complex problems. CAL is the broad framework encompassing the techniques of computer-assisted instruction (CAI) and computer-managed instruction (CMI) (Hannah, Ball, & Edwards, 1994).

Computer-assisted instruction uses the computer to communicate information to the learner without direct interaction between the student and the human instructor. Umlauf (1990) describes the use of CAI enhanced with interactive video to provide teaching and review of cardiopulmonary resuscitation (CPR) to hospital staff nurses who wished to become certified in CPR according to the standards of the American Heart Association (AHA). The CAI program was a rousing success for staff nurses, since it allowed them to use the system at any time of the day or night and allowed instantaneous feedback measuring the nurse's skills against the range of acceptable performance according to AHA standards. Nurses also were able to use the system to brush up on their skills as needed.

Computer-managed instruction refers to a broad system of educational management designed to develop unique programs of instruction for individual students (Hannah, Ball, & Edwards, 1994). Here, instructors may use the computer to maintain detailed student records; complete curriculum data, including course schedules; and information about available learning resources. Using CMI, a nursing student might be pretested for knowledge of diabetes management in the elderly, and then, based on the pretest score, a "prescription" of learning might be developed. The computer might be used to suggest certain textbooks, available clinical experiences at local hospitals and nursing homes, and a series of CAI modules dealing with diabetes in the elderly. The student would perform the required activities until the standard level of competency required by the school was met. The computer could also maintain records of each student's progress for individual evaluation. Instructors would be able to summarize all students' progress in the area of diabetes management of the elderly client and, as a result, could evaluate the learning program using objective data.

Computer Adaptive Testing

Computer adaptive testing is a method of testing using computer technology and measurement theory. Computerized testing provides criterion-based tests in which questions can be generated at random. Because of the rapid processing capabilities of the computer, the examinees' performance on the test generally are available on completion of the examination. An example of computer adaptive testing is the National Council Licensure Examination (NCLEX) whereby graduate nurses take the registered nurse licensure examination by computer (Weinert, 1993).

An innovative use of computerized testing is that of computerized *clinical simulation testing* (CST), which tests the clinical decision-making skills of nurses (Bersky & Yocom, 1994). Presented with case scenarios, nurses must identify the problems presented by the client and specify their choices of nursing interventions. Through computer simulation, the client's condition changes as a result of the nurse's choice of action and the underlying condition. For example, a client experiencing chest pain is described on initial examination and again as the chest pain is alleviated or increased. Nurses simulate the provision of care as the client's condition changes. This type of computerized examination offers an opportunity to test nurses' clinical skills under simulated conditions, thereby preparing them for actual client care.

Bibliographic Retrieval Systems

Medical and other health-related libraries are a rich source of material that can be used by nurses to enhance their practice. The most important element in obtaining information is the ability to organize and retrieve information easily. The *Cumulative Index to Nursing and Allied Health Literature* (CINAHL) is an example of a database that has organized bibliographic materials for the sciences of nursing and allied health. This index is a source of nursing and allied health journals and uses the National Library of Medicine's Medical Subject Headings (also known as MeSH) as the model for its thesaurus. MeSH incorporates subheadings for nursing ethics, nursing laws, and the nursing profession. The MeSH language was developed to search the *Medical Literature Analysis and Retrieval System* (MEDLARS) database. MEDLARS contains 1800 headings and provides access to citations and abstracts of articles in over 3700 journals, including nursing. Approximately 70% of the headings searched using CINAHL are MeSH headings; however, CINAHL also incorporates into its database more than 2000 unique headings for nursing and allied health, including NANDA nursing diagnoses, the Iowa Nursing Interventions Classification (NIC), major nursing models, and terms for all recognized nursing specialties (Levy, 1993).

Using CD-ROM technology, which allows storage and retrieval of vast amounts of information (Hannah, Ball, & Edwards, 1994), nurses can search for and retrieve information on a variety of topics. For example, if a nurse is interested in finding articles related to the use of "decision support" in nursing, CINAHL may be searched electronically. After the CINAHL database program has been accessed, a search may be conducted by entering the term "decision support" directly when asked to by the program. By entering the term "decision support" followed by a command key, the nurse retrieves 47 articles dealing with the subject of "decision support." Examples of these articles include ones dealing with the future of computer-aided diagnosis in the laboratory, decision support and outcomes of nurses' care planning, and a comparative study of manual versus computerized automated drug delivery. Another strategy is to use the thesaurus that is embedded in the CINAHL database program. When the thesaurus is used to search the term "decision support," several similar terms are retrieved by the system. For example, "decision making, computer assisted" and "decision making, clinical" are called up by using the thesaurus. The thesaurus is valuable to nurses because it provides them with the ability to retrieve articles on the topic of interest that are catalogued under a different term that has the same or a similar meaning. CINAHL also permits nurses to search by age group, by year of publication, and by type of document. Examples of types of documents are research and review articles, or articles that display a questionnaire in the text. A powerful database such as CINAHL assists nurses in accessing bibliographic materials on a topic of interest quickly and thoroughly. Several other self-service databases are available to nurses. These include MEDLINE, AIDSLINE, PsycLIT, Computer Select, Micromedex CCIS, and Bioethicsline. Descriptions of these databases are presented in Table 21-2.

Information Resources On-line

Nurses have access to the "information superhighway," another name for the *Internet,* which is a large, global association of government, academic, and research computer networks (DuBois & Rizzolo, 1994; Taira, 1993). Originally called the ARPAnet, the network was an experimental project developed in 1969 by the Advanced Research Projects Agency in the U.S. Department of Defense. ARPAnet was designed so that research could be shared between military and university sources and, more important, so that such communication could be sustained in the event of a nuclear attack.

Not long after ARPAnet was designed, the Defense Department developed a standard protocol called *Transmission Control Protocol/Internet Protocol* (TCP/IP), a data communications standard that determines how two computers will exchange information. By using TCP/IP, other networks could also establish a gateway to the Internet. A *gateway* is a computer system that transfers data between normally incompatible computer networks. With these technologies, the Internet has become available for everyone's use.

Table 21-2 **Bibliographic Databases**

Database	Description
AIDSLINE	Citations of published literature and audiovisuals on AIDS and related topics
Bioethicsline	Information on ethical and public policy issues in health care and biomedical research
Computer select	Full-text computer product reviews, analyses, buyer's guides, and manufacturer's listings; specifications for hardware, software, and data communications
CINAHL	References from English language nursing journals, American Nurses' Association and National League for Nursing publications, and primary journals in more than a dozen allied health disciplines
Micromedex CCIS	Full-text and emergency care information providing evaluative monographs on current therapeutic products, acute care treatment of disease and trauma, and more
MEDLINE	The data of the National Library of Medicine, which includes citations from approximately 3700 biomedical journals
PsycLIT	References and abstracts to over 1300 journals in psychology and the behavioral sciences

Courtesy Health Sciences Library, University of Maryland at Baltimore.

Popular features of the Internet are its e-mail, List Serv, and conferencing ("chat") features. Nurses can gather information on a variety of subjects using the file transfer protocol (FTP) and information-searching tools such as Gopher. A glossary of terms applicable to Internet use are presented in the box below.

Internet e-mail is much like the electronic mail a person might have on the local area network at his or her workplace. This feature allows a person to send a message from any place and at any time by computer. It enables one to log off and then return to the computer when it is convenient to check for an answer.

Another of the Internet's most desirable features is the potential for discussion on a variety of subjects. One of the easiest ways to get involved is to join a mailing list. The most well known type of mailing list application on the Internet is a *List Serv,* an application that makes sending mail to a group of people as simple as sending it to a single designated group, without the need to enter each recipient's name. Once the group is specified, the mail is distributed to each individual on the list. List Servs for several nursing specialty groups are available. Table 21-3 shows examples of List Servs that may be of interest to nurses. Information about List Servs is catalogued on-line on the Internet or in the reference section of academic libraries (Hancock, 1994).

An innovation in on-line communications of particular interest to nurses is the AJN Network, a federally funded project of the American Journal of Nursing Company. The *AJN Network* is designed to provide a variety of formal and informal continuing education services to nurses in medically underserved communities (DuBois & Rizzolo,

---

Glossary of Internet Terms

Conferencing (chatting) "Talking" live to other network users from any and all parts of the world.

Electronic mail (e-mail) An Internet feature that allows one to send messages to anyone in the world by computer.

File transfer protocol A protocol that transfers files from one computer to another.

Gopher A menu-based system for exploring Internet resources.

Hypermedia A combination of hypertext and multimedia.

Hypertext Documents that contain links to other documents; selecting a link automatically displays the second document.

List Serv An application making it possible to send an electronic message to a group of people who subscribe to the list.

Multimedia Documents that include different kinds of data (e.g., plain text and audio; text in several languages; plain text and a spreadsheet).

Protocol A definition of how computers will act when "talking" to each other. Standard protocols allow computers from different manufacturers to communicate.

TELNET The Internet's remote "login" protocol that allows one to sit at a keyboard connected to one computer and log on to a remote computer across the network.

Data from Krol, E. (1994). *The whole Internet* (2nd ed.). Sebastopol, CA: O'Reilly & Associates; and Levine, J.R., & Young, M.L. (1994). *More Internet for dummies.* San Mateo, CA: IDG Books Worldwide.

Table 21-3 **Sample Nursing List Servs**

List Serv	Description
SNURSE-L	Student nurse conference list
GRADNURSE	Discussion group for practicing nurses
NURSE-L	Nursing school project
NURSENET	Global forum for nursing issues
NURSING-L	Nursing informatics

1994). The AJN Network provides nurses with a number of valuable services, such as continuing education offerings in text and CAI formats, client care information, news related to health care, and nursing resource databases. Using the AJN Network, nurses are able to reach nurse experts and consultants through e-mail, and they can even have a live "chat" with nurse consultants on a variety of professional nursing topics.

Nurses are also fortunate to have Sigma Theta Tau International's Virginia Henderson Nursing Electronic Library (Hudgings, 1992) available to them on the Internet. Included in its holdings is *The On-Line Journal of Knowledge Synthesis for Nursing,* which is available only in electronic format (DuBois & Rizzolo, 1994).

Using the Internet

The Internet is a source of vast amounts of information and has sophisticated capabilities for searching. Two tools of the Internet that increase the ease of obtaining information useful to nurses are Gopher and file transfer protocol (FTP). *Gopher* is a menu-based system of searching for information that works much like a card catalog in a library. There are two parts to Gopher software: a server and a client. A *Gopher server* is a program and database that provide services to the *client,* in this case, the nurse. Gopher services include the availability of menus from which one may select items using very few key strokes. Once a nurse is connected to a Gopher server, information is obtained by simply using the "arrow keys" to select a menu item and then pressing the "enter" key to retrieve the item. Gopher also can be used to obtain text files stored in the database. Once the information is found, it can be downloaded to the user's personal computer using FTP. *File transfer protocol* is an efficient way to obtain files electronically and then use one's own computer to manipulate the file and print information. Gopher allows users to make connections to other Gopher servers and computer systems.

Nightingale, the University of Tennessee, Knoxville, College of Nursing Gopher, is an example of a Gopher for searching information specific to nursing. Nightingale provides information about nursing research, education, and practice. Professional issues such as nursing policies at the national, state, and local levels also are addressed. Nightingale allows nurses to TELNET to other on-line computer networks, such as the AJN Network (University of Tennessee, Knoxville, College of Nursing, 1995).

Another major source of information that may be accessed using Gopher is the National Library of Medicine (NLM), the world's largest biomedical and health-related research library. Using the NLM Gopher, nurses can enjoy access to information from the library's more than 5 million books, journals, technical reports, manuscripts, microfilm, and pictorial materials. The NLM Gopher also provides information about programs at the National Institutes of Health, such as grant and contract programs for nurses who wish to conduct research or initiate innovations in nursing. A resource of particular interest to nurses who wish to see the results of a comprehensive assessment of a technology using the technology assessment framework is Health Services/Technology Assessment Texts (HSTAT). This electronic resource provides full text reports of technology assessments, such as an assessment conducted recently on extracorporeal membrane oxygenation (ECMO). This file provides information on standards of care, practice guidelines, and abstracts of major studies conducted on ECMO. HSTAT also provides access to the full text of clinical practice guidelines and other documents useful in health care decision making (National Institutes of Health, 1994).

Accessing the Internet differs according to the type of computer hardware and software available. Good sources for assistance in logging on to the Internet are the computer/information services department at the university with which the nurse is affiliated or the public library. Commercial services such as Compuserve, Prodigy, and America Online make the Internet available for a fee. Reference manuals to assist in learning the how-tos of connecting to the Internet are available (Krol, 1994; Levine & Young, 1994).

The World Wide Web

The most recent addition to the world of the Internet is the World Wide Web. The *World Wide Web* is a system of interlinked information that lets one use Mosaic for Windows or any of its clones, such as Netscape, to work with multimedia information on the Internet. *Mosaic* and its clones are graphical user interfaces that transform the Internet into a rich world of pictures, sounds, and colors to display information of interest. Nurses can use Mosaic to develop their own Web documents as a means of establishing a presence on the World Wide Web. For example, a nurse specializing in therapeutic touch may use a Web document to introduce the concept and techniques, as well as to advertise his or her services to other Web users. A unique feature of the Web is the use of hypertext to allow a person to "click" onto a highlighted word or phrase to link or "jump" automatically to another layer of information about the topic of interest. The nurse's Web document page may give an overview of therapeutic touch and then use a phrase such as "therapeutic techniques" to link to other documents that describe in more detail the step-by-step techniques associated with therapeutic touch. The strength of the Web is that the techniques, which may sound foreign to nurses who are unfamiliar with therapeutic touch, can be viewed as a demonstration using color, sound, and video.

As nurses begin to explore the Web, more nursing Web documents will become available. Web documents can provide a valuable resource for nurses. However, since these documents have the potential to be viewed by millions of people from around the world, care should be exercised in producing such a document.

The Web is also a rich source of information for the nurse. For example, nurses can obtain information on several of the nursing programs offered at universities around the country. Also, nurses can access a document called *Virtual Nursing,* developed at the University of Iowa, which provides information on client treatments for a variety of conditions, such as chronic wound care and pain management. Nurses are able to view actual color photographs of wounds and learn how to care for these wounds. Nurses can obtain information on a variety of other professional issues, such as preparation for certification examinations and information on standards of practice. Health question-and-answer services are also available to nurses on the Web.

Nurses can venture outside the health care field and access Web sites such as the White House, where governmental information is made available to citizens across the country. Recently, several colleges have begun publishing computerized versions of their school newspapers that can be accessed on the Web (Wanat, 1994). The Web offers lots of sites, either educational or entertainment oriented, that are of particular value depending on one's interests.

The World Wide Web appears to be gaining inroads into providing timely, interesting information and will, no doubt, change the way in which information is processed and disseminated. Shortcomings of the Web include the requirement for high-speed telecommunications, limited available support, and frustration in locating information because of the lack of a uniform system for organizing information (Vaughan-Nichols, 1994). Reference manuals on the hardware and software requirements, and instructions on how to connect to the World Wide Web are available (Angell & Heslop, 1995; Gilster, 1995).

EVOLUTION OF NURSING INFORMATICS AS A SPECIALTY

A vast array of information technologies is being used to support and enhance nursing practice. As these technologies continue to develop and proliferate, it is important that nurses be educated in the technologies to ensure their role in subsequent developments and discoveries related to information technology. Because of this need, the specialty of nursing informatics has emerged.

As nursing evolves as a science and art, its practice becomes differentiated into specialization. In addition, education, research, and representation by a professional group may increase the likelihood of a specialty being recognized within nursing (Styles, 1989). *Nursing informatics* has been defined as a combination of computer science, information science, and nursing science designed to assist in the management and processing of nursing data, information, and knowledge to support the practice of nursing and the delivery of nursing care (Graves & Corcoran, 1989).

As a specialty, nursing informatics develops applications, tools, processes, and structures that assist nurses in managing data in taking care of clients or in supporting the practice of nursing. Nursing informatics supports client care, either directly or indirectly, by supporting nursing education, research, and administration (American Nurses Association [ANA], 1994).

Nursing informatics continues to gain momentum in the clinical setting. Graduate programs in nursing that provide formal education in this field have been developed (Heller et al., 1989; "University of Utah," 1990). Recognizing the increasing need for nurses to incorporate information technology into their practice, a recent trend is to introduce nursing informatics formally into baccalaureate programs in nursing (Vanderbeek et al., 1994).

Nursing informatics has been recognized as a specialty by the ANA. Most recently, the American Nurses' Credentialing Center (ANCC) (1995) has provided a formal mechanism for recognizing specialization in nursing informatics at the generalist level through its certification program. *Certification* assures the public that an individual has mastered a body of knowledge and acquired skills in a particular specialty. Certification of nursing practice has been used as a credentialing mechanism for nearly 50 years to signify the achievement of predetermined skills and knowledge in a specific field of study (Parker, 1994).

• • •

In this age of high-technology client care, nursing practice requires vast amounts of information to formulate plans of care and uses sophisticated technologies to provide care. Nurses must synthesize information efficiently to support and enhance their practice. To strengthen their practice, nurses must evaluate technologies within the context of the technology assessment framework. Nurses must be educated consumers of information technology and active participants in developing practice innovations resulting from the use of information technology. These actions ensure that nurses have a leadership position in the provision of client care in the information age.

Key Points

- Technology, the practical application of science, can be described as either therapeutic or information oriented in nature.

- The technology assessment framework is a useful tool to evaluate the risks and benefits associated with specific technologies.

- Nursing will experience rapid developments in information technology and integrate these developments into practice.

- Nursing will continue to be challenged to develop its nursing language, as in the Nursing Minimum Data Set, the North American Nursing Diagnosis Association Taxonomy, the Nursing Interventions Classification, the Omaha Problem Classification, and the Home Health Care Classification of Nursing Diagnoses and Interventions.

- Information systems are used to support nurses' clinical decision making and critical thinking.

- Integrated management systems are used to support the effective administration of nursing practice in a variety of settings.

- Nurses will communicate globally using the Internet to enhance education, practice, and research.

- Nurses will use information technologies in conjunction with the art and science of nursing to promote society's health.

 ## Critical Thinking Exercises

1. Apply the technology assessment framework to an information-handling/managing technology in your practice setting. Is the technology safe, effective, economical, and associated with a positive social impact? If not, what alterations can be made in (a) the technology itself, (b) the organizational structures supporting it, or (c) the uses of the technology to ensure consistency with the objectives of the technology assessment framework?

2. Use the technology assessment framework to evaluate a therapeutic technology in use in your health care organization. According to the framework, what are the strengths and limitations of this technology?

3. Review the nurse's role in maintaining privacy and confidentiality of client information. Discuss the nurse's responsibility for upholding confidentiality. Can you identify potential data security problems in your setting?

4. What are your information needs for clinical decision making in the management of clients in your clinical practice setting? Categorize your needs in relation to their source (e.g., database management systems, expert systems, List Servs, etc.). Discuss the design of a clinical information system that would meet the needs of your clients.

References

American Nurses' Association. (1994). *The scope of practice for nursing informatics.* Washington, DC: The Association.

American Nurses Credentialing Center. (1995). *Informatics nurse certification catalog.* Washington, DC: The Center.

Andrew, W.F. (1994). Point-of-care technology: The "window" into the integrated clinical database (Pt. 9). *Computers in Nursing, 12*(5), 171-173.

Angell, D., & Heslop, B. (1995). *Mosaic for dummies.* San Mateo, CA: IDG Books Worldwide.

Bersky, A.K., & Yocom, C.J. (1994). Computerized clinical simulation testing—Its use for competence assessment in nursing. *Nursing and Health Care, 15*(3), 120-127.

Blum, B.I. (1986). *Clinical information systems.* New York: Springer-Verlag.

Brennan, P. (1985). Decision support for nursing practice: The challenge and the promise. In K.J. Hannah, E.J. Guillemin, and D.N. Conklin (Eds.), *Nursing uses of computer and information science: Proceedings of the IFIP-IMIA international symposium* (pp. 315-319). Amsterdam: Elsevier.

Brennan, P. (1988). DSS, ES, AI: The lexicon of decision support. *Nursing and Health Care, 9*(9), 500-503.

Capron, H.L., & Perron, J.D. (1993). *Computers & information systems: Tools for an information age* (3rd ed.). Redwood City, CA: Benjamin Cummings.

Chang, B.L., Roth, K., Gonzales, E., Caswell, D., & DiStefano, T. (1988). CANDI: A knowledge-based system for nursing diagnosis. *Computers in Nursing, 6*(1), 13-21.

Chapman, R.H., Reiley, P., McKinney, J., Welch, K., Toomey, B., & McCausland, M. (1994). Implementing a local area network in a large teaching hospital. *Computers in Nursing, 12*(2), 82-88.

Dillon, T.W., McDowell, D., Norcio, A.F., & DeHaemer, M.J. (1994). Nursing acceptance of a speech-input interface:

A preliminary investigation. *Computers in Nursing, 12*(6), 264-271.

DuBois, K., & Rizzolo, M.A. (1994). Cruising the "information superhighway." *American Journal of Nursing, 94*(12), 58-60.

Fitzpatrick, J.J., Kerr, M.E., Saba, V.K., Hoskins, L.M., Hurley, M.E., Mills, W.C., Rottkamp, B.C., Waren, J.J., & Carpenito, L.J. (1989). Translating nursing diagnosis into ICD code. *American Journal of Nursing, 89*(4), 493-495.

Gilster, P. (1995). *The Mosaic navigator.* New York: John Wiley & Sons.

Gordon, M. (1982). *Nursing diagnosis: Process and application.* New York: McGraw-Hill.

Graves, J., & Corcoran, S. (1989). The study of nursing informatics. *Image: Journal of Nursing Scholarship, 21*(4), 227-231.

Hadden, S.G. (1986). Intelligent advisory systems for managing and disseminating information [special issue]. *Public Administration Review, 46,* 572-578.

Hancock, L. (1994, March 26). Listserv lists. *Internet/Bitnet Health Sciences Resources.*

Hannah, K.J., Ball, M.J., & Edwards, M.J.A. (1994). *Introduction to nursing informatics.* New York: Springer-Verlag.

Hanson, A., Foster, S.M., Nasseh, B., Hodson, K.E., & Dillard, N. (1994). Design and development of an expert system for student use in a school of nursing. *Computers in Nursing, 12*(1), 29-34.

Heller, B.R., Romano, C.A., Moray, L.R., & Gassert, C.A. (1989). Special follow-up report: The implementation of the first graduate program in nursing informatics. *Computers in Nursing, 7*(5), 209-213.

Hudgings, C. (1992). The Virginia Henderson International Nursing Library: Improving access to nursing research databases. In Arnold, J.M., & Pearson, G.A. (Eds.), *Computer applications in nursing education and practice.* New York: National League for Nursing.

Krol, E. (1994). *The whole Internet* (2nd ed.). Sebastopol, CA: O'Reilly & Associates.

Levine, J.R., & Young, M.L. (1994). *More Internet for dummies.* San Mateo, CA: IDG Books Worldwide.

Levy, J.R. (1993). *Mastering the database search: Self-study and class guide to the use and understanding of the CINAHL database.* Glendale, CA: CINAHL Information Systems.

Martin, K.S., & Scheet, N.J. (1992). *The Omaha system: Applications for community health nursing.* Philadelphia: W.B. Saunders.

McCloskey, J., & Bulechek, G.M. (Eds.) (1996). *Iowa intervention project: Nursing interventions classification* (NIC) (2nd ed.). St. Louis: Mosby.

McCormick, K.A. (1991). Future data needs for quality of care monitoring, DRG considerations, reimbursement and outcome measurement. *Image: Journal of Nursing Scholarship, 23*(1), 29-32.

McDaniel, G. (1994). *IBM dictionary of computing.* New York: McGraw-Hill.

Meikle, S.M. (1993). Local area network: Preparing for installation in the operating room. *AORN: Official Journal of the Association of Operating Room Nurses, 58*(4), 708-713.

Nashimoto, M., Kobayashi, Y., Kuribayashi, S., Takabayashi, K., Yoshida, S., & Satomura, Y. (1994). YUMIS: Computer assisted instruction for diabetic patients using multimedia environment on a Macintosh computer. In S.J. Grobe & E.S.P. Pluyter-Wenting (Eds.), *Nursing informatics: An international overview for nursing in a technological era* (pp. 423-426). Amsterdam: Elsevier.

National Institutes of Health. (1994). *National Library of Medicine fact sheet.* Bethesda, MD: U.S. Department of Health and Human Services.

Parker, J. (1994). Development of the American Board of Nursing Specialties (1991-93). *Nursing Management, 25*(1), 33-35.

Pillar, B., Jacox, A.K., & Redman, B.K. (1990). Technology, its assessment, and nursing. *Nursing Outlook, 38*(1), 16-19.

Saba, V.K. (1994). *Home health care classification (HHCC) of nursing diagnoses and interventions.* Washington, DC: Georgetown University.

Saba, V.K., & McCormick, K.A. (1986). *Essentials of computers for nurses.* Philadelphia: J.B. Lippincott.

Saleem, N., & Moses, B. (1994). Expert systems as computer assisted instruction systems for nursing education and training. *Computers in Nursing, 12*(1), 35-45.

Sandelowski, M. (1993). Toward a theory of technology dependency. *Nursing Outlook, 41*(1), 36-42.

Simpson, R.L. (1993). Client/server technology: A new way to manage information. *Nursing Management, 24*(5), 30, 32.

Simpson, R.L. (1994). Ensuring patient data, privacy, confidentiality, and security. *Nursing Management, 25*(7), 18-20.

Styles, M.M. (1989). *On specialization in nursing: Toward a new empowerment.* Kansas City, MO: American Nurses' Foundation.

Sweeney, M.A., Mercer, A., Lester, J., & Opperman, C. (1994). Multimedia interventions in maternal-infant community-based clinics. In S.J. Grobe & E.S.P. Pluyter-Wenting (Eds.), *Nursing informatics: An international overview for nursing in a technological era* (pp. 427-431). Amsterdam: Elsevier.

Taira, F. (1993). Driving down the electronic highway. *Computers in Nursing, 11*(5), 219-221.

Umlauf, M.G. (1990). How to provide around-the-clock CPR certification without losing any sleep. *The Journal of Continuing Education in Nursing, 21*(6), 248-251.

University of Tennessee, Knoxville, College of Nursing (1995, July 20). *Nursing Gopher* [On-line]. Available Gopher: nightingale.con.utk.edu

University of Utah to open nursing informatics program. (1990). *Input/Output, 6*(2), p. 7.

Vanderbeek, J., Ulrich, D., Jaworski, L.W., Hergert, D., Beery, T., & Baas, L. (1994). Bringing nursing informatics into the undergraduate classroom. *Computers in Nursing, 12*(5), 227-231.

Vaughan-Nichols, S.J. (1994). The Web means business. *Byte, 19*(11), 26-27.

Wanat, T. (1994, November 30). *The Chronicle of Higher Education,* pp. A22, A24-25.

Weinert, R.L. (1993). NCLEX using CAT [Special edition on computerized adaptive testing]. *Issues* (National Council of State Boards of Nursing).

Werley, H.H. (1988). *Identification of the nursing minimum data set.* New York: Springer.

Zielstorff, R.D. (1994). National data bases: Nursing's challenge. In R.M. Carroll-Johnson & M. Paquette (Eds.), *Classification of nursing diagnoses: Proceedings of the Tenth Conference of the North American Nursing Diagnosis Association* (pp. 34-41). Philadelphia: J.B. Lippincott.

Zielstorff, R.D., Hudgings, C.I., Grobe, S.J., & The National Commission on Nursing Implementation Project on Nursing Information Systems. (1993). *Next-generation nursing information systems: Essential characteristics for professional practice.* Washington, DC: American Nurses' Association.

Index